Superjustice

Superjustice

Law in the Age of Artificial Intelligence

SAMUEL I. BECHER

Professor of Law, Victoria University of Wellington, Wellington, New Zealand

BENJAMIN ALARIE

Osler Chair in Business Law, University of Toronto, Toronto, Canada

OXFORD
UNIVERSITY PRESS

OXFORD
UNIVERSITY PRESS

Great Clarendon Street, Oxford, OX2 6DP,
United Kingdom

Oxford University Press is a department of the University of Oxford.
It furthers the University's objective of excellence in research, scholarship,
and education by publishing worldwide. Oxford is a registered trade mark of
Oxford University Press in the UK and in certain other countries.

Published in the United States of America by Oxford University Press
198 Madison Avenue, New York, NY 10016, United States of America.

British Library Cataloguing in Publication Data
Data available

Library of Congress Control Number: 2025950250

ISBN 9780198991908

DOI: 10.1093/9780198991885.001.0001

The manufacturer's authorized representative in the EU for product safety is
Oxford University Press España S.A. of Parque Empresarial San Fernando de Henares,
Avenida de Castilla, 2 – 28830 Madrid (www.oup.es/en or product.safety@oup.com).
OUP España S.A. also acts as importer into Spain of products made by the manufacturer.

MIX
Paper | Supporting responsible forestry
FSC® C013604

Acknowledgments

This book is the product of many years of collaborative work, sustained by the generosity, insight, and encouragement of a remarkable scholarly community.

Our intellectual homes have provided the fertile ground for this project to flourish. Wellington School of Business and Government (Dean Jane Bryson) and the Faculty of Law at the University of Toronto (Dean Jutta Brunnée) offered environments of rigorous debate, encouragement, and practical support. We are fortunate to work in institutions that nurture curiosity and innovation.

We have been enriched by the engagement of our academic colleagues. We thank Abdi Aidid, David Beatty, Uri Benoliel, Lee Andrew Bygrave, Anthony Duggan, David Dyzenhaus, Mindy Herzfeld, Edward Iacobucci, Hans-Wolfgang Micklitz, Anthony Niblett, Jeannie Paterson, Taki Sarantakis, Jeff Sovern, Michael Trebilcock, Albert Yoon, and Tal Zarsky for engaging conversations, thoughtful critique, and exacting standards. David Dyzenhaus provided incisive editorial guidance on our journal article *LexOptima* (University of Toronto Law Journal, 2025), shaping several dimensions of this book. Ongoing conversations with Abdi Aidid, Anthony Niblett, and Albert Yoon—as academic colleagues at the University of Toronto and, for Benjamin, as collaborators at Blue J—have played a pivotal role in testing arguments and broadening our perspectives.

Samuel also thanks the organizers and participants at the many conferences and institutions where he presented early versions of *LexOptima* and parts of this book, including the Annual Australasian Consumer Law Roundtable (Melbourne, 2024), SMU Yong Pung How School of Law Seminar (Singapore, 2024), Future-proofing Businesses with AI, Proactive Law and Clear Communication (Aalto University, 2024), AI Regulation and Governance Conference (Oslo Faculty of Law, 2024), the International Academy of Commercial and Consumer Law (Fordham Law School, 2025), City University of Hong Kong School of Law seminar (2025), Chinese University of Hong Kong Faculty of Law seminar (2025), Kyoto University workshop (2025), and Hitotsubashi University workshop (Tokyo, 2025). Special thanks to colleagues and reviewers such as David Beatty, Anthony Duggan, Jaco Jooste, Kwan Ho Lau, Michael Trebilcock, and Jan Trzaskowski, whose thoughtful, generous feedback sharpened the arguments and helped to clarify the book's core claims.

Benjamin thanks Blue J for cultivating a unique environment at the crossroads of legal scholarship and technology. He is especially grateful to his colleagues at Blue J—Avi Brudner and Brett Janssen—for their openness, challenge, and creativity, which provided essential intellectual energy and practical insight throughout the development of this project.

The intellectual foundation for *Superjustice* was laid by our earlier work, particularly *The Legal Singularity* (University of Toronto Press, 2023) and the journal article *LexOptima*. The feedback and debate that followed these projects directly informed the questions and structure of this book.

We are grateful for the financial support that made this research possible. Samuel acknowledges the generous financial support of Victoria University of Wellington. Benjamin's contributions were supported by the Osler Chair in Business Law at the University of Toronto, as well as the supportive communities at the Vector Institute and the Schwartz Reisman Institute for Technology and Society, whose resources and collaborative spirit were invaluable throughout this project—especially the leadership and encouragement of Gillian Hadfield.

We thank Peter Daniell and Mirza Rizwaan Ahmad at Oxford University Press and Reyman Joseph at Newgen KnowledgeWorks for their support and astute editorial guidance throughout the publication process, and the anonymous reviewers of the book proposal for their valuable feedback. The manuscript also benefited from the expert freelance developmental and copy editing of Hugh Barker, whose meticulous attention to detail was invaluable. Any remaining errors are our own.

We are deeply appreciative of the contributions of our research assistants, all JD students at the University of Toronto, during this project. Omar Alikhan conducted foundational research on decentralized systems. Ben Elhav provided legal research and case study analysis. CeCe Li verified references and contributed critical feedback on drafts. Their dedication and diligence have left a lasting mark on the finished work.

We owe a special debt to Yale Law School, whose community during the 2002–03 academic year brought us together. The friendships and scholarly culture fostered in the Sterling Law Buildings became the foundation for this collaboration, demonstrating how formative environments can shape intellectual lives for decades.

Finally, we owe our deepest gratitude to our families. Samuel thanks Michal, Leehee, Mai, and Gal for their steadfast love, patience, and encouragement. Benjamin thanks Khrista, Charlotte (Charley), and Frances (Frankie) for their constant support, humor, and inspiration. Their understanding and resilience made the demanding work of research and writing not only possible but joyful.

We offer *Superjustice* as an invitation to collective imagination, critical engagement, and the ongoing pursuit of a fairer legal future.

To all who have traveled with us on this journey—thank you for believing that better is possible, and for helping us make it real.

Contents

Superjustice: Law in the Age of Artificial Intelligence

Samuel I. Becher and Benjamin Alarie

Introduction

Inclusive, democratic institutions are the bedrock of human prosperity.[1] Yet, today's justice systems remain slow, opaque, and inaccessible to many. This book introduces Superjustice—a paradigm shift that envisions legal systems harnessing artificial intelligence (AI) to become more democratized, efficient, participatory, and equitable. Realizing this promise, however, will require more than technical ingenuity; it demands a wholesale reimagining of justice itself.

Not everyone sees the use of AI in law in the same way. Optimists hail AI as the key to a more accessible, efficient, and fair legal system. At the same time, critics warn it could facilitate totalitarianism and erode due process, accountability, and the human soul of justice. To be sure, while the premise of this book is a call to leverage technological tools to advance justice, some may wish to use AI as a tool to pursue their own nefarious aims rather than justice. But this debate, while crucial, misses another important point: The transformation is not on the horizon—it is already underway. Within five years, artificial general intelligence (AGI)—AI systems that can match or exceed human cognitive abilities across most domains—may emerge, bringing capabilities that will fundamentally redefine how we understand and operationalize justice. With thoughtful design and governance, technology can drive greater transparency, curb abuses, and tilt outcomes toward justice transformation that truly serve humanity.

The need for such a transformation is evident given the growing disconnect between rapid technological progress and legal stasis—a gap that creates both extraordinary risk and unprecedented opportunity. As AI transforms everything from how we work to how we create, our legal systems remain tethered to frameworks designed for a technologically more primitive era. The cost of this misalignment is staggering. Billions of people lack meaningful access to justice, legal services remain unaffordable for most,

[1] See, for example, James A Robinson and Daron Acemoglu, *Why Nations Fail: The Origins of Power, Prosperity and Poverty* (Profile 2012); Daron Acemoglu and James A Robinson, *The Narrow Corridor: States, Societies, and the Fate of Liberty* (Penguin 2019); Adam Przeworski and others, *Democracy and Development: Political Institutions and Well-being in the World, 1950–1990* (Cambridge University Press 2000).

Superjustice. Samuel I. Becher and Benjamin Alarie, Oxford University Press.
 DOI: 10.1093/9780198991885.003.0001

and even wealthy nations struggle with overwhelming case backlogs and declining public trust.

It is understandable that people have concerns about new technologies and systemic changes. Yet, we often fail to consider the mounting costs of inaction and inertia. The question is not whether legal systems will change, but whether we will shape that change proactively or let dysfunction force reactive and suboptimal responses.

This technological disruption extends far beyond the law to virtually all professional domains. AI is fundamentally reshaping how specialized expertise is developed, accessed, and applied across fields like medicine, education, accounting, architecture, and consulting. Although Superjustice focuses specifically on legal transformation, many of the challenges and opportunities we explore reflect broader patterns of professional disruption.

The legal profession is not exceptional in facing AI-driven change, but it is distinctive in its role as a mechanism for political decision-making and social governance. Law's unique function in establishing societal norms and rules, resolving disputes with binding authority, and translating democratic values into enforceable principles makes its transformation particularly consequential for social order and human welfare. Thus, our analysis offers insights relevant to other professional domains, yet we concentrate on legal systems because of their foundational importance to democratic institutions and social trust.

The pace of this transformation in law is accelerating rapidly. In 2023, AI passed the bar exam (the Uniform Bar Examination in the United States), reportedly outperforming most human lawyers.[2] This milestone reflects more than technological prowess; it portends a radically transformative era for justice. Indeed, we stand at a crossroads. If legal systems embrace this transformation, they could dramatically improve access to justice, reduce costs, and better serve their communities. Those systems that resist change risk becoming increasingly irrelevant to how people resolve their disputes and navigate legal challenges.

Yet, for most people, these profound changes still feel distant from their daily experience of the law. Consider an ordinary Tuesday morning: you wake up, brush your teeth, and head out the door. Throughout the day, you habitually and instinctively follow social norms—letting a driver merge in traffic, thanking the barista for your coffee—without ever pausing to think about the law. Unless something unusual happens, the law remains all but invisible, part of the background fabric of your life.[3] Outside of those for whom the law is their professional occupation, it is normal (and arguably preferable) to not give much thought to the law until we encounter serious or unfortunate circumstances.

[2] See Debra Cassens Weiss, "Latest Version of ChatGPT Aces Bar Exam with Score Nearing 90th Percentile" *ABA Journal* (March 16, 2023); John Koetsier, "GPT-4 Beats 90% of Lawyers Trying To Pass The Bar" *Forbes* (March 15, 2023); "GPT-4" *OpenAI* (March 14, 2023) <www.openai.com/index/gpt-4-research/>.

[3] On the importance of the social norms that govern much of our lives see Robert C Ellickson, *Order Without Law: How Neighbors Settle Disputes* (Harvard University Press 1994). For a fascinating analysis of the diverse ways in which people in different countries respond to norms and disobey or comply with rules see Michelle Gelfand, *Rule Makers, Rule Breakers: How Tight and Loose Cultures Wire Our World* (Scribner 2018).

What situations, then, bring the law into focus? Perhaps our marriage has broken down, and we have been served with divorce papers. Or maybe we find ourselves with an exploded automobile airbag in our face after a collision. Or perhaps we have been called into a boardroom with our manager and a representative from Human Resources, who solemnly regret to inform us that our employment is being terminated. Or maybe we find ourselves stopped by the police for a traffic law violation. Even worse, perhaps we have been unjustly charged with a criminal offense or just heard of such a horrifying story.[4] Or the trigger for thinking about the law might have been something else entirely. However, what is common to these scenarios is that something unusual has happened, giving rise to questions about how the law affects the situation we find ourselves in.

When these kinds of situations arise, the importance of the law comes into sharp focus and features prominently in our lives. Suddenly, what was once taken for granted and habitually relegated to the background rises to occupy our attention, becoming a crucial framework for decision-making. In such moments, the law transitions from a distant abstraction to an intangible instrument, guiding our actions and shaping the outcomes. In these instances, individuals often find themselves grappling with deep uncertainty, relying on law in action and a host of unfamiliar legal actors to provide a sense of direction and reassurance.

Most of us are unfamiliar with the law and feel powerless when confronted with it. We may be fearful of the unknown and feel somewhat disoriented. We may naturally dread the uncertain process of trying to find (hopefully) effective help, and then equally fear the expected exorbitant cost of paying for that. We likely feel that we need to get up to speed on legal terminology and processes, to grapple with relevant legal rights and responsibilities, and to scrutinize the potential consequences of our possible next actions. In these circumstances, the law—often perceived as a top-down, distant, marble and oak enterprise—can impact our lives directly and profoundly, sometimes haphazardly and unreasonably, but almost never delightfully.

This shift in our attention reflects a broader truth: Whether in mundane or unusual situations, the law is integral to societal order, guiding our actions even when we are not consciously aware of it. Throughout our lives—whether we are driving, insuring our cars, signing a lease, filing our taxes, agreeing to terms and conditions online, filling out an application for a credit card, or negotiating the purchase of a new house—we are *presumed* to know the law and to understand the legal consequences of our actions. Nonetheless, access to justice remains a challenge, trust in legal institutions is declining, and the legal system is struggling to keep pace with the rapid technological advances of our modern world.

Consider the case of new technologies. As society becomes increasingly digitized and globalized, traditional legal frameworks and institutions are wrestling with novel challenges, such as protecting digital rights, mitigating hate speech and misinformation,

[4] For one powerful example see Piper French, "The Human Cost of Jeff Landry's Drive to Resume Executions" *Bolts* (March 20, 2025).

ensuring data privacy, protecting intellectual property, and resolving cross-border disputes. When it comes to AI, current legal systems are ill-equipped to regulate emerging developments and to optimally leverage their potential benefits.

Access to justice is another pressing issue. Our legal systems struggle to provide affordable and equitable access to justice. Worldwide, estimates suggest that over a billion people have unmet civil or administrative justice needs, and countless others are excluded from the opportunities for redress that the law provides.[5] A significant number of people do not seek legal advice to understand or resolve their problems, with a large proportion reporting severe difficulties in dedicating the necessary resources of time and money to address their legal issues.[6]

The complexity and high cost of legal processes create significant barriers for individuals seeking justice. For many, the system's intricacies prove overwhelming, leading them to avoid seeking legal assistance altogether. The complexity of the legal system can ultimately lead to severe delays and tragic outcomes. This challenge, compounded by the system's inherent inertia, creates legal gridlock. This is a problem. After all, "Justice delayed is justice denied."[7]

What if, in the future, no one feels this uncertainty, dread, or lack of confidence about the law? What if our legal systems were highly dynamic, constantly evolving, and adeptly representing societal values and views? What if we could take it for granted that there will be *no* gotchas, that justice *will be* served, that all stakeholders *will be* treated fairly, and that the policies advanced by the law will be as efficient and reasonable as possible, all things considered?

For one thing, this would constitute a sharp departure from our current experience. Even in the world's most effective legal systems, legal advice is invaluable. It helps us to protect our interests, work within legal frameworks, and apply them to our specific circumstances. However, essentially all the world's legal systems fail to provide affordable and high-quality access to justice. Even as the world becomes more interdependent and intricate, the world's best legal systems struggle to accommodate the current dynamics of our increasingly complex societal and technological environment.[8] And the world is not magically going to become simpler with rapid advances in new technology; precisely the opposite is almost certainly our direction of travel.

These systemic challenges demand a fundamental rethinking of how the law operates. In this book, we explore how emerging technological developments are poised to revolutionize the world's legal systems. We argue that these technological innovations provide us with "a moment of opportunity" that could lead us to a perpetually evolving

[5] SC Long and A Ponce, *Measuring the Justice Gap: A People-Centered Assessment of Unmet Justice Needs Around the World* (*World Justice Project*, 2019) <www.worldjusticeproject.org/sites/default/files/documents/WJP_Measuring%20the%20Justice%20Gap_final_20Jun2019_0.pdf>.

[6] CG Patiño and others, *Global Insights on Access to Justice: Findings from the World Justice Project General Population Poll In 101 Countries* (*World Justice Project*, 2019) <www.worldjusticeproject.org/sites/default/files/documents/WJP-A2J-2019.pdf>.

[7] Widely attributed to William E Gladstone.

[8] On the inadequacies of our current legal institutions and the need for a system revamp see Gillian K Hadfield, *Rules for A Flat World: Why Humans Invented Law and How to Reinvent It for a Complex Global Economy* (Oxford University Press 2017).

and radically improved AI-enabled legal system.[9] Optimistically—and plausibly—we envision a future system where the law is more accessible, transparent, tailored to community demands, and responsive to changing circumstances and individual needs.

Enter Superjustice. A data-driven, decentralized, participatory, real-time model for dynamic, fair, and efficient law.

What will drive this paradigm shift, and how might it unfold? The answers to these questions lie at the heart of this book. To set the stage, imagine that the legal systems and institutions of the future will be characterized by their use of decentralized, community-driven data and algorithms to generate context-aware law, personalized law, and carefully tailored legal services in real time. If executed well, Superjustice would improve access to justice, reduce bias in legal processes, empower communities, and democratize our legal institutions.

This transformation will not happen overnight. In fact, the process will likely face resistance from entrenched interests and could take decades. It will also raise various concerns, including data privacy, the rule of law, algorithmic transparency, accountability, and equitable implementation. However, these challenges present an opportunity to build a legal system that balances technological innovation with ethical oversight and human values. Current legal systems have not been designed with AI capabilities in mind. Legal systems are far from fully prepared to leverage technological developments or distribute their benefits equitably. While concerns over data privacy, cybersecurity, algorithmic transparency, comprehensive planning, adequate oversight, and opposition from incumbent interests are real, it is essential to recognize that they will also be co-opted by those who resist change for a variety of reasons of their own.[10]

Ultimately, the promise of Superjustice lies in its potential to leverage technology to positively redefine how law serves society. Superjustice offers a vision of a legal system that is both technologically sophisticated and deeply humanistic. As we stand at the cusp of this revolution, it falls upon us to thoughtfully harness the power of AI and proactively shape the future of law to better our societies.

The Plan of the Book

This book explores the revolutionary potential of AI in law, proposing key considerations for a dynamic approach to legal transformation. We argue that, by thoughtfully integrating AI technologies and adopting a multidisciplinary, inclusive approach, we can harness a golden opportunity to transform our legal systems, making them more just, efficient, and democratic.

Part I of this book consists of four chapters, collectively providing the conceptual underpinnings and the foundations of Superjustice. Chapter 1 introduces the

[9] We are inspired here by Yochai Benkler, *The Wealth of Networks: How Social Production Transforms Markets and Freedom* (Yale University Press 2006) and his views on the immense potential of the internet to impact our society.

[10] See Michael J Trebilcock, *Dealing with Losers* (University of Toronto Press 2014).

conceptual framework for Superjustice. It focuses on the objectives, approaches, and values that ground the concept of transformative justice in the age of AI. As an introductory chapter, it seeks to make complex ideas accessible to readers from diverse backgrounds, including those without extensive prior knowledge of the law, AI, or legal theory.

The following chapters explore specific features of legal systems in detail. Chapter 2 begins by exposing the limitations of current centralized legal systems, focusing on their inefficiencies and the need for a more dynamic, responsive approach. It categorizes the faults and ailments of modern legal systems into ten key areas, which we call the "Ten Pillars of Legal Dysfunctionality." Identifying these challenges is a necessary first step in developing an effective framework for mitigating them.

After discussing the main problems of current legal systems, Chapter 3 examines the shift toward decentralized models of governance, offering a framework for understanding the role of decentralized authority in law. The chapter defines legal centralization and highlights its historical roots. It then explores the potential rise of decentralized models, drawing on case studies and examples from various fields to demonstrate the benefits of distributing legal authority. The chapter addresses key challenges to decentralization, such as ensuring consistency and accountability. The chapter concludes by proposing ways that hybrid legal systems could strike a balance between centralization and decentralization.

Chapter 4 considers the role of data and technology in shaping a new legal paradigm. It outlines the different types of data crucial for implementing Superjustice, including traditional legal data and macro- and micro-extralegal data. This discussion highlights the importance of data quality, data governance, and data ethics. The chapter further explores the concept of elicited input, highlighting the importance of integrating public opinion and diverse perspectives into the legal system. Chapter 4 also introduces the idea of personalized laws in the era of powerful AI. It describes how Superjustice could revolutionize legal systems by making traditional legal standards and rules obsolete.[11] This discussion highlights the transformative impact of technology on legal processes, underscoring how data-driven methods can enhance the efficiency, inclusivity, and adaptability of legal systems.[12]

Part II, comprising Chapters 5–7, tackles the implementation of Superjustice. We begin this exploration in Chapter 5, which scrutinizes the shifting equilibrium between AI's capabilities and the intrinsic human character that underpins justice and the legal system. The chapter investigates the opportunities presented by integrating advanced technology into legal processes while emphasizing the need to ensure justice

[11] Legal standards are vague norms (such as "reasonable") that allow flexible application but do not provide concrete guidance. Legal rules are concrete and specific norms (such as exact dates, speed limits, and minimum ages). They are inflexible and do not account for specific circumstances, yet they provide clear guidance with little need for interpretation. See, for example, Duncan Kennedy, "Form and Substance in Private Law Adjudication" (1976) 89 Harvard Law Review 1685; Pierre J Schlag, "Rules and Standards" (1985) 33 UCLA Law Review 379.

[12] For examining the relationship between technology, legal processes, and access to justice in the near to medium term see David Freeman Engstrom (ed), *Legal Tech and the Future of Civil Justice* (Cambridge University Press 2023).

is perceived as fair. The chapter proposes a gradual shift and blend of innovation and tradition, guaranteeing that legal systems continue to reflect human values, by humans, and for humans—with AI.

Chapter 6 introduces the concept of "Justice as a Service." It explores how Superjustice would facilitate legal accessibility and equity through AI integration. The chapter presents the design and implementation of technologies, aiming to expose wider audiences to fundamental legal resources. It further demonstrates how equitable access to legal services can be achieved in practice, underscoring Superjustice's commitment to a more democratic and fair legal system.

Chapter 7 explores how Superjustice will reshape legal education and the legal profession. In doing so, it analyzes the necessary changes in curricula and teaching methods, with a focus on legal employability and the new competencies lawyers must acquire. It also examines the evolving nature of legal practice, including shifts in traditional roles and the rise of new specialties. It emphasizes the importance of interdisciplinary collaboration in preparing legal professionals for the era of Superjustice. It concludes by discussing how Superjustice could democratize legal knowledge and practice, making the legal profession more accessible and efficient.

Part III, which includes Chapters 8–10, adopts a holistic perspective, addressing future implications, applications, and challenges. Chapter 8 examines how AI will reshape the legal profession, driving the emergence of new roles like AI auditors and legal engineers, while transforming judicial decision-making. It explores how AI-augmented legal processes can enhance efficiency and reduce bias, while also raising concerns about judicial independence. The chapter also considers how legal business models will evolve, with value-based pricing and subscription-based services gaining prominence.

Chapter 9 introduces the concept of CRISPR-J, a legal system design that pursues Cost-effective, Rapid, Inclusive, Smart, Predictive, and Resilient Justice (CRISPR-J). It explores how data-driven law could personalize legal rules without sacrificing clarity or equity. Beyond rulemaking, we further demonstrate how CRISPR-J principles can be applied in the contexts of enforcement, compliance, and judicial decision-making. Through various case studies drawn from multiple domains, we illustrate how smart regulation and legal analytics—such as real-time monitoring and predictive tools—could bridge the gap between law in books and law in action.

Finally, Chapter 10 considers multifaceted challenges that accompany the implementation of AI in legal systems. To this end, Chapter 10 introduces a dynamic challenges matrix and investigates the impact of Superjustice on procedural justice and social trust. It also tackles the challenges and risks relating to privacy and data security, AI bias, fairness, the digital divide, and AI inaccuracies and explainability. The analysis underscores that, while some developments may seem inevitable, the choices we make today will significantly influence the path our future legal systems take.

Overall, this book will equip readers with a comprehensive framework for addressing a critical question: How can we shape legal systems to seize this unprecedented technological moment? AI provides powerful tools that can serve vastly different ends. The path we choose depends entirely on our collective decisions. It is not technology alone but humans collectively who will determine how equitably its benefits are distributed, and how its potential materializes. We hope that the vision we offer in this book will inspire and guide the thoughtful integration of technology into legal systems in ways that reflect our highest values and aspirations.

PART I
THE FOUNDATIONS OF SUPERJUSTICE

1
A Paradigm Shift

The Library of Alexandria 2.0

The ancient Library of Alexandria was more than a collection of scrolls: It was civilization's boldest attempt to assemble universal wisdom in one place.[1] Yet, its gradual disappearance through calamity and neglect remains one of history's great intellectual tragedies. It is a stark reminder of how knowledge, even when meticulously preserved, is a precious resource that we must handle with constant vigilance.

Today's legal landscape embodies a similar paradox: Vast repositories of legal knowledge exist, yet they remain inaccessible to most. Like the original Library—where wisdom was centralized and available only to an elite—modern legal information is locked behind commercial databases, buried in arcane structures, and incomprehensible to the average person. For many, the law is not a resource but a labyrinth, navigable only by those with privilege or specialized training.

Now, imagine a different paradigm—the Library of Alexandria 2.0. In this reimagined institution, intelligent guides appear beside each visitor, instantly translating legal texts, pinpointing the most relevant precedents, and even anticipating unasked questions. The library's walls dissolve, granting unrestricted access to knowledge from anywhere in the world, regardless of wealth or status. Rather than a static repository, the library becomes a living, responsive ecosystem—serving individuals, communities, and legal systems that are struggling to bridge the gap between the law and those it is meant to serve.

This transformation from an impenetrable archive to an open, dynamic knowledge network mirrors the paradigm shift that Superjustice represents for law. Rather than digitizing outdated hierarchies, Superjustice reshapes how law itself is approached, practiced, and enforced. It is not just about increasing access, but also about reshaping the foundations of justice. It represents a fluid, intelligent, and adaptive legal system that evolves with collective participation, moving beyond the limitations of centralized control. This shift—from a static collection accessible to few to a living knowledge network that serves societies worldwide—embodies the fundamental reimagining of justice at the heart of this book.

[1] See Luciano Canfora, *The Vanished Library: A Wonder of the Ancient World* (University of California Press 1990); Roy MacLeod (ed), *The Library of Alexandria: Centre of Learning in the Ancient World* (IB Tauris 2000).

Superjustice. Samuel I. Becher and Benjamin Alarie, Oxford University Press.
 DOI: 10.1093/9780198991885.003.0003

What is Superjustice?

The integration of artificial intelligence (AI) into legal systems has begun. AI-driven tools already assist with tasks like legal research, analysis, document drafting, and contract review, yet these remain incremental enhancements rather than fundamental changes. True transformation demands a paradigm shift. As AI technology advances and becomes deeply embedded in the legal landscape, we stand at the threshold of a radically different legal framework: AI-transformed legal systems that break from traditional hierarchies, reimagine accessibility, and redefine legal processes. This shift sets the stage for Superjustice: A legal paradigm that harnesses AI, decentralized governance, large-scale data integration, and participatory processes to fundamentally reshape the law.

Accurately predicting the trajectory of AI is challenging, if not impossible. However, a few observations are straightforward. The technology is already impressive and powerful. Consider how GPT-3.5, an AI large language model (LLM), took the world by storm in 2022, demonstrating a remarkable advance in natural language processing. Yet, in just a few years, GPT-3.5 has become a distant memory of an anachronistic system, supplanted by more capable and powerful AI models.

Technology is advancing at a remarkable pace, faster than humanity has previously experienced. Moore's Law predicted an exponential rise in computing power, and this principle has propelled cutting-edge developments, particularly in AI. Increasing computational capabilities continue to fuel the evolution of AI technologies; however, the precise rate at which the timescale for training LLMs is growing remains uncertain. Some observers have estimated that the required computing power doubles approximately every six to nine months, although this figure is not definitively confirmed and may vary by source or timeframe.[2] Even so, if such an exponential trend were to persist for a few more years, the associated processing power could plausibly have increased many times over. By extrapolation (though we note this is speculative), AI might require up to 1,000 times more computational power by 2030 than it does in 2024. This power, combined with algorithmic innovation and vast amounts of data, is a major driving force behind AI progress. Increased computing power complements algorithmic advances, resulting in improved performance. Thus, rapid growth in computing power and algorithmic efficiency also fuels predictions about the exponential growth in AI strength and capabilities.

Some believe that foundational LLMs like Claude, Gemini, DeepSeek, and GPT have already developed a form of "world model"—a structured internal representation that enables them to implicitly understand relationships, cause-and-effect dynamics, and contextual nuances, thus generating responses that resemble human comprehension. For example, their ability to answer complex legal queries with contextually

[2] For some data see, for example, OpenAI, "AI and Compute" (May 16, 2018) <www.openai.com/index/ai-and-compute/>; Epoch AI, "Machine Learning Trends" (January 13, 2025) <www.epoch.ai/trends>; Stanford Institute for Human-Centered Artificial Intelligence, *AI Index Report 2024* <www.aiindex.stanford.edu/>.

appropriate responses suggests a deep understanding of intricate concepts. Others argue that LLMs are simply advanced pattern predictors, relying on statistical probabilities rather than a true understanding of underlying concepts. This perspective highlights the absence of genuine reasoning or awareness in these systems.[3]

The combination of an accelerated pace of technological development and innovation will probably eventually lead to the emergence of artificial general intelligence (AGI)—possibly the most powerful tool humankind has ever created. While there is no single agreed-upon definition, AGI can be broadly understood as highly capable AI systems with the ability to match or surpass human intelligence. This revolutionary breakthrough will present both immense opportunities and profound challenges, extending far beyond mere progress in computational power, speed, or data processing.

As AI continues to evolve, it will assist in more than procedural tasks, making significant contributions in areas that require human-like judgment, emotional intelligence, and ethical reflection. AI will probably develop "soft" capabilities, such as exhibiting apparent empathy and demonstrating adept moral reasoning. This shift opens new opportunities for meaningful advances and collaboration between humans and AI, particularly in domains like creativity, complex problem-solving, ethical decision-making, and self-improvement. We will thus have to reconsider the roles and activities that provide us with purpose.[4]

AGI may achieve these "soft" capabilities sooner than anticipated, with some estimates predicting it by 2027. AGI and related technological developments are expected to drive real-world progress, achieve unprecedented efficiencies, supplement human input, and overtake our cognitive limitations. The rate of advancement would be unparalleled, potentially condensing fifty to a hundred years of progress into the next five to ten years. This presents both an extraordinary opportunity and a stark challenge for legal systems. Those who adapt could dramatically improve access to justice and institutional effectiveness. Those who fail to adapt risk becoming increasingly irrelevant.

In light of this expected trajectory, we believe it is critical to have an inspiring vision for a positive legal future enabled by powerful AI.[5] We employ the term "powerful AI," envisioning a system more capable than law professors across domains of relevant knowledge, more adept than seasoned lawyers across areas of legal practice, and more able to complete open-ended and complex legal tasks autonomously. We also believe this capability will be scalable to millions or billions of parallel instances in multiple jurisdictions and languages.

[3] See Kenneth Li, "Do Large Language Models Learn World Models or Just Surface Statistics?" *The Gradient* (January 21, 2023); Emily M Bender and others, "On the Dangers of Stochastic Parrots: Can Language Models be Too Big?" (2021) Proceedings of the 2021 ACM Conference on Fairness, Accountability, And Transparency 610 [10.1145/3442188.3445922]; Rishi Bommasani and others, "On the Opportunities and Risks of Foundation Models" (2021) arXiv preprint arXiv 2108.0725.

[4] See Nick Bostrom, *Deep Utopia: Life and Meaning in a Solved World* (IdeaPress Publishing 2024).

[5] We are informed here by Dario Amodei, "Machines of Loving Grace: How AI Could Transform the World for the Better" (October 2024) <https://darioamodei.com/machines-of-loving-grace#basic-assumptions-and-framework>. Amodei prefers the term "powerful AI" over "AGI."

The evolving relationship between AI and law can thus signal the rise of a new legal framework. The dominant assumption today envisions a future of AI-human collaboration, where machines augment human decision-making. We posit that this model probably underestimates the full potential of AGI. As AI continues to evolve, its role could extend beyond merely assisting legal professionals to filling existing gaps in legal services and enabling entirely new processes. More controversially, it may also assume more autonomous decision-making roles in areas traditionally reserved for judges, lawyers, and legal scholars, such as adjudication, case management, and legal analysis.

This progress will not occur in isolation. Global powers such as the United States and China are already locked in a high-stakes race to dominate AI capabilities. The outcomes of this race could reshape geopolitical structures, with AGI becoming a tool for international influence or dominance. To address such risks, international regulatory frameworks could be established to promote the ethical use of AGI. These frameworks could draw from historical precedents like the nuclear non-proliferation treaties, which established collaborative mechanisms to prevent the misuse of nuclear technologies, and the Paris Agreement, which emphasized shared global responsibility. Global collaboration is essential to mitigate the risks of authoritarian regimes or rogue actors exploiting AGI for harmful purposes.

This book seeks to advance and advocate for the prospect that AGI will ultimately be used to foster democracy, justice, and human rights. AI holds immense promise and is advancing at an extraordinary pace, but transforming the global justice system comes with high stakes. The process that takes us toward an AI-driven legal system should be swift and determined, but not hasty. To that end, the legal system should adopt a "fast follower" strategy.

In management parlance, "first movers" are the pioneers who adopt new technologies early, taking on high risks but potentially reaping significant rewards.[6] Meanwhile, "fast followers" wait for the initial problems and challenges to be worked out by the first movers, learning from their successes and mistakes. Fast followers then adopt the technology with a more refined approach. Finally, "late movers" come in afterward, avoiding most of the risks but potentially missing out on opportunities to shape the innovation and reap its benefits earlier. Superjustice, as a legal paradigm, should position itself as a fast follower. This would entail that governments and legal institutions keep a close watch on legal tech, adopting (and adapting) innovation as soon as it is proven in the private sector.

Being a first mover in legal AI carries significant risks, such as ethical concerns, unintended biases, and potential harm to public trust if the technology is not sufficiently mature. Moreover, as we explain in Chapter 2, law is slow to adapt and often resists innovation. The legal system is not designed to foster innovation, promote market competition, or maximize value. However, adapting too late may lead to missed

[6] See Marvin B Lieberman and David B Montgomery, "First-Mover Advantages" (1988) 9.S1 Strategic Management Journal 41; Steven P Schnaars, *Managing Imitation Strategies* (Simon & Schuster 2002); Heidrun C Hoppe, "Second-Mover Advantages in the Strategic Adoption of New Technology Under Uncertainty" (2000) 18(2) International Journal of Industrial Organization 315.

opportunities to improve efficiency and access to justice, as well as undermining the ability to shape global AI standards in law. In taking the fast-follower approach, legal institutions should adopt AI technologies through careful iteration, leveraging all lessons learned to avoid premature implementation, while ensuring ethical and operational readiness. With stronger AI arriving, even a "fast follower" strategy must be executed with speed. Legal systems cannot afford to lag if they wish to harness AI's immense transformative potential.

With this general vision in mind, let us now step back to contextualize and explore the meaning and implications of this transformation. The remainder of this chapter briefly presents the framework of Superjustice, describing its emergence and future trajectory. It also briefly discusses some mitigation strategies designed to address potential risks and challenges as we navigate the path toward radically better legal systems.

The Emergence of AI-transformed Legal Systems

AI-enabled legal systems will capitalize on artificial intelligence and advanced technologies to improve the efficiency, accessibility, and fairness of legal processes. These systems will automate routine legal tasks, bridge existing gaps, assist in legal decision-making, enhance legal processes, and provide personalized legal guidance. The initial integration of AI in the legal domain aims to address the persistent limitations of traditional legal systems, including high costs, inefficiencies, delays, and inconsistencies.[7]

The success and potential demonstrated by AI-enabled legal systems will pave the way for further innovations, leading to the emergence of Superjustice. This new paradigm represents a significant leap forward, building upon the core principles of AI-enabled legal systems while introducing cutting-edge technologies and novel approaches to legal problem-solving. These technologies will allow the system to process vastly greater amounts of data, identify more complex patterns, generate highly accurate predictions and recommendations, prevent and resolve disputes, and profoundly change litigation. Leveraging these advanced capabilities will allow Superjustice to create a legal system that is not only more efficient and effective but also more adaptable and responsive to the ever-changing needs of society. This will facilitate deep legal and institutional reforms, spanning new legislation, constitutional amendments, rapid new policy and regulatory responses, and dynamic, real-time reforms to legal processes.

One of the key distinguishing features of Superjustice is its emphasis on decentralization and community-driven legal processes. While AI-enabled legal systems focus primarily on the *application* of AI within the existing legal framework, Superjustice envisions *new models* of decentralized legal governance. For example, Superjustice responds to the concern that centralized law often ignores or silences marginalized communities and the most vulnerable people.[8] As Chapter 3 illustrates, Superjustice

[7] Chapter 2 provides a detailed exposition of these failures and limitations.

[8] Public choice theory and the concept of regulatory capture provide a compelling framework explaining why the traditional law- and rulemaking processes do not properly reflect the public's voice, interests, and needs. See

envisions a future where legal norms are often shaped by the collective input and participation of individuals and communities rather than being solely determined by centralized authorities.

At the same time, Superjustice will place a strong emphasis on personalization, recognizing that the one-size-fits-all approach of traditional legal systems often fails to address individuals' unique circumstances and needs. By leveraging advanced data analytics and AI algorithms, Superjustice will aim to provide context-aware law and legal services tailored to individuals' specific characteristics, preferences, and situations. This personalized approach can reinforce engagement and trust, and ensure that legal norms are more relevant, effective, and equitable.

In summary, Superjustice marks a pivotal shift in the role of AI in the legal domain. It transitions from a mere *enabling* tool to a *transformative* force that reshapes the foundations of our legal systems. This technological evolution not only refines existing tools but also introduces novel capabilities central to the development of Superjustice. As we investigate the transformative potential of Superjustice throughout this book, we will systematically explore the specific technologies, frameworks, and implications of this groundbreaking approach to legal evolution.

The Landscape of Technological Evolution

The rapid advances in AI and related technologies will fuel the emergence of Superjustice, enabling the development of sophisticated systems that process vast amounts of data.[9] At the forefront of this technological revolution is the field of machine learning. Machine-learning algorithms enable computers to learn from data and continually improve their performance over time without requiring explicit programming. This capability is particularly significant in the legal domain, where vast amounts of legal data, including case law, statutes, and regulations, can be analyzed to identify patterns and provide insights that would escape human attention.

Deep learning, a subset of machine learning, underpins progress in AI-driven legal systems by enabling more sophisticated and accurate analyses. Deep learning algorithms can automatically extract high-level features and representations from raw data. This allows AI systems to uncover complex relationships and make even more sophisticated predictions, surpassing traditional capabilities. LLMs have massively accelerated progress in natural language processing (NLP). NLP enables computers to understand, interpret, and generate human language, facilitating automated analysis of legal documents, contracts, and other text-based sources. As we explain in Chapter 5,

Daniel Carpenter and David A Moss (eds), *Preventing Regulatory Capture: Special Interest Influence and How to Limit It* (Cambridge University Press 2014).

[9] Some scholars predict that technological progress will result in more fundamental and irreversible changes in the law in the coming two decades than we have experienced in the past two centuries; see Richard Susskind, *Tomorrow's Lawyers: An Introduction to Your Future* (3rd edn, Oxford University Press 2023).

advanced NLP techniques can extract valuable insights from unstructured legal data, thereby facilitating tasks such as document classification, information retrieval, and legal reasoning.

But this is just the beginning. AI-powered NLP systems can work with multiple languages, breaking down linguistic barriers and enabling the processing and analysis of legal documents from various jurisdictions. Speech translation systems already possess the competence to provide simultaneous spoken language conversion, like the fictional, universally translating Babel fish from Douglas Adams's 1979 novel, *The Hitchhiker's Guide to the Galaxy*.[10] This multilingual capability enhances the system's potential in navigating international law and cross-border legal matters. It also allows for the exchange of knowledge and insights between legal systems across different languages. By facilitating the sharing of legal expertise and experiences from diverse linguistic, jurisdictional, and cultural backgrounds, AI technologies can help enrich and harmonize legal practices on a global scale.

The integration of current and emerging cutting-edge AI technologies enables the legal system to automate routine legal tasks, such as document review and contract analysis. This frees up legal professionals to concentrate on the more complex and strategic aspects of their work. Additionally, AI-powered predictive analytics can assist in forecasting legal outcomes, risk assessment, and decision support, enhancing the efficiency and accuracy of legal processes. The potential impact of these capabilities is immense. For example, highly accurate predictions can render most litigation superfluous, as parties will often be able to forecast reliably *ex ante* what a court will rule on their dispute *ex post*.

As we explore in more detail in subsequent chapters, the technological landscape driving Superjustice extends beyond AI and machine learning. With its decentralized and immutable ledger system, blockchain technology offers new possibilities for secure and transparent record-keeping, smart contracts, and digital identity management. The integration of blockchain in Superjustice can enable the creation of tamper-proof legal records, automate the execution of legal agreements and judicial or arbitral decisions, and facilitate secure data sharing among stakeholders.

Furthermore, the proliferation of IoT devices and advanced sensors will provide a wealth of real-time data that Superjustice can leverage. For instance, IoT devices could be used to monitor compliance with environmental regulations by tracking emissions in real time or detecting building code violations through embedded sensors. An even more advanced infrastructure—collaborative sensing—could move beyond conventional IoT by linking devices, AI models, and data streams into a shared, context-aware network.[11] Alongside these sensing networks, physically embodied AI systems, such as robots, drones, or autonomous vehicles, represent an advanced form of IoT infrastructure. Unlike passive sensors, these agents engage directly with physical spaces,

[10] Douglas Adams, *The Hitchhiker's Guide to the Galaxy* (Harmony Books 1979).

[11] See Daniel Dossenbach, David Parekh, and Karen Hallberg, "Collaborative Sensing: Empowering Connected Systems to Make Context-Aware Decisions" in *Top 10 Emerging Technologies of 2025* (World Economic Forum 2025) 33–35.

exploring complex terrains or testing structural integrity, thereby refining their world model in unique ways.

Equipped with onboard intelligence, these devices can move through and interact with the environment to gather novel data, conduct inspections, and detect potential breaches of legal norms or violations more effectively. Rather than merely reporting raw data, these systems could actively integrate and interpret information from diverse sources, enabling predictive compliance monitoring, proactive regulatory adjustments, and dynamic legal enforcement. A futuristic version of this architecture—an "AI of Things" (AIoT)—could combine collaborative sensing with advanced AI analytics to trigger automated legal actions based on predefined rules and evolving conditions. This integrated ecosystem would respond promptly to changing circumstances, expand its enforcement capabilities, and continuously adapt its underlying frameworks based on firsthand, real-time observations.

Thus, the technological landscape driving Superjustice is not limited to individual technologies; instead, it encompasses the convergence and synergy among them. The combination of AI, blockchain, AIoT, advanced sensors, and other emerging technologies creates a powerful ecosystem that can transform the legal system in ways previously unimaginable. As Superjustice evolves, it will continue to harness the latest technological advances to enhance its capabilities. The rapid pace of technological progress suggests that the future of Superjustice will be shaped by a continuous stream of innovations, pushing the boundaries of what is possible in legal technology.

The Conceptual Framework Behind Superjustice

With a robust technological foundation in place, we next consider the values and the framework that guide the operation and governance of Superjustice. At its core, Superjustice is built upon three fundamental components: (1) AI-driven decision-making, (2) decentralized governance, and (3) accessible and personalized legal norms and services. We will flesh out these three foundational components throughout the book; however, the following paragraphs offer a general overview.

AI-Driven Decision-Making

AI algorithms in Superjustice will be trained on extensive datasets of legal precedents, statutes, and regulations, enabling the system to develop a comprehensive understanding of legal principles and their application in rich and varied contexts. AI algorithms within Superjustice could leverage this knowledge base to provide intelligent recommendations, predict potential outcomes, and assist legal professionals in making well-informed decisions. As we elucidate throughout the book, the integration of AI in legal decision-making processes offers several advantages. It can help reduce bias, ensure consistency, and improve the speed and accuracy of legal analysis.[12]

Superjustice will also be trained on an enormous corpus of non-legal data and information, either directly or indirectly. It will use leading foundational AI models that encompass a broad range of capabilities, including large-scale, multimodal systems for text, audio, and video analysis. These foundational models are trained on vast, multimodal datasets encompassing text, audio, and video sourced from across the internet. These models, including those now powering LLMs such as ChatGPT, Claude, and Gemini, are continually evolving to integrate emerging technologies and data modalities. As we explore in Chapter 4, the use of non-legal or extralegal data will allow Superjustice to better contextualize legal principles and ensure they are aligned with social, economic, and technological developments. It will also enhance lawmaking and open new possibilities for legal innovation.

Decentralized Governance

Unlike traditional legal systems, which rely on centralized authorities and hierarchical structures, Superjustice will embrace a more distributed and participatory approach to legal governance. It will enable decentralized governance by employing blockchain technology, which provides a secure and transparent scheme for recording and verifying legal transactions and agreements. Smart contracts, meaning self-executing contracts with terms directly written into code, can automate the enforcement of legal obligations and reduce the need for intermediaries.

As we emphasize in Chapter 3, the decentralized nature of Superjustice facilitates greater participation and collaboration among stakeholders, including legal professionals, policymakers, regulators, and the public. It will enable the creation of community-driven legal ecosystems, in which individuals can contribute to developing and refining legal norms. Decentralized governance can also promote transparency and accountability in legal processes. With blockchain-based record-keeping, legal transactions and decisions will be immutably stored and easily auditable, reducing the risk of corruption and enhancing public trust.[13]

Central to the conceptual framework of Superjustice and an inherent part of its decentralized ethos is the notion of community-driven law, which draws on the collective wisdom and participation of the populace.[14] Accordingly, Superjustice recognizes the

[12] The literature that explores the irrationality of and inconsistencies in human judgment and decision-making and how to respond to them is voluminous. For two prominent books see Daniel Kahneman, *Thinking, Fast and Slow* (Farrar, Straus and Giroux 2011); Richard H Thaler and Cass R Sunstein, *Nudge: The Final Edition* (Penguin Books 2021).

[13] For a general exploration of the importance of integration, engagement, and trust and their decline in modern societies see Robert D Putnam, *Bowling Alone: Revised and Updated: The Collapse and Revival of American Community* (Simon & Schuster 2020).

[14] The law and politics of decentralization have received scant scholarly attention. For a recent book offering a comparative account of decentralization see Aslı Ü Bâli and Omar M Dajani (eds), *Federalism and Decentralization in the Contemporary Middle East and North Africa* (Cambridge University Press 2023).

importance of community engagement and participatory justice in creating a legal system that truly reflects the values, needs, and aspirations of society and its diverse voices. Superjustice will thus foster a more inclusive, visible, and responsive legal system, empowering individuals and communities to actively participate in the legal process.

One way in which Superjustice furthers community engagement is through the *crowdsourcing of legal knowledge*. By leveraging the community's collective intelligence, Superjustice can tap into a vast pool of expertise, experiences, and perspectives to enrich legal development. Through online platforms and collaborative tools, individuals from diverse backgrounds can contribute their insights, opinions, and suggestions on various legal issues. Crowdsourcing legal knowledge would democratize access to legal information, ensuring that the legal system remains responsive to society's evolving needs and values. It would enable the identification of emerging legal issues, the generation of innovative solutions, and the incorporation of diverse viewpoints into the legal discourse.

Another way to facilitate a community-driven law is through *participatory policymaking*, where citizens have a direct say in shaping the rules and regulations that govern their lives. Through digital platforms and collaborative tools, Superjustice would enable individuals to engage in the policymaking process at various levels, from local communities to national and international arenas. Such engagement can take various forms, including online public consultations, deliberative forums, and virtual citizen assemblies. These mechanisms could allow individuals to provide feedback, propose amendments, and vote on policy proposals, ensuring that the resulting policies reflect the will and priorities of the people. This, in turn, will increase the legitimacy and effectiveness of legal norms, while cultivating a sense of ownership and buy-in among the public.

A third form of community-driven law pertains to *dispute resolution mechanisms*. By empowering communities to resolve conflicts at the local level, Superjustice can alleviate the burden on formal legal institutions and provide more tailored, context-specific solutions. Community-driven dispute resolution in Superjustice can take the form of online mediation, peer-to-peer arbitration, and community justice panels. These mechanisms better respect local cultures and build on community members' knowledge, skills, and social capital. To that end, Superjustice will provide the necessary technological infrastructure and support. This will include, among other things, AI legal agents that can advise and assist individuals; secure platforms for communication and evidence sharing; and fair, open, and accessible decision-making processes.[15]

Superjustice recognizes the importance of empowering individuals to participate in, understand, and assert their legal rights and responsibilities. Thus, *citizen legal education* is the fourth manifestation of community-driven law in Superjustice. By providing

[15] For a general discussion of online courts and their ability to deliver justice see Richard Susskind, *Online Courts and the Future of Justice* (Oxford University Press 2021). See also Tara Vasdani, "Robot Justice: China's Use of Internet Courts" *The Lawyer's Daily, LexisNexis* (2020).

accessible, user-friendly legal resources, Superjustice seeks to bridge the knowledge gap between the legal system and the public. This approach will promote a more legally empowered and engaged citizenry, reducing the power imbalance between legal professionals and lay individuals. Consequently, more people will be able to make informed decisions and effectively advocate for their rights and interests.

Moreover, Superjustice will harness state-of-the-art tools such as interactive legal guides, video tutorials, and gamified learning experiences to ensure effective citizen legal education. These resources will demystify complex legal concepts, provide practical guidance on common legal issues, and equip individuals with the confidence and tools needed to navigate the legal system effectively. To accommodate diverse user backgrounds, we imagine a system in which each tool will be tailored to match individual traits such as language proficiency, prior experience, and educational level. To guarantee the reliability and effectiveness of these educational resources, Superjustice will commit to rigorous, evidence-based research, including user testing, data analysis, and expert review. This approach will help ensure that each component is scientifically validated and precisely adapted to meet the practical needs of users. In the longer term, AGI will be able to generate tailored information, recommendations, and tools for everyone, communicating in a way that the specific individual readily understands.

Through these various mechanisms of community engagement and participation, Superjustice aims to leverage communities' collective wisdom, energy, and creativity. In doing so, it seeks to create a legal system that is truly of the people, by the people, and for the people. The concrete examples we analyze in Chapter 9 will showcase the practical implementation of making the law more bottom-up and reflective of society's needs.

Personalized Law and Accessible Legal Services

Superjustice recognizes that every individual's legal needs are unique and that a one-size-fits-all approach is often inadequate.[16] Therefore, a core component of Superjustice is the provision of personalized legal services tailored to each user's specific circumstances and preferences. By leveraging advanced data analytics and AI algorithms, Superjustice can gather and analyze a wide range of data points about an individual, including their legal history, personal characteristics, subjective preferences, and specific legal issues. This data-driven approach will facilitate customized legal advice, recommendations, and solutions that are most relevant and effective for each user.

In many (if not all) jurisdictions, most legal disputes are resolved through negotiation rather than formal litigation. Harnessing personalized AI agents on each side of a dispute can streamline these negotiations by identifying common ground, mapping

[16] The idea of personalized law was powerfully introduced by Omri Ben-Shahar and Ariel Porat, *Personalized Law: Different Rules for Different People* (Oxford University Press 2021). We argue that AI capabilities make this idea even more fascinating and allow its expansion to legal services and beyond.

out optimal settlement ranges, and suggesting fair compromises. This "smart" negotiation process would expedite dispute resolution and increase the overall social surplus, yielding more efficient outcomes that benefit all parties involved. Throughout, humans remain at the center—empowered by AI agents.[17]

Personalized legal services in Superjustice extend beyond tailored negotiations and legal advice. AI legal agents can automate the generation of legal documents, such as contracts and agreements, based on user-specific inputs and preferences. This system will also provide interactive tools and platforms that allow users to navigate complex legal processes with ease and confidence. Overall, the personalization of legal services in Superjustice aims to empower individuals by providing them with accessible, affordable, and user-friendly legal support. Tailoring legal solutions to individual needs, Superjustice will bridge the gap between the legal system and the people it serves.

Challenges and Risks

While Superjustice could create a more responsive and inclusive legal system, it also faces a range of potential challenges and risks that must be carefully addressed. Failing to address such concerns could lead to potential miscarriages of justice and severe erosion of public trust in the legal system. The following discussion flags some of the key risks and challenges that will be echoed throughout the book and dealt with more systematically in several chapters, particularly Chapter 10. For the sake of brevity, we focus here on three categories of concerns: (1) technological and substantive challenges, (2) privacy and data security risks, and (3) ethical and social responsibility.

Technological and Substantive Challenges

Legal decision-making often involves fact-finding and nuanced reasoning, requiring the ability to analyze data, understand humans, consider social norms and cultures, interpret legal principles, and apply them to specific cases. Legal reasoning often involves weighing competing narratives, interpreting abstract concepts, balancing competing interests, and exercising discretion. Developing AI algorithms that can effectively replicate human-like reasoning and judgment is a significant challenge. Given the inherent complexities and ambiguities of the legal domain, one of the primary technological challenges in implementing Superjustice is ensuring the reliability, accuracy, and robustness of AI algorithms.

AI systems can make errors, with grave implications, such as misinterpreting data or failing to capture the nuances of human behavior and intent. Therefore, there must be clear and robust mechanisms for accountability and redress when AI systems produce

[17] See Samuel I Becher and Benjamin Alarie, "Legal Order in the Age of AI Agents" (forthcoming, 2026) University of Toronto Law Journal.

erroneous or harmful outcomes.[18] Without robust accountability measures, such as audits, oversight, and clear liability rules, these errors may go unchecked and lead to serious injustice. To mitigate such risks, it is essential to consider the need to keep humans in the loop.[19]

Superjustice will include legal and regulatory frameworks that assign responsibility to the relevant stakeholders, such as the designers, developers, or operators of the AI systems. It will also provide avenues for individuals to challenge or appeal AI-generated decisions. As part of this strategy, there would be ongoing monitoring, evaluation, and adjustment of AI systems. This may involve conducting impact assessments and engaging in public consultations to identify and address any mistakes, injustices, or unintended consequences. On a related point, capacity building and training for legal professionals will be vital. This entails integrating AI and data science into legal education and fostering collaboration among legal experts, ethicists, and technologists.

Irrespective of the risk of AI errors, it remains essential for individuals to receive and to understand the substantive reasoning underlying the decisions that affect them in a legal context. At the same time, the complex and opaque nature of current AI algorithms makes it impossible to provide clear explanations for their outputs. As a result, the use of AI in the legal system raises questions about the explainability and transparency of AI-generated decisions. As the discussions throughout the book illustrate, explainability and interpretability are essential for maintaining public trust and confidence in Superjustice.

A related challenge is the potential impact of AI on the role of human judgment and discretion in the legal system. While AI can assist in decision-making processes, it is necessary to strike a balance between the efficiency and consistency that AI provides and the value of human expertise and contextual understanding. Balancing AI automation with human judgment is a critical challenge that requires a nuanced approach to determine the appropriate level of human engagement. As we explore in Chapter 5, the key lies in developing a dynamic, context-dependent framework that optimizes the strengths and mitigates the weaknesses of both AI and humans. Toward that goal, Superjustice must carefully determine and continuously evaluate the importance of human oversight, discretion, and contextual understanding. Over time, rather than merely assisting human decision-makers, AI should be positioned as a primary decision-maker, with human oversight diminishing as AI capabilities advance and prove reliable.

The integrity of AI systems in legal contexts relies heavily on the accuracy and authenticity of the data they are trained on, which can be ensured through robust data provenance and validation frameworks. Here, a key concern is that data could be tampered with to manipulate AI-driven decisions and outputs. To mitigate this risk, Superjustice

[18] For a proposal advancing AI legal neutrality and not discriminating between AI and human behavior see Ryan Abbott, *The Reasonable Robot: Artificial Intelligence and the Law* (Cambridge University Press 2020).

[19] For interesting discussions of the "human in the loop" concept see Eduardo Mosqueira-Rey and others, "Human-in-the-Loop Machine Learning: A State of the Art" (2023) 56(4) Artificial Intelligence Review 3005; Rebecca Crootof and others, "Humans in the Loop" (2023) 76 Vanderbilt Law Review 429.

would require comprehensive data validation frameworks and the integration of blockchain technologies to ensure data traceability and immutability. Implementation of regular audits and monitoring by independent third-party organizations could further safeguard against manipulation, thereby maintaining the system's credibility and trustworthiness. Moreover, collaborative efforts among legal experts, data scientists, and cybersecurity professionals could be essential to develop and maintain these technical safeguards against data manipulation and system tampering.

Privacy, Data Security, and Power Imbalances

One of the most pressing criticisms of integrating AI into legal systems is the potential for privacy violations and the ways that online information can undermine human agency and exacerbate power imbalances.[20] The collection, storage, and analysis of vast amounts of personal data—ranging from legal records to personal communications—necessitate stringent safeguards to protect sensitive information. However, there is an inherent tension or trade-off between transparency measures and tools (such as blockchain) that reduce the risk of corruption, and the need to protect individuals' privacy.

Adopting privacy-preserving technologies could enable AI to learn from data without accessing it directly, thereby maintaining confidentiality while still benefiting from data insights. Such technologies may include federated learning, a method where AI algorithms are trained across decentralized devices. They may also incorporate differential privacy, which introduces random noise to data, effectively obscuring sensitive information while preserving overall utility. Likewise, Superjustice must be protected against potential breaches, cyberattacks, or tampering attempts that could compromise its integrity. Here, Superjustice should employ measures such as robust encryption methods, multifactor authentication, strict access controls, and transparent data-handling policies. Intrusion detection systems, data backup and recovery mechanisms, and regular security audits and updates will be necessary to promptly identify and address vulnerabilities. We will return to this important topic in Chapters 4 and 10.

Socially and Ethically Responsible Innovation

The role of AI in legal decision-making introduces complex ethical and societal challenges.[21] One significant issue here is the reliance on algorithms that may inadvertently perpetuate or amplify existing biases.[22] Biases can manifest in various forms,

[20] For an influential account see Shoshana Zuboff, *The Age of Surveillance Capitalism: The Fight for a Human Future at the New Frontier of Power* (PublicAffairs 2019).

[21] For scholarly work bringing together the seemingly divergent fields of AI and Ethics see Markus D Dubber, Frank Pasquale, and Sunit Das (eds), *The Oxford Handbook of Ethics of AI* (Oxford University Press 2020). The recent rise of generative AI underscores the importance of AI ethics.

[22] Compare Sandra G Mayson, "Bias In, Bias Out" (2019) 128 Yale Law Journal 2218.

such as racial, gender, or socioeconomic biases, and can profoundly impact individuals' access to justice and the fairness of legal decisions. AI's training data often reflects historical prejudices, despite efforts to design fair and impartial systems. Addressing such challenges requires a proactive approach to identifying and mitigating sources of bias through transparent AI design. Such design features should safeguard diverse and representative training data, implement fairness metrics and review mechanisms, and continuously monitor and regularly adjust algorithms for potential biases. These challenges also merit gradual adoption and rigorous testing, introducing temporary schemes and regular checkpoints to reevaluate modalities.

Another concern is that an AI-powered legal system may exacerbate the digital divide. Individuals without access to technology or the internet may find themselves disproportionately disadvantaged, unable to benefit from and contribute to AI-enhanced legal services. Elderly people, for example, may struggle to access or effectively use digital platforms, leaving them excluded from essential legal services. To narrow this gap, policymakers should support initiatives that expand digital literacy and access to technology, particularly in underserved and rural communities. Public-private partnerships could facilitate the installation of the necessary infrastructure. At the same time, community-driven programs could offer training and support to ensure that all members of society can navigate and benefit from the new legal landscape. Public assistance—possibly in the form of public advocates who will support elderly individuals and other vulnerable groups—would help bridge this gap and ensure equitable access to AI-enhanced legal resources.

Proactively addressing such concerns will help ensure that the vision of Superjustice does not inadvertently create new forms of inequality or compromise widely accepted ethical standards. To achieve this, Superjustice will incorporate robust governance frameworks and ethical guidelines for the development and use of AI in the legal domain. These frameworks should be advanced through multi-stakeholder collaboration involving legal professionals, technologists, ethicists, and representatives from diverse communities.[23]

Future Trajectory

The trajectory of Superjustice will be shaped by a confluence of technological advances, shifting societal expectations, and the pursuit of more efficient, equitable, and accessible legal systems. It will thus be characterized by continuous innovation and adaptation. In what follows, we recap previous discussions and provide further insight into the major components of this confluence. These insights will be echoed and developed further in subsequent chapters.

[23] A somewhat similar approach has been suggested for advancing transparency more generally. See Archon Fung, Mary Graham, and David Weil, *Full Disclosure: The Perils and Promise of Transparency* (Cambridge University Press 2007).

Integration of Emerging Technologies

As the pace of technological innovation accelerates, Superjustice will continue to harness the power of cutting-edge tools and platforms to enhance its capabilities and expand its reach. Superjustice will benefit from advances in natural language processing, enabling more sophisticated analysis and understanding of legal texts and documents. Machine-learning algorithms will become increasingly accurate and efficient in predicting legal outcomes, identifying relevant precedents, generating recommendations, and assisting with negotiations. This continuous evolution entails the employment of AI systems to perform tasks that traditionally require human intelligence. At a minimum, this includes analyzing legal documents, evaluating cases, predicting their outcomes, and providing personalized legal advice. As advanced technologies materialize, this may expand to more complex and autonomous decision-making.

Blockchain is often associated with cryptocurrencies, but its use in Superjustice is more about securing data. Picture it as a digital ledger that is publicly accessible and capable of recording legal data in a manner that is highly secure against tampering. These ledgers ensure transparency and prevent tampering by maintaining a permanent and verifiable record of legal transactions, like legal decisions, patents, or contracts. The use of smart contracts will automate the execution and enforcement of legal obligations, reducing the need for intermediaries and increasing the speed and efficiency of legal processes.

Integrating AIoT devices and sensors will enable real-time monitoring and data collection, facilitating evidence gathering, compliance tracking, and proactive legal interventions. IoT involves various devices, ranging from smartphones to sensors in buildings, all of which are connected online. These devices collect and share data in real time. In Superjustice, the IoT could be combined with AI capabilities to amplify compliance monitoring and provide evidence in legal cases. The AIoT could be described as a network of eyes and ears that helps the legal system stay informed, accurate, and reactive.

Immersive technologies such as augmented reality (AR) and virtual reality (VR) will transform the ways that legal information is presented and interacted with. These technologies will create immersive and engaging experiences for legal professionals and the public alike. For example, AR could be used to overlay relevant legal information, such as case law or statutory provisions, onto real-world objects or locations. This could provide instant access to crucial data during negotiations, legal proceedings, or investigations. VR, at the same time, could enable users to explore crime scenes virtually. Likewise, it could reconstruct accidents or simulate court scenarios, facilitating a deeper understanding of complex scenarios. As AR and VR advance, they will probably play an increasingly significant role in enhancing accessibility and transparency, ultimately contributing to the overall effectiveness and fairness of Superjustice.

Furthermore, advanced robotics and embodied intelligence—the ability to learn through physical interaction with the environment—will further expand Superjustice's capabilities, combining physical presence with sophisticated cognitive abilities. These systems will utilize robust world models (i.e., comprehensive frameworks that understand physical space, human behavior, and social dynamics) to interact meaningfully in real-world legal scenarios. For instance, robots could secure crime scenes, collect evidence with precision, or assist in reconstructions. When integrated with other technologies like AIoT and AR/VR, these systems will create a seamless blend of physical and digital legal operations. This convergence of embodied and virtual intelligence represents a significant step toward a unified, intelligent legal ecosystem that can perceive, understand, and act in both physical and digital realms.

Adoption: Training and Service Delivery Models

As we will see in Chapters 5–8, Superjustice will significantly alter the roles of human lawyers, judges, law professors, and legal professionals.[24] In the short to medium term, legal professionals will need to collaborate with AI systems, leveraging their unique capabilities while maintaining oversight and governance over these platforms. Mundane and routine tasks, such as document review and legal research, will be increasingly automated, freeing human legal professionals to focus on more complex, strategic, and creative aspects of their work. Accordingly, legal professionals must be prepared to work alongside AI systems, providing oversight and guidance while leveraging the efficiency and analytical power of these technologies.

At the same time, legal professionals must resist the temptation to prematurely defer to AI-driven decisions. In the early years of Superjustice, legal professionals should maintain a critical role in ensuring that legal processes remain fair, ethical, and aligned with widely accepted human values.[25] Accordingly, encouraging collaboration between technologists and legal professionals will be essential in shaping the development and deployment of Superjustice systems, ensuring they are designed with appropriate safeguards, transparency, and accountability measures.

The transformation to Superjustice necessitates the development of cross-disciplinary knowledge and the nurturing of soft skills, such as critical thinking, problem-solving, and emotional intelligence, which are less susceptible to automation. In the long run, however, advanced technologies will probably exhibit many so-called "soft skills" and will be capable of outperforming most humans even in more sensitive and complex legal domains. It will thus become pivotal to develop

[24] See also Abdi Aidid and Benjamin Alarie, *The Legal Singularity: How Artificial Intelligence Can Make Law Radically Better* (University of Toronto Press 2023); Richard Susskind, *The End of Lawyers?: Rethinking the Nature of Legal Services* (Oxford University Press 2010).

[25] See also Mireille Hildebrandt and Kieron O'Hara (eds), *Life and the Law in the Era of Data-Driven Agency* (Edward Elgar Publishing 2020); Marcelo Corrales, Mark Fenwick, and Nikolaus Forgo (eds), *Robotics, AI and The Future of Law* (Springer 2018); Mireille Hildebrandt, *Smart Technologies and the End(s) of Law: Novel Entanglements of Law and Technology* (Edward Elgar Publishing 2016). On the importance of preserving human dignity when algorithmic systems shape decision-making environments see, for example, Jan Trzaskowski, *Your Privacy Is Important to Us!—Restoring Human Dignity in Data-Driven Marketing* (Ex Tuto Publishing 2021).

comprehensive training programs tailored to legal practitioners. Such training programs should emphasize not only technical proficiency but also the art of translating AI-driven decisions into clear, meaningful explanations that build public trust and understanding.

Moreover, a phased implementation approach can facilitate a smoother transition, allowing for iterative feedback and adjustments. Starting with more mundane and less critical legal domains or voluntary opt-in pilot projects can help build trust and demonstrate effectiveness. Each phase should prioritize transparency and explanation, assisting stakeholders to understand not just what decisions are being made, but why, and how they serve justice. Engaging with professional legal bodies to co-develop these initiatives will ensure that the transition respects the nuances of legal practice. This co-development will also help set ethical standards that align with professional values and responsibilities, while maintaining a focus on clear communication and public understanding.

Ergo, Superjustice will foster, if not necessitate, a culture of lifelong learning and professional development among legal professionals. Lawyers will become the human face of a justice system that is increasingly powered by AGI and other technologies. This change will necessitate access to cutting-edge legal education and training programs, equipping legal professionals with the skills and knowledge needed to thrive in an increasingly technology-driven legal environment. Superjustice's robust information infrastructure will facilitate peer-to-peer learning, mentorship, and collaboration, enabling legal professionals to learn from one another more effectively and collectively advance the field.

As Superjustice evolves and matures, it will also transform the way that legal services are delivered, accessed, and experienced. All things considered, Superjustice will drive a significant expansion of legal service delivery models. In Chapter 6, we explore how increased automation and self-service capabilities will empower individuals and businesses to access legal services in more convenient, cost-effective, and personalized ways. Online legal platforms and marketplaces will proliferate, seamlessly and efficiently connecting legal service providers with clients. These platforms will apply AI-powered matchmaking algorithms to pair individuals with the most suitable legal professionals and service providers based on their specific needs, preferences, and budgets.

Additionally, Superjustice will elevate the growth of alternative legal service providers, such as legal process outsourcing firms, legal tech startups, and community-based legal clinics. These providers will leverage technology to offer unbundled legal services, fixed-fee arrangements, and subscription-based models, making legal assistance more accessible and affordable to a wider range of clients. Beyond that, Superjustice will enable the development of self-help legal tools and resources, empowering individuals to navigate common legal issues independently. Chatbots, virtual legal agents, and interactive legal guides will provide personalized advice and support, helping individuals understand their rights, obligations, and legal options in a user-friendly and effective manner.

Globalization and Cross-Border Collaboration

As commerce expands, legal issues increasingly transcend national boundaries and become more complex and interconnected. As a result, greater cooperation and coordination among legal systems worldwide will be beneficial and essential. Superjustice's decentralized and networked architecture will foster seamless data sharing, knowledge exchange, and collaborative problem-solving among legal professionals and institutions across jurisdictions, cultures, and languages.

To support this globalized collaboration, Superjustice will facilitate the creation of international legal databases and knowledge repositories. These resources could include shared case law libraries, comparative legal analyses, and best practice guides. This body of knowledge will, in turn, enable the identification of common challenges and solutions, and nurture the development of innovative legal approaches that draw from diverse legal traditions and perspectives. This will eventually encourage the development of global legal standards, best practices, and harmonized approaches to legal issues.

Employing its cross-cultural, multilingual, and multi-jurisdictional competencies, Superjustice will support the growth of international dispute resolution mechanisms, such as online AI arbitration and mediation platforms. These platforms will provide efficient, fair, and cost-effective means for resolving cross-border disputes, reducing the barriers to access to justice in a globalized world. In this respect, Superjustice has the long-run potential to facilitate a more open, trusting, and collaborative geopolitical environment.[26] Most likely, the realization of this potential will require coordinated efforts from governments, academia, and private providers, each bringing their unique capabilities and interests to this challenge.

Concluding Remarks

Our laws and legal institutions are the product of recent centuries and have largely coevolved with the rise of the Industrial Revolution. Laws were forged, hammered, and human-crafted by many minds and hands over dozens of decades to regulate physical entities, tangible assets, human labor, and human behavior. The design of legal systems did not, however, account for the advent of AI capabilities. Unsurprisingly, then, our laws and legal systems are not well-positioned to leverage the immense potential of new technologies that transcend the boundaries of traditional legal constructs. As we move into an era where AI, machine learning, and other cutting-edge technologies are reshaping various aspects of society, it becomes increasingly evident that our existing legal frameworks could benefit from a deep overhaul.

[26] For an insightful historical treatment linking and analyzing the present-day revolutions of globalization, technology, identity, and geopolitics see Fareed Zakaria, *Age of Revolutions: Progress and Backlash from 1600 to the Present* (Penguin Random House UK 2024).

The core components of Superjustice—AI-driven decision-making, decentralized governance, and personalized law and legal services—provide the foundation for a paradigm shift. AI enables intelligent analysis, prediction, recommendation, and decision-making capabilities that enhance the speed, consistency, and fairness of legal processes and dispute resolution practices. Decentralized governance, powered by blockchain, encourages greater participation, collaboration, and accountability among stakeholders. Personalized legal services, tailored through data analytics, empower individuals with accessible, affordable, and user-friendly legal support.

The path to realizing the full potential of Superjustice is not without challenges. Technological issues around algorithmic bias and algorithmic justice; substantive concerns regarding human discretion and judgment; and thorny questions related to fairness, transparency, explainability, and accountability must all be thoughtfully navigated. Superjustice will need to adopt proactive strategies to mitigate risks, such as establishing governance frameworks, monitoring impacts, implementing regular auditing, building capacity, and maintaining human-centricity where appropriate. In pursuing a more just and efficient legal system, we must strive to create a deeply symbiotic relationship between human wisdom and AI. Carefully designing this symbiotic relationship will be the key to ensuring that our legal system remains grounded in the rich tapestry of human experiences that give it meaning.

We began with the Library of Alexandria, so let's return to its lessons. Whereas the ancient Library stood as an impressive physical monument to human wisdom, it was accessible only to the privileged few and vulnerable to destruction. Superjustice, however, offers the opportunity to build something that cannot be lost to fire or decay: a resilient, distributed network of justice that transcends physical limitations and bridges divides of privilege and access. In reimagining our legal systems through the lens of powerful AI, we may yet fulfill the original ostensible purpose of Alexandria: not merely to hoard knowledge, but to transform it into enduring and ever-growing wisdom that serves humanity.

2

Ten Pillars of Legal Dysfunctionality

The Case for Change

Picture Jane, an ordinary citizen with a spotless record, always mindful of complying with the law, who has just moved to a new town. Unfortunately, Jane finds herself entangled in a bureaucratic web while contesting what she believes is an unfairly issued parking ticket. The signage was unclear, causing her to misunderstand the parking regulations. As she is convinced that the ticket was issued in error, Jane decides to challenge it.

What should have been a simple, straightforward process quickly spirals into a frustrating ordeal. Jane spends hours on the phone, being passed from department to department, only to be redirected repeatedly without resolution. Another call yields no result. Her written appeal is rejected. Eventually, she is forced to litigate her case and take time off work to appear in court, which is located a few hours' drive from her new town. The system is slow, rigid, emotionally draining, and unresponsive, offering little flexibility for someone unfamiliar with the legal system who is juggling a busy life.

Now, imagine an alternative. In a Superjustice system, partially decentralized and powered by advanced technology, Jane could have addressed her issue through a user-friendly app on her phone. This app, powered by blockchain and smart contracts, would give her instant access to relevant legal resources, provide a transparent and automated review process, and enable her to resolve the dispute without ever leaving her home. No long waits, no frustrating phone calls, no complex forms to submit, no need to take time off work—just a quick, efficient resolution, tailored to her circumstances and easily accessible from her personal device.

This narrative captures the essence of the challenges faced in today's complex, centralized legal structures, which move slowly, frequently break down, and cost far more to run than they should. Centralized legal systems are like an old, creaky car. Better than a horse and carriage and serviceably reliable in its day, but now constantly in need of maintenance, struggling to meet the demands of modern life. By contrast, imagine Superjustice as an agile, autonomous vehicle that seamlessly navigates complex terrains and city streets. It is responsive, efficient, and can adapt smoothly to changing conditions.

You might feel comfortable sticking with your familiar "legal vehicle" for now or wonder how this proposed legal agility applies to your specific circumstances. These reactions are entirely natural. People tend to prefer the status quo and can become

Superjustice. Samuel I. Becher and Benjamin Alarie, Oxford University Press.
 DOI: 10.1093/9780198991885.003.0004

loss-averse and uncomfortable when faced with a novel and transformative change.[1] Yet, our legal systems are rooted in the past and, in many respects, fail to meet contemporary demands.

Make no mistake: Our legal systems offer significant strengths and have many virtues. Modern law plays a fundamental role in advancing social order, reducing violence, and providing a relatively structured framework that seeks to facilitate predictable and civilized human interactions. It safeguards individual rights, promotes equality, and advances human rights, contributing to justice and fairness. Additionally, the legal infrastructure supports economic growth by providing the predictability necessary for trade and commerce. Law also fosters innovation through intellectual property protections and promotes environmental sustainability by regulating the use of natural resources. On a global scale, legal frameworks enable cooperation between nations, addressing transnational issues and resolving conflicts. Through these functions, the law serves as a cornerstone of societal stability and human advancement.

However, these strengths coexist with significant and persistent weaknesses. Despite its virtues, the law—both as a concept and a tool—falls short of a utopian ideal. Most notably, while the law's aspirations are lofty, its reality is often rudely sobering. This chapter delves into these negative aspects, focusing on the persistent challenges that continue to afflict modern legal systems.

Unlocking Legal Surplus

No system is perfect, and readers may question the value of dedicating a chapter to the flaws of current legal systems in a book focused on the transformative power of artificial intelligence (AI). The answer to this question lies in the untapped potential, or "legal surplus," that could be realized by addressing systemic weaknesses. Centralized legal systems, burdened by bureaucracy and tradition, experience inertia and struggle to evolve at the pace required to meet these demands. While traditional legal systems continue to grapple with backlogs and inefficiencies, the rapid advancement of AI provides a striking contrast.

As AI progresses toward superhuman capabilities, design, production, and information costs are falling dramatically, creating new opportunities to reimagine the future of legal systems. Meanwhile, each day of delay compounds these systemic costs—cases pile up, people are denied justice, and the gap between technological capability and legal delivery widens. By tapping into the underutilized surplus of the legal system and redistributing it more equitably, we can significantly enhance the overall value of the system.

[1] See, for example, William Samuelson and Richard Zeckhauser, "Status Quo Bias in Decision Making" (1988) 1 Journal of Risk and Uncertainty 7; Daniel Kahneman, Jack L Knetsch, and Richard H Thaler, "Anomalies: The Endowment Effect, Loss Aversion, and Status Quo Bias" (1991) 5(1) Journal of Economic Perspectives 193.

However, even the most revolutionary technology is merely a tool. To understand how to use it wisely, we must adopt a strategic vision that acknowledges the deeply rooted issues undermining our current legal systems. Redesigning legal systems is not solely a technological endeavor; it is a profound societal challenge. The undertaking encompasses a vast ecosystem of actors and is deeply influenced by the complex social, cultural, economic, technical, and institutional contexts in which these systems operate. As technology evolves and interacts with these forces, public values shift in response to new realities, power dynamics, and people's engagement with the legal and technological landscape. Thus, integrating AI and computational infrastructures into legal systems involves more than rethinking the technical capabilities of law. To maximize the legal surplus, we must also consider the institutions that enforce the law, the decision-making processes that underpin it, and the roles of the professionals and citizens who interact with it. Technological innovation is key to unlocking its untapped surplus, but so too is the integration of user and community perspectives through participatory design processes, stakeholder consultations, and ongoing feedback mechanisms.

As we will argue in Chapter 3, AI capabilities and legal decentralization can work in tandem; together, they are critical elements in designing the future of legal governance within the broader existing societal framework. Decentralization can harness technologies to reduce the cost of law and increase the legal surplus, while further democratizing legal systems. Unlike today's costly and centralized systems, Superjustice would integrate both centralized and decentralized elements. This, in turn, promises a more affordable, accessible, inclusive, and efficient justice system, which addresses many of the current shortcomings.

The Cost of Tradition

With this vision in place, let's examine the primary limitations of centralized legal systems through a structured typology. We now turn to ten distinct categories, referred to as "The Ten Pillars of Dysfunction." Together, these pillars illustrate how centralization and high costs burden the legal system, resulting in inefficiencies and suboptimal outcomes that undermine its core objectives.

Pillar 1. Prohibitive Costs and Access to Justice

One of the most pressing issues of centralized legal systems is the exorbitant costs that burden every stage of the legal process. The mere existence of legal systems entails inescapable costs. Transacting with information, enacting and enforcing regulation, becoming informed about the law, adjudicating disputes, and compensating legal system actors are costly undertakings. Moreover, the issues in the other pillars of dysfunctionality—such as legal complexity, administrative inefficiencies, and a lack of transparency—further compound these costs, leading to injustice and disproportionately affecting vulnerable populations. However, the entire life cycle of law incurs significant costs. Drafting laws, revising them, administering the legal system, ensuring compliance, enforcing regulations, and litigating cases are all costly, inefficient, and slow.

These rising costs are partly attributable to what economists call Baumol's cost disease, a phenomenon whereby, over time, labor-intensive services like legal work become more expensive relative to goods and services that benefit from technological automation.[2] Unlike manufacturing, where productivity gains have dramatically reduced costs, legal services remain fundamentally human-centered, requiring significant time from highly trained professionals. Even as technology advances, the core activities of legal reasoning, advocacy, and judgment still demand skilled human attention. While this economic reality does not excuse inefficiencies or justify barriers to justice, it helps explain why legal costs persistently outpace inflation, despite modernization efforts. The challenge, then, is to reimagine how legal services are delivered to overcome these structural economic constraints.

Indeed, centralized legal systems worldwide are notorious for their high costs, significantly impeding access to justice. Attorney fees, court costs, and associated legal expenses often make the legal process extraordinarily expensive and unattainable for many. High legal fees reduce access to justice, disproportionately affecting vulnerable populations, exacerbating societal inequalities, and undermining the fundamental principles of justice. The complexity of extensive legal procedures, principles, and systems, combined with the cost of legal advice and formal representation, creates multiple burdens and barriers that distance ordinary citizens from the justice system that is presumed to serve them.

The costs and complexities that make access to justice such a thorny issue manifest themselves in every aspect of the law. Laypeople frequently encounter barriers in navigating the legal system. Laws are often lengthy, complicated, and filled with jargon, rendering them incomprehensible to non-experts and, at times, even to seasoned legal professionals.[3] This is true for almost any type of legal document, from written judgments to insurance policies, from consumer contracts to privacy agreements, and from tax forms to lease and employment agreements.

Moreover, even when laws and regulations seem straightforward, they often come entangled with local ordinances, legal jargon, and forms that require expertise to complete. This complexity forces individuals to seek expert legal counseling, further increasing their financial burden. For example, a litigant must often wade through a complex web of laws, administrative rules, and statutes, sometimes spread across multiple jurisdictions. The complexity is further exacerbated by various layers of

[2] See the seminal work by William J Baumol and William G Bowen, *Performing Arts—The Economic Dilemma: A Study of Problems Common to Theater, Opera, Music and Dance* (Twentieth Century Fund 1977).

[3] See Eric Martínez and others, "Even Laypeople Use Legalese" (2024) 121 Proceedings of the National Academy of Sciences e2405564121 [10.1073/pnas.2405564121].

precedents, interpretive conventions, general principles, and enforcement norms, all of which increase the difficulty of navigating the legal system without expert assistance.

Jane's experience illustrates this clearly: What should have been a straightforward dispute over a parking ticket unnecessarily escalated into an expensive and arduous experience. To resolve her grievance, Jane was forced to invest time, emotional energy, and money. This barrier deters many from engaging with the legal system, while others opt for informal resolutions or abandon legal recourse altogether. In essence, Jane's case is emblematic of a broader problem: The legal system's reliance on complex and expensive procedures often turns uncomplicated and minor issues into disproportionately burdensome operations.

The reader may have reasonably assumed that the police or the local council issued Jane's parking ticket. However, a small tweak to the story further demonstrates how seemingly straightforward legal matters like parking tickets can become unexpectedly complex. Interestingly, the following case variation is based on a common experience of many car users in New Zealand.[4]

Imagine Jane had parked her car in a private parking garage and paid for two hours. Returning a few minutes late, Jane receives a "breach notice" from the garage operator, demanding $60 for overstaying. The garage operator cites its standardized terms and conditions, which customers are presumed to accept by entering the car park. This scenario raises a barrage of legal questions, extending far beyond a simple parking dispute: Is Jane legally obliged to pay the $60? Can Jane challenge the owner's practice as unfair? Could this fee be considered an unlawful penalty under contract law? Would Jane be safe in simply ignoring the notice? The complexity of contract law, enforcement mechanisms, and consumer protection norms transforms this seemingly small infraction into an intricate legal puzzle. Even seasoned lawyers may find this scenario far from trivial.

Alarmingly, the disproportionate impact of legal costs and complexity on marginalized populations is one of the most glaring failures of centralized systems. For marginalized communities, the high cost of navigating legal systems effectively closes the door to justice, reinforcing cycles of exclusion and inequality. Administrative inefficiencies, lengthy procedures, and the high fees for legal assistance further discourage these groups from accessing justice in a timely and affordable manner.[5] Yet, access to justice is a fundamental human right. When significant portions of the population cannot afford

[4] See, for example, Rachel Moore, "Why Won't the Commerce Commission Investigate Wilson Parking?" *Stuff* (May 21, 2024) <www.stuff.co.nz/nz-news/350281579/why-wont-commerce-commission-investigate-wilson-parking>; Tom Hunt and Frances Chin, "Wellington Waterfront Stoush Ends with Fine Waived" *The Post* (August 26, 2024) <www.thepost.co.nz/nz-news/350390588/wellington-waterfront-parking-stoush-ends-fine-waived>; Steve Williams, "Auckland Driver Stunned to Cop a Fine When the Empty Clearing She Regularly Parked in Suddenly Turned into a Car Park" *Daily Mail* (May 1, 2024) <www.dailymail.co.uk/news/article-13369699/Auckland-driver-stunned-fine-gravel-clearing-turned-car-park.html>; Sonya Bateson, "Shopping Centre, McDonald's Parking Fines Frustrate Bay of Plenty Customers" *NZ Herald* (May 7, 2024) <www.nzherald.co.nz/rotorua-daily-post/news/shopping-centre-mcdonalds-parking-fines-frustrate-bay-of-plenty-customers/OEZNERAWTRBFZGF7XT3C7EZHRA/>.

[5] See Hazel Genn, *Paths to Justice: What People Do and Think about Going to Law* (Bloomsbury Publishing 1999); Rebecca L Sandefur, "Access to Civil Justice and Race, Class, and Gender Inequality" (2008) 34(1) Annual Review of Sociology 339.

legal services or navigate the legal system, it undermines the principle of equality before the law. This lack of access perpetuates social inequities, alienates citizens from the justice system, and erodes public trust in its ability to deliver fair outcomes.

Pillar 2. Geographic Barriers and Global Legal Fragmentation

Financial and procedural barriers to accessing justice are widely recognized. However, geographic and jurisdictional challenges often receive less attention, despite their significant impact. These barriers can be just as insurmountable, limiting people's ability to protect their rights and fully engage with legal institutions and processes.

Traditional centralized legal systems frequently impose significant obstacles due to physical distance and location-based limitations. In many regions, particularly rural or remote areas, individuals may struggle to access legal institutions. This is because they are located a long way from courthouses, legal aid offices, or other essential legal services. Distance, inadequate infrastructure, and limited public transportation make it difficult for people to engage with the legal system. In more remote or isolated areas, the time and costs associated with traveling to participate in legal proceedings or access legal advice can be prohibitive. These challenges also create a justice gap, exacerbating inequalities between those in urban centers and those in more isolated locations.

Unlike Jane, many people in small towns lack the time, motivation, resources, and energy to drive hours to a courthouse to contest an unjust parking ticket. Furthermore, many standardized contract terms further complicate things and deter people from taking legal action. For example, in *Uber Technologies Inc v Heller*, 2020 SCC 16, the Supreme Court of Canada dealt with a dispute over mandatory arbitration clauses in Uber's contracts with its drivers. The term in question required drivers to resolve disputes through arbitration in Amsterdam of all places, effectively barring many from accessing justice. Such terms are prevalent in employment and consumer contracts and can have a chilling effect on laypeople, even if they may be—at least in some jurisdictions—unfair or unconscionable.

While technology offers potential solutions to some of these issues—such as online dispute resolution platforms and virtual courtrooms—the adoption of these innovations has been slow.[6] Many centralized systems rely on outdated processes that require the physical presence of the parties, even when technology could simplify or expedite proceedings. Furthermore, access to digital infrastructure, like stable and fast internet connections, remains far from universal. This digital divide is particularly acute in marginalized communities, where investment in infrastructure and digital literacy remains minimal.[7]

[6] See, for example, Richard Susskind, *Online Courts and the Future of Justice* (Oxford University Press 2021); Ethan Katsh and Orna Rabinovich-Einy, *Digital Justice: Technology and the Internet of Disputes* (Oxford University Press 2017).

[7] For a discussion of the digital divide and its impact on access to justice see Jane Bailey, Jacquelyn Burkell, and Graham Reynolds, "Access to Justice for All: Towards an 'Expansive Vision' of Justice and Technology" (2013)

While geographic barriers highlight the localized challenges of physically accessing justice, centralized legal systems also face challenges at the global level. As the world becomes more interconnected, legal systems encounter increased complexities that extend beyond physical borders. This leads to what is often referred to as legal fragmentation, whereby centralized systems, built primarily for domestic governance, struggle to address both local and global demands. Legal fragmentation occurs when different jurisdictions impose diverse and sometimes contradictory legal frameworks, complicating the legal landscape for multinational corporations, cross-border trade, and international digital transactions.

Centralized systems, primarily built for domestic governance, tend to focus on addressing national legal concerns, often struggling to accommodate the transnational demands of modern society and achieve international legal coherence. As a result, centralized systems often struggle to adapt to the increasingly global nature of commerce, migration, and digital interactions. Just as physical distance limits access to legal institutions, legal fragmentation creates barriers to justice in an increasingly interconnected world. This fragmentation can lead to legal uncertainty, delays, and additional costs.[8]

For example, consider the fact that international businesses are often required to comply with the regulatory frameworks of multiple countries, each with its own legal standards for taxation, data protection, and consumer rights. A company might find itself in full compliance with domestic law, only to face legal challenges abroad due to differing regulations. This fragmentation complicates legal compliance for international businesses and individuals, resulting in legal uncertainty, increased legal costs, and more disputes. While organizations such as the World Trade Organization (WTO) or United Nations Commission on International Trade Law (UNCITRAL) aim to promote legal harmonization across borders, progress has been slow, international cooperation is partial (or absent), and enforcement mechanisms are often weak. Consequently, centralized legal systems can become barriers to legal harmony across borders.

The challenges posed by geographic and legal fragmentation represent missed opportunities for legal harmonization and broader access to justice. While technology holds the potential to bridge some of these divides, it remains underutilized in most centralized legal systems. Legal reforms aimed at improving access to justice should move beyond economic barriers and address the physical and jurisdictional divides that complicate commerce and limit people's ability to engage with the law. In an

31(2) Windsor Yearbook of Access to Justice 181; James E Cabral and others, "Using Technology to Enhance Access to Justice" (2012) 26(1) Harvard Journal of Law & Technology 241.

[8] For the contention that the traditional, state-centric model of law is increasingly inadequate in a world where legal norms come from multiple state and non-state sources see Paul S Berman, *Global Legal Pluralism: A Jurisprudence of Law Beyond Borders* (Cambridge University Press 2012). Likewise, scholars argue that the emergence of transnational law challenges the traditional understanding of law as tied to the nation-state. See Peer Zumbansen, "Transnational Legal Pluralism" (2010) 1(2) Transnational Legal Theory 141. However, scholars also argue that the chances of extensive harmonization in various domains are slim, and for various persisting reasons. See, for example, Lee A Bygrave, *Data Privacy Law: An International Perspective* (Oxford University Press 2014) and particularly ch 7 (Prospects for Global Consensus).

increasingly interconnected world, legal systems must integrate both domestic and international perspectives to effectively address global challenges. Comprehensive reforms should focus on creating cohesive legal frameworks that span national borders while also improving accessibility for all individuals, regardless of their physical location.

Pillar 3. Over- and Under-Prescription

Beyond the exorbitant costs of the law and its limited universality, the mere creation of laws is fraught with difficulty. The fundamental nature of legal norms often contributes to inefficiencies and inequities. Legal norms tend to fall into two extremes: Some are grossly underspecified, relying on ambiguous standards like "fair" or "reasonable." Other legal norms, such as speed limits, are rigidly prescriptive, lacking the flexibility required for real-world circumstances. The binary nature of many legal norms—either too vague or overly prescriptive—creates endemic inefficiencies.

Laws relying on indeterminate standards, such as "fair use" (eg, in copyright law), "reasonable efforts" (eg, in contract law), "cruel and unusual punishment" (constitutional law and human rights), "substantial transformation" (in custom and trade law), or "good faith" (eg, in employment law), leave too much discretion to judicial or administrative interpretation. This, in turn, introduces unpredictability into the application of the law. For instance, employment laws that mandate "good faith" in employment relationships, "reasonable accommodations" to employees with disabilities, or "just cause" for termination often create uncertainty for both employers and employees.

Indeterminacy and unpredictability impose costs on individuals and organizations who find it difficult to manage risk and align their actions with legal expectations. Additionally, unpacking the meaning of these ambiguous legal norms requires judicial determination and formulation, with lengthy and intricate litigation adding considerably to the high costs of producing legal information. The judicial process of interpreting and applying vague legal norms may lead to bias and further harm marginalized groups. For example, judges may envisage the "reasonable person" to be WEIRD[9] and view terms such as "good faith" through their own cultural, subjective prism.

Conversely, highly prescriptive rules, such as speed limits or tax codes, often lack the flexibility needed to respond to contextual factors or evolving circumstances.[10] For example, tax codes that do not account for emerging business models, such as digital platforms and the sharing economy, can result in anomalies and hinder legal compliance.

[9] The WEIRD problem refers to the oversampling of Western, Educated, Industrialized, Rich, and Democratic populations in research, which limits the generalizability of findings. See Joseph Henrich, Steven J Heine, and Ara Norenzayan, "The Weirdest People in the World?" (2010) 33(2)–(3) Behavioral and Brain Sciences 61.

[10] For classic discussions see Duncan Kennedy, "Form and Substance in Private Law Adjudication" (1976) 89 Harvard Law Review 1685; Lewis Kaplow, "Rules Versus Standards: An Economic Analysis" (1992) 42 Duke Law Journal 557.

The rigidity of legal rules can lead to inefficiencies, where the rules are either too restrictive (ie, constraining behavior when adaptability is needed) or quickly become outdated in rapidly changing environments. These inflexibilities represent another systemic flaw, imposing costs on society through suboptimal legal norms.

Excessive legal prescription can also manifest itself in the expansion of laws criminalizing minor offenses. Such an expansion can be detrimental to individuals and society, wasting resources on minor infractions while more serious crimes often fail to receive adequate attention. It can contribute to high incarceration rates, overcrowded prisons, and strains on the justice system. It also disproportionately affects marginalized communities, contributing to cycles of poverty, imprisonment, and disenfranchisement.

Jane's situation exemplifies this flaw: Her experience highlights how rigid, one-size-fits-all regulations failed to account for her unique circumstances. As a newcomer to the town with no history of infractions, she was still subject to inflexible rules and confusing signage governing parking violations. The rigid system left no room for discretion, forcing Jane to navigate an unyielding system.

Pillar 4. Inconsistencies and Discretion Issues

While formulating legal norms poses significant challenges, the way these norms are applied and enforced brings another set of problems. Human discretion plays a central role in enforcement decisions, often resulting in unpredictable and variable outcomes. Human discretion can be valuable in unique circumstances or complex situations, but it frequently results in a paradox of under- and over-enforcement: Some laws are (mostly) strictly enforced, others are (largely) ignored, and many fall into a gray zone of discretionary enforcement.

Police, tax authorities, and regulators often use their judgment to decide whether to enforce or pursue minor infractions, such as petty traffic violations or informal employment arrangements like babysitting.[11] At the same time, authorities often face pressure to either ignore minor, technically illegal behavior (such as trivial breaches of zoning regulations), or strictly enforce laws in ways that may contradict their spirit (as seen in areas like taxation). This results in some infractions going unnoticed or unpunished, creating variability where illegal behavior may be ignored in one instance but penalized in another. Depending on the enforcer's discretion, two individuals in similar circumstances may receive considerably different penalties.

Discretion is an unavoidable feature of centralized systems, in which human decision-makers manage, enforce, interpret, and apply laws. Laws cannot foresee every possible scenario. Therefore, human judgment is necessary to navigate complex or unforeseen circumstances, such as evaluating the intent (or lack thereof) behind a

[11] For a book-length analysis see Michael Lipsky, *Street-Level Bureaucracy: Dilemmas of the Individual in Public Services* (Russell Sage Foundation 1980).

minor infraction or the context in which it occurred. However, this reliance on human judgment often results in inconsistent and unfair outcomes, highlighting the difficulty centralized systems face in applying legal norms equitably, systematically, and predictably. For instance, certain groups, such as minorities or marginalized communities, are more likely to be targeted by law enforcement and often face more severe punishments relative to non-marginalized groups.[12] In corporate regulation, large corporations often circumvent laws or frequently negotiate settlements for infractions that would result in severe penalties for smaller entities.[13] The variability in enforcement leads to unfair outcomes and erodes public trust.

A stark illustration of how discretionary powers can enable systematic discrimination emerged in 2024 from the Alameda County District Attorney's office in California.[14] Prosecutors' notes from death penalty cases, spanning decades, revealed explicit discrimination in jury selection based on race, religion, and ethnicity. Index cards used by prosecutors documented strategies to exclude Jewish and Black potential jurors, with comments like "Must Kick, too Risky" next to Jewish candidates. The discovery led to the review of thirty-four death penalty convictions and ultimately the resentencing of fourteen defendants. This case exposed the way that discretionary powers in jury selection, ostensibly designed to ensure fair trials, instead enabled prosecutors to systematically exclude certain groups from capital juries—precisely the practice that the US Supreme Court had aimed to prevent in *Batson v Kentucky*.[15] The incident demonstrates how discretionary powers, without proper oversight and transparency, can perpetuate bias and erode the fundamental right to a fair trial.

In Jane's case, the inconsistency might become apparent if her minor infraction were rigorously pursued, while similar issues in her community were overlooked, or if others in her situation were erratically excused. Selective enforcement creates a perception of unfairness. It burdens individuals like Jane with consequences that others may never face for similar infractions.

While discretion may be an inherent feature of legal systems, there are often insufficient mechanisms to address the inconsistencies it creates. Individuals faced with uneven enforcement are rarely able to challenge these disparities due to the high costs, procedural hurdles, and obstacles in proving selective enforcement or inconsistent treatment. Even when discretion is exercised consistently, enforcement gaps can undermine public trust and lead to a diminished respect for the law.

[12] See, for example, Sharad Goel, Justin M Rao, and Ravi Shroff, "Precinct or Prejudice? Understanding Racial Disparities in New York City's Stop-and-Frisk Policy" (2016) 10(1) The Annals of Applied Statistics 365; M Marit Rehavi and Sonja B Starr, "Racial Disparity in Federal Criminal Sentences" (2014) 122(6) Journal of Political Economy 1320.

[13] Mihailis E Diamantis and William S Laufer, "Prosecution and Punishment of Corporate Criminality" (2019) 15 Annual Review of Law and Social Science 453.

[14] Jennifer Gonnerman, "An Investigation into How Prosecutors Picked Death-Penalty Juries" *New Yorker* (November 18, 2024).

[15] *Batson v Kentucky* [1986] USSC 476.

Pillar 5. Resistance to Innovation and Change

Inconsistencies in enforcement and discretion are symptomatic of a broader problem: the inherent rigidity of centralized legal systems. This inflexibility does not just affect day-to-day operations; it also manifests as a profound resistance to innovation and change. As society evolves and technology advances, legal frameworks struggle to keep up, often clinging to outdated methods, norms, and procedures. Historical examples include the lag in updating data privacy regulations to keep pace with technological progress.

Institutional actors, including judicial bodies, law firms, and regulatory agencies, frequently resist innovation. This resistance stems from conservatism and concerns over losing status or revenue streams. The fear that technology may upset long-standing power structures exacerbates this resistance. Bureaucratic inertia, a preference for "proven" methods, and an aversion to risk within legal institutions all intensify this resistance. Bureaucratic culture prioritizes stability over efficiency, and the fear of disruption often overrides the need for change. Historical resistance to e-filing systems in US courts illustrates this, where initial opposition delayed widespread adoption despite the clear benefits.

Automation tools, such as AI-driven document review and text analysis, threaten to displace legal jobs. With automation already outperforming humans in some legal tasks, legal professionals fear job displacement and the devaluation of their expertise.[16] As a result, the legal profession and legal institutions are often actively working to maintain the status quo, reinforcing resistance to new technologies.

Jane's case offers a good illustration of how resistance to innovation affects individuals. Suppose her parking dispute occurred in a city that had adopted smart parking systems. These systems, using integrated signage and default automatic payment options, could have prevented Jane's unfortunate experience altogether. Such a system could have provided Jane with real-time clarity on parking rules and signage, prompting her to pay for the additional parking time and offering her convenient or automatic payment options.

The reluctance to adopt innovations within centralized systems leaves individuals like Jane trapped in antiquated frameworks that serve questionable institutional interests. Instead of benefiting from such a smart parking system, Jane was forced to navigate an outdated, cumbersome scheme. The slow, manual processes delayed her case, perpetuating inefficiencies that benefited the fining authority, which profits from parking tickets. Beyond Jane's case, this resistance to change is evident in the slow adoption of technologies like technology-enhanced judicial decision-making, online dispute resolution, and AI-driven legal analysis. Such innovations could dramatically reduce the

[16] See, for example, Richard Susskind, *The Future of Law: Facing the Challenges of Information Technology* (Oxford University Press 1996).

time and costs associated with legal processes, but they remain underutilized in most centralized legal systems.

Moreover, once laws are codified, they are often difficult to amend, and the slow-moving nature of legislative bodies means that legal frameworks can quickly become outdated. As Guido Calabresi observed decades ago, statutory rigidity often leads to legal systems becoming encumbered by obsolete laws that no longer serve their intended purpose.[17] This problem is even more pronounced in today's rapidly changing technological landscape. Time and again, statutory rigidity and slow adaptation prevent the law from keeping pace with advances in fields such as AI, blockchain, fintech, drones, gene-editing, nuclear fusion, and autonomous vehicles.

Pillar 6. Unresponsiveness to Real-time Data

Closely related to the phenomena of resistance to innovation is the inability of centralized systems to effectively utilize live data. There is a systemic disconnect between technological potential and current practices. This unresponsiveness leads to decisions based on outdated or incomplete information. Legal norms are typically static and slow to adapt, relying on outdated methods of assessment and decision-making. This hampers their ability to respond effectively to new information, novel insights, and technological developments.

Centralized systems' reliance on fixed norms reflects their resistance to technological advances and perpetuates inefficiencies. Speed limits, for example, are presumably imposed uniformly, without accounting for specific traffic or environmental conditions. Similarly, environmental regulations often rely on periodic reporting rather than real-time pollution monitoring, leaving authorities without the timely data needed to act swiftly when standards are breached.

The slow adoption of technological tools and real-time data analytics is not surprising. Legal systems were not built to be dynamic and highly adaptive.[18] Law is traditionally a slow-moving enterprise, in which gradual and incremental progress is often considered a feature rather than a flaw. However, slow and rigid centralized legal systems can be inefficient, allowing sophisticated actors to gain considerable advantages over ordinary actors, exploit legal loopholes, circumvent oversight, and undermine intended safeguards or protection mechanisms.[19]

As one example, consider fintech companies, which often present themselves as user-friendly alternatives to traditional banks, offering quick and seamless services.

[17] See the insightful discussion in Guido Calabresi, *A Common Law for the Age of Statutes* (Harvard University Press 1982).

[18] For an interesting discussion on the rigidity of the law and its struggle to keep up with the fluid nature of societal changes and needs see, for example, Lon L Fuller, *The Morality of Law* (Yale University Press 1964).

[19] See, for example, Robert A Kagan, *Adversarial Legalism: The American Way of Law* (Harvard University Press 2001); Marc Galanter, "Why the 'Haves' Come Out Ahead: Speculations on the Limits of Legal Change" (1974) 9 Law & Society Review 95.

However, unlike conventional banks, fintech apps frequently operate outside stringent regulatory frameworks designed to protect consumers' financial interests. In one notable instance in 2024, a fintech company went bankrupt, leaving thousands of users without access to their funds.[20] This case highlights the hidden risks within such unregulated financial systems.

The absence of tailored, dynamic oversight enables fintech companies to expose consumers to risks they may not fully understand. Companies may create a false sense of security, while exploiting regulatory gaps that allow them to operate with fewer safeguards. As a result, consumers are drawn to using fintech products without fully understanding how they differ from more secure, traditionally regulated investment tools and platforms such as banks. Consequently, consumers are left vulnerable to greater risks, including fraud, cyberattacks, or limited legal recourse in the event of bankruptcy or disputes. This highlights the need for a more responsive legal system and the importance of striking the right balance between the centralization of legal frameworks and the decentralization of financial products.

The failure to harness real-time data leaves centralized legal systems out of step with the rapid developments in other sectors. As industries increasingly rely on dynamic analytics and adaptive decision-making, the legal system's continued reliance on outdated frameworks keeps it reactive and inefficient. The gap between societal needs and legal oversight demands urgent reform to create a more adaptive and proactive legal infrastructure.

Pillar 7. Slow Response Times and Case Overload

Lack of agility and responsiveness isn't just a matter of missed opportunities for informed decision-making. It also creates systemic inefficiencies, most notably in slow response times and overwhelming case backlogs. A measured processing time can reduce unwarranted emotional responses and facilitate deliberation and exploration. However, too many mundane cases take months or even years to resolve, causing prolonged uncertainty and hardship for those involved.[21]

The problems of slow adaptation and case overload are endemic to centralized systems, where bureaucratic procedures, coupled with an under-resourced public service, stifle innovation and contribute to inertia and significant backlogs. Legal institutions and enforcement entities are overburdened with cases, leading to lengthy delays in delivering justice, which often forces decision-makers to rush case closures. This overload compromises both the timeliness and quality of legal decisions; overworked

[20] See Hugh Son, "Nearly $109 Million in Deposits Held for Fintech Yotta's Customers Vanished in Synapse Collapse, Bank Says" *CNBC* (June 21, 2024) <www.cnbc.com/2024/06/21/synapse-collapse-nearly-109m-in-yotta-customer-deposits-vanish.html>.

[21] See, for example, Brian J Ostrom and others, *Delivering Timely Justice in Criminal Cases: A National Picture* (National Center for State Courts 2020); Hazel Genn, "When Law is Good for Your Health: Mitigating the Social Determinants of Health through Access to Justice" (2019) 72(1) Current Legal Problems 159.

decision-makers frequently lack the time to adequately consider the complexities and unique circumstances of each case.[22]

Additionally, slow response times reflect a larger inability of centralized systems to react to the increased pace of technological, social, demographic, and economic changes. When legal frameworks cannot keep up with demand, costs rise, people are denied their day in court, and criminal defendants can languish in detention for extended periods without trial. In extreme cases, delays can lead to tragic outcomes, such as that of Adam Capay, who spent more than 1,500 days in solitary confinement awaiting trial.[23] Capay's prolonged isolation in a cell with constant artificial light violated his basic human rights and exacerbated his mental health issues.[24] His case underscores the harsh reality of the saying, "Justice delayed is justice denied."

At the other end of the spectrum, Jane's case illustrates how even minor disputes can become frustrating experiences within slow, centralized systems. In her case, contesting a simple parking ticket spiraled into a drawn-out saga due to inefficient and bureaucratic administrative processes. Where such delays persist, they prevent justice from being delivered and impose unwarranted emotional and financial burdens on those involved—often those least equipped to bear them.

Pillar 8. Opaque Processes and Accountability Gaps

While efficiency and timely responses are major concerns, transparency and accountability are equally crucial for maintaining trust in legal systems. However, centralized models often fall short in these areas. Judicial deliberation, legislative processes, and regulatory enforcement frequently occur behind closed doors, leaving the public with little understanding of how decisions are made or who is responsible. Franz Kafka's *The Trial* powerfully illustrates this nightmare scenario, with a protagonist trapped in an incomprehensible legal system, unable to identify the charges against him or understand the processes that will determine his fate. The novel's enduring resonance suggests how deeply humans fear being subjected to opaque authority, and how dehumanizing unaccountable and incomprehensible systems can be.

Lack of transparency fuels perceptions of arbitrariness and favoritism, especially in high-stakes cases involving corporate interests or government actions. When the public is excluded from decision-making processes, faith in the system erodes. In some cases, non-transparency can facilitate corruption, including bribery, manipulation of

[22] For a discussion of the possible link between time pressure, caseload, and the quality of judicial decision-making see, for example, Jeffrey J Rachlinski and Andrew J Wistrich, "Judging the Judiciary by the Numbers: Empirical Research on Judges" (2017) 13 Annual Review of Law & Social Science 203; Chris Guthrie, Jeffrey J Rachlinski, and Andrew J Wistrich, "Blinking on the Bench: How Judges Decide Cases" (2007) 93 Cornell Law Review 1.

[23] See Martin Patriquin, "Why Adam Capay Spent 1,560 Days in Solitary" *Maclean's* (November 2, 2016) <www.macleans.ca/news/why-adam-capay-has-spent-1560-days-in-solitary/>.

[24] Ibid.

evidence, and undue influence, thereby undermining the rule of law.[25] A legal system perceived as corrupt loses legitimacy, leading to social unrest and instability.

In addition to lacking transparency, centralized systems sometimes fail to ensure proper accountability mechanisms. Even when decisions are made public, citizens often have limited avenues through which to challenge, question, or rectify actions taken by centralized authorities. Too often, weak oversight mechanisms, vague guidelines, regulatory capture, and inadequate scrutiny lead to decisions that favor powerful actors while neglecting the public interest.[26] For instance, corporate entities may wield disproportionate influence over regulatory bodies, resulting in lenient rulings, lax enforcement of environmental violations, weak consumer protection measures, or tax rules that benefit powerful and wealthy actors.

Jane's experience illustrates the frustrations of dealing with opaque processes and weak accountability. In attempting to contest her parking ticket, Jane encountered a labyrinth of bureaucratic roadblocks. She was left in the dark about how her case was being handled, who was responsible for reviewing her claim, and when she could expect a resolution. This lack of clarity and responsibility typifies larger foundational issues: Without transparent, accessible, and accountable processes, individuals have little recourse to ensure their concerns are addressed fairly.

Jane's hypothetical case reflects a common frustration with bureaucratic opacity. But the dangers of unaccountable legal processes extend far beyond parking tickets. Consider Jasmine Mooney, a Canadian entrepreneur detained in 2025 by US immigration authorities despite holding a valid visa.[27] Confined for nearly two weeks in harsh conditions and denied clear information or legal access, Mooney's experience underscores the human cost of systems that operate behind closed doors. Unlike Jane, Mooney was not navigating a local grievance but facing confinement by a transnational enforcement body. Her case is a chilling reminder that opaque procedures can escalate into serious rights violations, especially when individuals lack access to advocacy or public visibility.

To be sure, this opacity disproportionately affects individuals who lack the resources to navigate complex legal processes. While influential firms and wealthy individuals can hire expert counsel to challenge unfavorable decisions, marginalized groups often have neither the means nor the institutional support to understand their rights or seek redress. This power imbalance further entrenches existing social inequities in how justice is accessed and administered.

[25] For example, an investigation in Brazil revealed systemic judicial bribery; judges across six state courts had accepted payments to alter rulings. See Arkady Petrov, "Corruption Allegations Shake Brazil's Judicial System" *The Rio Times* (November 25, 2024) <www.riotimesonline.com/corruption-allegations-shake-brazils-judicial-system-to-its-core/>.

[26] For a comprehensive discussion see Daniel Carpenter and David A Moss (eds), *Preventing Regulatory Capture: Special Interest Influence and How to Limit It* (Cambridge University Press 2014).

[27] Jasmine Mooney, "I'm the Canadian Who Was Detained by Ice for Two Weeks. It Felt Like I Had Been Kidnapped" *The Guardian* (March 19, 2025).

Transparency is essential for fairness and accountability. Simplifying and demystifying legal proceedings is crucial for an engaged and informed citizenry. The opacity of legal processes can make it difficult for individuals to understand their rights, obligations, and the progress of their cases. When individuals cannot comprehend the legal processes that affect them, it diminishes their ability to participate effectively and undermines confidence in the system.

Pillar 9. Concentration of Power and Bias

The opacity and weak accountability mechanisms in centralized legal systems are not merely procedural flaws. Instead, they are symptoms of a more fundamental problem: the concentration of power. Centralization perpetuates a lack of transparency and reinforces a top-down approach to justice, further alienating the legal system from the realities and needs of those it is meant to serve.[28]

When authority and power are consolidated, a select few hold immense influence over how laws are created, applied, and enforced. As Lord Acton observed, "Power tends to corrupt and absolute power corrupts absolutely." In many contexts, judges, regulators, law enforcement, and legislators may exert disproportionate power, which can facilitate systemic imbalances or biases. These, in turn, erode equality before the law and lead to unjust outcomes and social divisions.

Biased dynamics often reinforce existing social hierarchies and mirror the interests of the elite. Likewise, the imposition of uniform rules on diverse populations fails to account for the specific needs and legitimate expectations of different communities.[29] Even well-intentioned policymakers may advance laws with unforeseen consequences, as they often lack the necessary perspective, expertise, or insight into the realities of the people they govern.

Centralized frameworks tend to prioritize uniformity over flexibility, offering little opportunity for communities to influence how rules are established, designed, or enforced. As individuals increasingly confront the rigidity of centralized systems, they begin to question whether decision-makers are genuinely acting in their best interests. Over time, this doubt erodes the foundational principle that justice should be a shared societal resource.

[28] For a classic attack on centralized legal systems and top-down lawmaking that often fail to capture the complexity of society see Friedrich A Hayek, *Law, Legislation and Liberty*, vol 1: *Rules and Order* (University of Chicago Press 1973). For a powerful and more general argument against centralized power structures see Elinor Ostrom, "Beyond Markets and States: Polycentric Governance of Complex Economic Systems" (2010) 100(3) American Economic Review 641.

[29] Presumably, lawmakers, policymakers, and regulators should reflect the will of the public. Some are publicly elected. However, the reality is often more complex, and many decision-makers are insulated from public influence, exposed to lobbying and interest groups, and advance the interests of the powerful elite rather than the broader population. See, for example, Martin Gilens and Benjamin I Page, "Testing Theories of American Politics: Elites, Interest Groups, and Average Citizens" (2014) 12(3) Perspectives on Politics 581; Larry M Bartels, *Unequal Democracy: The Political Economy of the New Gilded Age* (Princeton University Press 2016).

Pillar 10. Informal Justice

Due to the many deficiencies inherent in centralized legal systems, a growing number of parties opt for alternative means of resolving disputes. Alternative mechanisms—such as negotiation, mediation, conciliation, and arbitration—allow individuals and organizations to sidestep the complexities, expenses, and delays associated with formal legal processes. For instance, private arbitration in corporate disputes or mediation in family conflicts can offer a broader spectrum of remedies and quicker resolutions, sidestepping the rigidity of the law and the need for lengthy court proceedings. By opting for these alternative mechanisms, parties can also better safeguard confidentiality and privacy, facilitating a resolution away from the public eye.

But despite their appeal, ADR methods are not without significant drawbacks. For one, ADR contributes to the long-term stagnation of legal development. Extrajudicial mechanisms often resolve disputes without setting legal precedents or contributing to the evolution of the broader legal framework. As a result, legal systems lose opportunities to adapt, develop, and evolve.[30] Moreover, like traditional judicial procedures, informal justice can disproportionately benefit powerful actors, such as large corporations or wealthy individuals, who are repeat players in arbitration or possess the resources to negotiate favorable outcomes.[31] The paucity of judicial oversight and the lack of public scrutiny can tilt the scales in favor of those with more knowledge, resources, and influence, leaving weaker parties at a disadvantage.

Some people, like Jane, elect to pursue formal channels to resolve their disputes. However, this is not the typical response. Rather than investing time and money in a slow, inefficient system, most people might simply pay the fine and abandon their claim—especially if they have failed to negotiate a better solution. The frequent use of (however imperfect) ADR mechanisms and people's tendency to forgo legal recourse altogether reflect a broader public mistrust in centralized legal institutions and their ability to provide accessible, timely, and affordable justice.

Where to From Here?

With these ten pillars of legal dysfunction in mind, we turn to Superjustice as a promising alternative. Let us visualize the differences between current legal systems and Superjustice, focusing on the two major aspects of costs and centralization. Figure 2.1 illustrates these differences. It shows that current legal systems are characterized by centralized authority structures, rigid hierarchies, and significant operational expenses due to their reliance on outdated processes and bureaucratic inefficiencies. By contrast,

[30] See the seminal work of Owen M Fiss, "Against Settlement" (1984) 93 Yale Law Journal 1073; see also David Luban, "Settlements and the Erosion of the Public Realm" (1995) 83 Georgetown Law Journal 261; Laura Nader, *The Life of the Law: Anthropological Projects* (University of California Press 2002).

[31] Lisa B Bingham, "Employment Arbitration: The Repeat Player Effect" (1997) 1 Employee Rights and Employment Policy Journal 189.

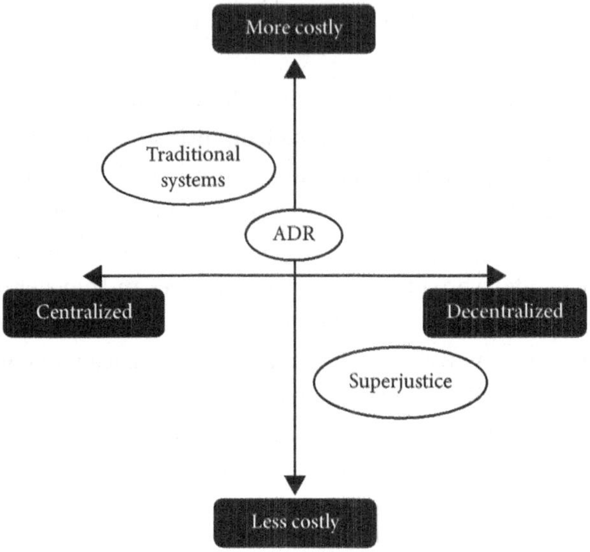

Figure 2.1 Comparison of Legal Systems: Decentralization and Costs

the graph suggests that Superjustice could balance centralization and decentralization while substantially reducing operational costs. The diagram positions ADR in between current legal systems and Superjustice.

Figure 2.2 provides an abstract framework for how Superjustice might address the deficiencies we outlined in this chapter. While the scores in Figure 2.2 are approximations, they nevertheless help capture the potential improvements that Superjustice can bring. Unsurprisingly, the most striking improvement is anticipated in the domain of innovation and flexibility. However, note the slightly less-than-perfect score for Superjustice on this dimension. Despite the technological advances driving Superjustice, it will still need to incorporate checks and balances to maintain integrity

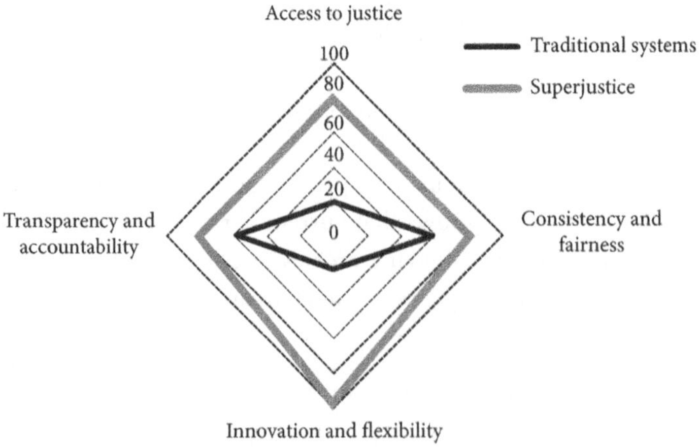

Figure 2.2 Multidimensional System Comparison

and ensure that innovation does not compromise fairness. We will explore these challenges in greater depth in Chapter 10.

Just as importantly, access to justice is projected to increase dramatically. Yet again, Superjustice does not score perfectly. Its imperfect score reflects ongoing challenges, albeit transitional ones, related to digital literacy, the digital divide, public participation, and trust in decentralized systems. We return to these challenges in Chapters 3, 6, and 7. In the mid to long term, however, we predict a sharper improvement in access to justice due not only to the transitional nature of some of the challenges but also to the rise of AI tools that will resolve most legal disputes through automated negotiations.

While the improvements in other domains are more moderate, they are no less important. Superjustice is expected to significantly enhance consistency and fairness. We note the relatively reasonable score of current legal systems on this dimension: Many traditional legal systems already incorporate mechanisms—such as appeals, sentencing guidelines, statutory limits, and fairness standards—that strive to maintain a degree of uniformity and fairness. In this context, Superjustice's imperfect score recognizes the challenges relating to algorithmic fairness and public perception. We will explore these challenges in detail in Chapters 5–6 and 8–10.

Similarly, transparency and accountability are also projected to improve. Here too, we note that current systems already implement measures—such as public access to court records, detailed and published judicial opinions, and regulatory transparency initiatives—that promote openness. We also accept that Superjustice will face its own challenges in ensuring transparency and accountability, at least in its early stages. We will explore this issue in greater depth in Chapters 3, 6, and 10.

Our current centralized legal systems have served us well in the past, but they are now breaking under their own weight. Polishing and fine-tuning current legal systems will be insufficient when everything around us is rapidly changing. If we focus too much on gradually improving our current systems, we will inevitably miss new and possibly powerful tools and capabilities that could revolutionize our legal systems. AI and decentralization offer these tools and can be instrumental in reimagining and restructuring the law.

Remember Jane's frustrating experience with that parking ticket? In a Superjustice system, her story would unfold very differently. Rather than taking time off work, driving hours to a courthouse, and navigating opaque bureaucracy, Jane might simply open an app on her phone, upload a photo of the unclear signage, ask her AI agent to appeal the fine, and receive a prompt, transparent decision. The system might recognize the legitimacy of her confusion and perhaps dismiss the fine or offer a reduced penalty appropriate to her circumstances. While this may seem like a distant, utopian vision, the next chapter will explore the practical transformations that could make Superjustice a realistic possibility.

3

Toward Hybrid Legal Decentralization

Foundations of Centralization

Sarah lives in a peaceful suburban neighborhood, but her mornings have been anything but serene lately. Every day, she is woken by the loud singing of birds nesting in her neighbor Tom's ancient oak tree. The branches hang over her garden, dropping leaves and fruit into her yard and becoming a haven for these early risers.

After weeks of enduring the mess and the noise, Sarah asks Tom to trim the branches. Tom, however, loves the birds and the shade from the tree and refuses to cut it back. Determined to resolve things amicably, Sarah tries multiple times to persuade Tom, even offering to split the cost. But each conversation ends the same way, with Tom firmly defending his tree and the habitat it provides. Sarah then tries various other approaches: She documents the noise and mess, seeks neighborhood mediation, and even suggests installing birdhouses elsewhere in Tom's yard—all to no avail. As a final effort, she consults other neighbors facing similar issues, hoping a collective appeal might sway Tom, but he remains adamant. Frustrated, Sarah contemplates taking legal action. Yet the thought of hiring a lawyer, paying steep fees, and enduring months of delays for something as simple as a few overhanging branches feels absurd.

If you have ever experienced a mundane neighbor dispute that you couldn't resolve amicably, you may sympathize with Sarah—or perhaps with Tom. This seemingly small conflict is the kind of issue that can end with an awkward stalemate or escalate into a drawn-out legal battle due to the rigid procedures and costs associated with centralized legal systems. These systems often lack accessible, low-cost alternatives for minor disputes, forcing individuals into formal channels that are disproportionate to the scale of their conflict. To understand why centralized legal systems operate this way, we briefly examine the idea of legal centralization, its historical roots, and the role it continues to play in shaping legal processes.

What is Legal Centralization?

Legal centralization refers to a system where authority, decision-making, and enforcement are concentrated within a limited number of institutions, such as courts, enforcement agencies, and regulatory bodies. These institutions are primarily responsible for enacting, interpreting, and enforcing laws and regulations. Their centralized control

Superjustice. Samuel I. Becher and Benjamin Alarie, Oxford University Press.
 DOI: 10.1093/9780198991885.003.0005

is designed to provide a cohesive legal framework that governs the entire territory uniformly. By concentrating authority, centralization seeks to apply laws consistently, preventing local variations or arbitrary enforcement. In its ideal form, this structure can foster trust in the rule of law and minimize legal uncertainty.

Being centralized, legal systems are supported and largely funded by the state, which maintains the infrastructure to secure law and order. In centralized legal systems, the state monopolizes the use of force, ensuring that legal decisions are enforced through state-controlled mechanisms such as the police and courts. This monopoly grants the state the exclusive power to compel compliance, reinforcing the central system's authority.

Accordingly, in many countries, national courts have the final say on constitutional matters, ensuring that fundamental legal principles, such as individual rights and governmental powers, are interpreted consistently across the nation. The top-down nature of centralization also creates clear lines of authority, simplifying decision-making processes and providing a stable framework for governance. In common law countries, the judicial hierarchy mandates that lower courts are bound by decisions of higher courts. This hierarchical structure allows for consistent legal interpretation across regions, further promoting similar rulings on similar legal issues.[1]

Despite this centralized framework, private law—particularly contract law—has long represented an important relaxation of legal centralization. Contracts allow individuals and organizations to create their own binding agreements, without immediate state involvement, effectively sidestepping centralization. However, this bypassing is somewhat limited. It functions smoothly until disputes arise, at which point parties typically need to return to centralized courts for resolution and enforcement. In fact, it is the *ex post* state backing that often gives the legal instrument of contracts its *ex ante* power. So even in the realm of contracts, the state provides the framework, supports its effectiveness, and serves as the ultimate arbiter and enforcer.

The Rise and Promise of Legal Centralization

Legal centralization emerged in response to societal needs for consistency, fairness, and accountability as communities expanded and governance systems became increasingly complex. With increasing population sizes and geographic dispersals, decentralized or localized governance systems have become insufficient to consistently and fairly manage disputes. A historical example is ancient Rome (8th century BCE to 5th century CE), where the *Lex Romana* provided a uniform code of law across the vast Roman Empire.[2]

[1] For a classic theoretical discussion of hierarchical legal systems see Hans Kelsen, *General Theory of Law and State* (Harvard University Press 1945).

[2] See David Johnston, *Roman Law in Context* (Cambridge University Press 1999) for further details on the uniformity and application of Roman legal codes.

Early states recognized that, without a single point of authority to interpret and enforce laws, communities were prone to conflicting legal norms, unequal enforcement, and local bias. In medieval Europe, localized feudal courts often produced inconsistent rulings based on local customs. Thus, Louis XIV of France (1643–1715) centralized legal authority under the monarchy to unify diverse provincial laws.[3] Similarly, the Norman Conquest of 1066 in England led to the consolidation of legal power under the Crown, establishing the King's Courts and the common law as a unified system across the kingdom. Over time, centralization played a key role in the British constitutional framework, concentrating decision-making within core institutions, while emphasizing the rule of law and parliamentary sovereignty.[4] The establishment of national courts and regulatory bodies with exclusive jurisdiction enabled states to apply a standardized legal framework that applied to all citizens.

Centralization also emerged as a mechanism for ensuring accountability and transparency in legal processes. In early decentralized systems, such as medieval Germanic tribal law, local rulers or judges often held unchecked power, leading to abuses, arbitrariness, or favoritism. Centralized systems, such as those developed under the Holy Roman Empire and later the Austro-Hungarian Empire, introduced oversight mechanisms. With such mechanisms in place, higher courts could review decisions made at lower levels, thereby offering a layer of accountability that reinforced public trust in the rule of law. In Revolutionary France, the creation of the *Cour de Cassation* in 1790 established a mechanism for ensuring uniform application of the law, with the power to quash lower court decisions that departed from national legal norms.

The push for centralization was closely tied to the need for consistency and predictability in legal outcomes. As states became more interconnected through trade, diplomacy, and military alliances, the demand for a cohesive legal framework that could address cross-regional issues grew. The creation of the Prussian Civil Code in the late 18th century and the Napoleonic Code of 1804 are prime examples of legal centralization aimed at unifying the law across regions. Centralized systems allowed states to create and enforce laws that transcended local customs, providing a stable legal environment conducive to economic growth and political stability.

In summary, the historical rise of centralized legal systems was driven by competition among states; increased public demand for justice; and the need to maintain order, ensure fairness, and provide a standardized and accountable framework for governance. From the Roman Empire to Napoleonic France and England, these systems offered a solution to the challenges of legal fragmentation, laying the groundwork for the legal structures we see today.[5]

[3] See James B Collins, *The State in Early Modern France* (Cambridge University Press 2009) for an analysis of this unification process.

[4] See Albert Venn Dicey, *Introduction to the Study of the Law of the Constitution* (Macmillan 1915).

[5] For a seminal analysis of the development of Western legal institutions and the rise of integrated legal systems see Harold J Berman, *Law and Revolution: The Formation of the Western Legal Tradition* (Harvard University Press 1983).

From Bottlenecks to Networks

Their historic roots notwithstanding, centralized legal systems resemble an outdated control tower, where every decision, whether big or small, must pass through a single point of authority. This represents a pendulum swing away from the fragmented feudal systems of medieval Europe, where justice varied widely from one location to the next. But centralization is far from a magic bullet. As detailed in Chapter 2, centralized legal systems often suffer from inefficiencies due to the bureaucratic nature of decision-making. Inaccessibility remains a major issue, with many individuals and communities struggling to navigate centralized legal systems. Today's networked society calls for neither feudal fragmentation nor rigid centralization, but for adaptable, connected systems.

While centralization has historically offered important benefits—such as consistency and accountability—there is a growing need for what we call "hybrid legal systems." Such systems would retain some of the advantages of centralization, particularly in maintaining oversight and uniformity. At the same time, they would also incorporate more decentralized elements to improve flexibility and responsiveness.

Understanding Decentralization

In contrast to centralized legal systems, decentralized legal systems distribute authority across multiple local or regional entities, allowing for more tailored approaches to governance and enforcement that reflect local needs and conditions. Decentralized legal systems can function like neural networks, where decisions are distributed across multiple nodes, allowing for a more efficient and effective approach to governance. Much like neurons communicating without a central command, a decentralized system enables legal decisions, dispute resolution, and regulatory processes to occur more fluidly and quickly. This setup eliminates the need to wait for approval or intervention from a central authority.

The neural network metaphor illustrates how decentralized systems can not only expedite decisions but also adapt organically to evolving legal needs, offering a responsive alternative to rigid centralized control. A notable success of a decentralized system was the establishment of the Gacaca courts in Rwanda. The *gacaca* process involved community-based courts that resolved tens of thousands of post-genocide cases efficiently by empowering local communities to take an active role in justice processes.[6]

[6] Human Rights Watch, "Justice Compromised: The Legacy of Rwanda's Community-Based Gacaca Courts" (May 31, 2011) <www.hrw.org/report/2011/05/31/justice-compromised/legacy-rwandas-community-based-gacaca-courts>. Gacaca courts were set up to deliver justice for the 1994 Rwandan genocide. The Human Rights Watch report illustrates the process, challenges, and achievements of the gacaca process.

Elements of decentralization already exist in many modern legal systems. This is particularly the case in federal structures, where authority is constitutionally divided between national, provincial/state, and local governments. These existing frameworks demonstrate both the benefits and challenges of distributed legal authority. Superjustice builds upon these established principles of power distribution, extending them further through technological innovations and public participation rather than proposing an entirely novel approach to legal governance.

Programs like South Carolina's Restoring Promise initiative demonstrate that, even in settings traditionally requiring the highest levels of centralized authority—such as prisons—decentralization is both feasible and beneficial.[7] Specifically, Restoring Promise creates housing units in which incarcerated young adults work alongside staff to develop community norms, resolve conflicts through dialogue, and participate in programming decisions. By empowering incarcerated individuals to shape aspects of their rehabilitative experience, Restoring Promise combines the structure of a centralized system with community-driven governance, fostering a more humane and responsive justice environment. This approach, akin to the hybrid system we suggest, has led to notable improvements. It has promoted a safer and more supportive environment within the prison by reducing violence, enhancing rehabilitative outcomes, and building rapport between staff and incarcerated individuals.

Superjustice envisages the coexistence of decentralized systems and centralized elements, creating hybrid legal models. In these models, local nodes—such as artificial intelligence (AI) arbitrators and random jurors—handle most everyday disputes. Central institutions, however, would oversee broader legal principles and provide national oversight for cases requiring a more centralized approach. This may include sensitive, complex, or high stakes issues, constitutional matters, or appeals where legal expertise is essential. Chapters 5, 6, and 9 will delve deeper into how these factors inform the model's nested hierarchical allocation of power, authority, and enforcement.

As a hybrid model, Superjustice would utilize powerful technological platforms, including AI-driven legal agents, blockchain for transparent dispute tracking, and crowdsourced data platforms that incorporate inputs from individuals and local communities. These tools would streamline the resolution of legal queries and disputes, offering rapid decision-making, secure documentation, and tailored solutions based on localized needs. By tapping into these diverse resources, Superjustice would amplify the social benefits of legal systems and optimize the use of limited resources. To illustrate this approach, we will next examine the concept of decentralization and its role in enhancing accessibility and adaptability within legal systems.

[7] For an interesting account see Maurice Chammah, "The Future of Prisons?" *The Marshall Project* (September 26, 2024).

Guiding Principles for Legal Decentralization

Decentralization represents a transformative shift in how legal systems can be structured, moving away from centralized control toward more distributed models of governance. In what follows, we explore the core principles of legal decentralization. We examine existing models that highlight the practical application of these principles and discuss the parallels between decentralized legal systems and other decentralization endeavors. Through this lens, we show how decentralization might enhance flexibility, access to justice, and citizen empowerment. We also explain how decentralized systems can coexist with centralized elements, forming hybrid models that can benefit from the best aspects of both centralization and decentralization.

As we have seen, legal decentralization refers to a system where authority, decision-making, and enforcement are distributed across multiple, often autonomous (and at times anonymous) elements. This model shifts power away from centralized bodies, allowing for more flexible and dynamic governance. Overall, we argue that this approach would create legal systems that are more accessible and responsive to the needs of diverse communities, addressing the ten pillars of legal dysfunctionality discussed in Chapter 2.

At the heart of legal decentralization are three core principles: democratization, access to justice, and empowerment. *Democratization* involves distributing legal authority, enabling wider participation in legal decision-making and dispute resolution. *Access to justice* is enhanced by reducing barriers through technology, making legal services more inclusive, affordable, and available. Lastly, *empowerment* is achieved when individuals and local entities gain greater autonomy in developing, implementing, and applying legal principles; handling legal matters directly; and using decentralized mechanisms to resolve their disputes.

Notably, decentralizing legal systems has profound implications that extend beyond technical or procedural improvements. Unlike decentralization in domains like technology or finance, legal decentralization directly impacts the way that democratically made decisions are implemented in society. Law serves a unique and distinctive function as the mechanism through which political decisions are transformed into policy implementation on the ground. When we decentralize legal processes, we necessarily redistribute political power—altering which voices influence how policies are interpreted and applied.[8]

This redistribution raises fundamental questions about democratic accountability and the way to ensure that decentralized legal mechanisms remain responsive to broader political processes and constitutional principles. As we explain throughout, the hybrid model of Superjustice attempts to navigate this tension by maintaining

[8] The work of Michael Trebilcock is particularly illuminating here. See Michael J Trebilcock, "The Choice of Governing Instrument" (1982) 2 International Review of Law and Economics 29; Michael J Trebilcock, *Dealing with Losers: The Political Economy of Policy Transitions* (Oxford University Press 2015).

centralized oversight for fundamental political decisions, while allowing for more decentralized implementation that better reflects local knowledge, norms, and preferences. This approach recognizes that effective implementation of political decisions often requires adaptation to specific contexts that centralized authorities may not fully understand, while also acknowledging that certain core principles and values must remain consistent across all nodes of the system.

Existing Models of Decentralization

Having explored the conceptual principles of decentralization, we now examine how these concepts have been successfully applied in non-legal domains. Specifically, we will explore blockchain technology, decentralized finance (DeFi), and open-source platforms to illustrate how decentralized models work. These existing models offer valuable insights for potential legal applications.

Blockchain, a type of distributed ledger technology (DLT), serves as a powerful example of decentralization in action.[9] Unlike traditional systems, in which central entities control data and authority, blockchain distributes control across a network of participants. A shared digital ledger (the distributed ledger) can be independently verified by participants, but no one person or group can alter the ledger without meeting the consensus threshold required by the network. Each transaction or record is added to this ledger only after it is validated under the network's rules by multiple nodes/validators. This process increases transparency, security, and resilience, making it difficult to tamper with its contents. Thus, blockchain distributes responsibility throughout its network, which can reduce reliance on a central intermediary and single points of failure, while simultaneously enhancing trust in data integrity.

A notable application of blockchain in governance is the rise of decentralized autonomous organizations (DAOs). DAOs are community-led organizations in which decisions are made through smart contracts—self-executing agreements with predefined rules coded into the blockchain. These contracts automatically enforce decisions once conditions are met. Participants, who are known as "token holders," use digital assets (tokens) to vote on proposals and governance issues.[10] This decentralized governance model allows for direct participation and eliminates the need for centralized leadership, as decisions are made collectively by the community.

Blockchain technology fundamentally disrupts centralized systems by making trustless transactions possible.[11] It reduces the reliance on centralized intermediaries, minimizing the potential for abuse of power. In the context of legal systems, blockchain

[9] For a foundational text on blockchain technology and distributed ledger systems see Satoshi Nakamoto, "Bitcoin: A Peer-to-Peer Electronic Cash System" (2008).

[10] For a book-length discussion about token-based governance models and the role of smart contracts in enabling DAOs see Shermin Voshmgir, *Token Economy: How the Web3 Reinvents the Internet* (Token Kitchen Publishing 2020).

[11] On the way blockchain creates "trustless" environments see Kevin Werbach, *The Blockchain and the New Architecture of Trust* (MIT Press 2018).

technology could enable decentralized contract enforcement, property registration, and dispute resolution through the use of smart contracts. For instance, blockchain can provide a robust and safe method of recording property ownership, reducing fraud, corruption, and disputes over ownership. Similarly, blockchain-based voting systems can provide an inclusive and secure method for community-driven legal participation.

The DeFi movement offers further insights into rethinking legal systems. DeFi operates on blockchain networks, allowing individuals to engage in financial transactions—such as lending, borrowing, and trading—without relying on traditional banks. One major example of DeFi's potential is smart contract lending platforms, where individuals can lend or borrow without the need for a centralized bank. DeFi's use of smart contracts could be adapted for legal agreements, streamlining contract execution and enforcement.

The guiding principles of transparency, accessibility, and resilience in DeFi resonate with those needed for decentralized legal systems.[12] In terms of transparency, all transactions in DeFi are recorded on the blockchain, providing full visibility and reducing the potential for corruption or manipulation. When it comes to accessibility, DeFi eliminates the barriers to entry associated with traditional finance (such as geography or high fees), making services available to anyone with the appropriate hardware, software, and an internet connection. DeFi systems are resilient, as they are resistant to single points of failure, just as decentralized legal systems would be resilient against corruption or manipulation.

Another successful decentralized model is Wikipedia, an open-source platform that operates on the principle of crowdsourcing knowledge from contributors worldwide. Wikipedia has no central editorial authority, allowing individuals to add, modify, or update content. This freedom comes with its challenges, including misinformation, bias, and content disputes. To address these issues, Wikipedia has developed robust community-driven moderation tools, employing volunteer editors to resolve conflicts and ensure content accuracy.[13]

Wikipedia's model demonstrates how a decentralized system can remain resilient while adapting to real-world challenges. Wikipedia relies on a reputation-based system, in which trusted editors have more influence over disputed content. This can be paralleled in decentralized legal systems that might count on trusted arbitrators or community jurors to resolve conflicts. Just as Wikipedia empowers its community to monitor and manage disputes, decentralized legal systems can enable individuals and communities to participate in law creation and dispute resolution without full dependence on centralized institutions.

Finally, the Linux operating system demonstrates a hybrid governance model that balances distributed development with structured leadership. While thousands of

[12] For an exploration of the core principles of DeFi and their potential application in other decentralized systems see Campbell R Harvey and others, *DeFi and the Future of Finance* (Wiley 2021).

[13] See Joseph M Reagle Jr, *Good Faith Collaboration: The Culture of Wikipedia* (MIT Press 2010), in which the author studies how Wikipedia operates as a decentralized community, using collaboration, crowdsourcing, and volunteer-driven moderation to maintain accuracy and resolve disputes.

developers worldwide contribute code and updates, the project maintains a hierarchical decision-making structure; founder Linus Torvalds retains final authority over the kernel, supported by trusted lieutenants who oversee specific subsystems. This "benevolent dictator" model has helped Linux maintain exceptional reliability and innovation over time. The system's success stems from its meritocratic principles—contributions from skilled developers are widely adopted based on technical merit rather than organizational position—and its efficient response to issues through collaborative problem-solving. Linux thus illustrates how open-source projects can effectively blend centralized leadership with distributed development, creating governance structures that are simultaneously authoritative, flexible, and inclusive enough to manage complex technical systems at scale.

These varied applications across sectors demonstrate the potential for decentralization in legal systems. While blockchain technology reduces reliance on central authorities, DeFi demonstrates how decentralization can remove barriers to access, Wikipedia illustrates the efficiency of decentralized moderation in resolving disputes, and Linux exemplifies how collaborative governance can sustain innovation over time. Taken together, these models provide important design principles for Superjustice. Building on these examples, we now explore how the foundations of legal decentralization could reshape lawmaking and dispute resolution, paving the way for Superjustice to leverage similar decentralized structures.

The Foundations of Legal Decentralization

We began this chapter with the dispute between Sarah and her neighbor, Tom, over the birds nesting in Tom's tree. After Tom refused Sarah's request to trim the tree, she considered legal action. In a traditional legal system, Sarah would probably face a lengthy and expensive court battle over this relatively minor issue. In a Superjustice legal system, however, Sarah would have other alternatives. One might be an AI arbitrator. As we explore in Chapters 5, 6, and 9, AI agents could resolve most discrepancies through negotiation, and AI arbitrators may end up being the leading mechanisms for resolving any remaining disputes. AI systems will be more effective, powerful, accurate, reliable, and trustworthy than humans, not to mention significantly less expensive.

Beyond AI or automated systems, decentralization presents another option that is more reliant on humans. Imagine legal advice crowdsourced at the touch of a button, with quality ensured through a reputation-based system where contributors with verified expertise provide guidance. Better yet, picture a decentralized legal system as a digital agora, in which individuals gather to create, share, and enforce laws in a virtual marketplace (see Figure 3.1).[14] Like the ancient Greek democracy, but powered

[14] Ober explores how the agora functioned as a central space for public discourse, lawmaking, and collective decision-making in ancient Athens, making it a valuable metaphor for decentralized, participatory systems. See Josiah Ober, *Democracy and Knowledge: Innovation and Learning in Classical Athens* (Princeton University Press 2008).

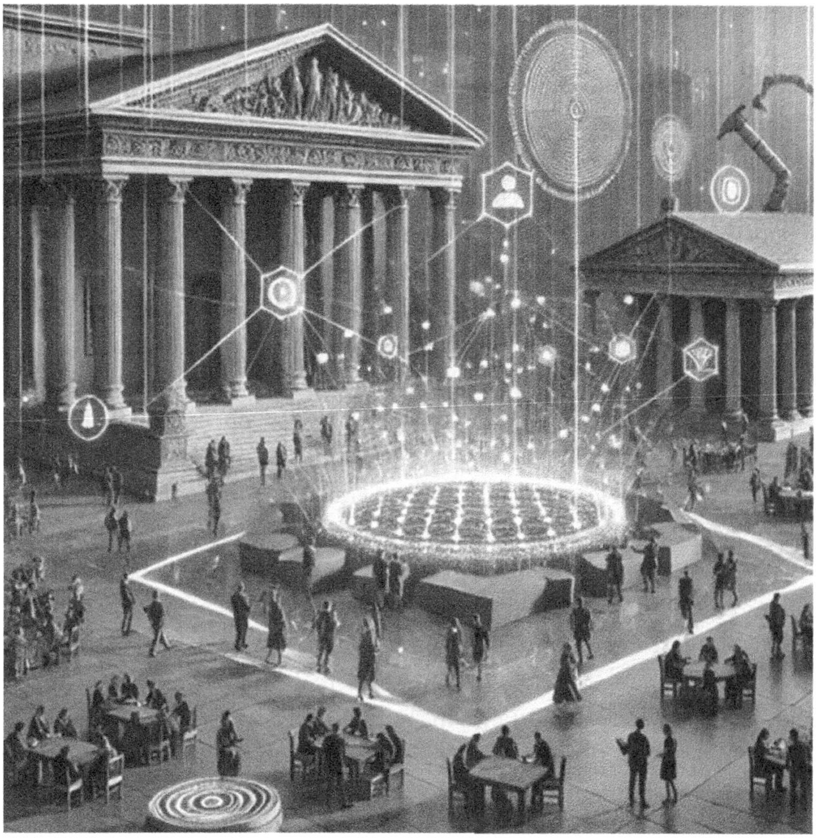

Figure 3.1 The Future of Lawmaking—A Modern Agora

by cutting-edge technology, this system would provide an alternative to the top-down legal frameworks we know today.

As we will see next, AI could play a crucial role in transforming human engagement with legal systems. Unlike traditional court systems, which often struggle with high caseloads and a lack of resources, hybrid legal models incorporate AI platforms to assist and augment human capacity. These AI systems can analyze vast amounts of legal data, including past cases, statutes, and regulations, to provide quick and consistent applications and interpretations of the law.

The potential of freeing up scarce judicial resources through decentralized, automated systems is promising. Courts around the world struggle with high caseloads and a lack of resources.[15] Acting as a virtual legal assistant, AI could manage thousands of cases simultaneously, reducing the burden on courts and increasing efficiency. In the initial implementation stages, AI tools could focus on resolving cases

[15] The strain on courts due to high caseloads and inefficiencies is a common challenge, impacting numerous jurisdictions. See, for example, Richard A Posner, *The Federal Courts: Challenge and Reform* (Harvard University Press 1985); Hazel Genn, *Judging Civil Justice* (Cambridge University Press 2010).

where the resolution is clear and straightforward and the stakes are relatively low. For certain types of disputes—such as small claims, consumer complaints, insurance claims, and tenant–landlord disputes—AI-powered systems could analyze case facts and relevant laws to propose solutions, reducing court backlogs and increasing access to justice.

Importantly, technologically enhanced hybrid systems could also prevent many legal disputes from arising or otherwise simplify them. For example, blockchain-based systems could create immutable records of intellectual property creation and ownership, potentially preventing some disputes over patent and copyright claims, and streamlining others. Furthermore, AI could help categorize and route legal issues to the most appropriate resolution method, whether that is mediation, arbitration, or a more formal court process. It could also assist in drafting legal documents, identifying relevant precedents, or suggesting fair settlements based on similar past cases.

Instead of enduring a lengthy court battle, Sarah and Tom could log into a platform designed for community disputes. Lay arbitrators—or AI systems—could assess the case, and a resolution could be reached almost instantly. AI might explain that the applicable law allows Tom's tree to grow despite Sarah's inconvenience, or it could clarify that the law supports Sarah's request to have the tree trimmed. Alternatively, community arbitrators could propose a compromise where the tree is partially cut, or Sarah is only allowed to take action to distance the birds. Either way, the community has its say. Both parties then move forward, having participated in a fair and timely resolution informed by property rights and stakeholders' preferences.

Kleros, a decentralized blockchain-based arbitration platform that utilizes smart contracts and crowdsourced jurors, offers an interesting operational example. The platform enables users to resolve conflicts outside of traditional courts, providing a faster and more accessible resolution process. Kleros leverages game theory to advance fairness: Jurors are chosen randomly to resolve disputes, and each juror stakes a token to participate in resolving one. If a juror's decision aligns with the majority, they are rewarded; however, if they vote differently, they risk losing their stake. However, Kleros has several limitations, including biases in juror selection, scalability issues when handling large or complex disputes, and its reliance on users staking tokens. Superjustice could address such issues by integrating advanced algorithms and developing scalable frameworks that leverage technological and human capabilities. We develop this further in Chapters 5, 6, and 8–9.

The Conceptual-Philosophical Foundations

Should we place our trust in a network of strangers or AI arbitrators, or even artificial general intelligence (AGI), to shape and interpret legal norms and decide legal disputes? This question warrants careful consideration, as it opens the door to examining the broader values embedded in decentralized systems. In this context, the move toward decentralized legal systems is grounded in key political and legal ideologies that emphasize diversity and local autonomy. Indeed, decentralized legal systems align with the political and legal philosophies of pluralism and subsidiarity.[16]

Pluralism allows multiple legal systems or norms to coexist within a broader framework, reflecting the diverse needs of communities. Subsidiarity holds that decisions should be made at the lowest, most local level capable of handling the issue. For instance, local municipalities in Switzerland have significant autonomy to manage education and public services, ensuring that decisions are tailored to the specific needs of the community.[17] In decentralized models, wherever possible, power is distributed to local entities, communities, and individuals, creating a system where legal authority is exercised closest to those affected.

These core principles of pluralism and subsidiarity find practical expression in modern technologies, which can allow decentralized systems to empower individuals and communities in legal decision-making. Through real-time data collection and transparent processes, technology can enhance this participatory governance and better reflect communal values and preferences. As the following discussion elucidates, initiatives of this nature are already being implemented, albeit sporadically.

Public Participation in Lawmaking

An interesting initiative that seeks to facilitate public participation in lawmaking is CrowdLaw, which aims to amplify public perspectives in legislative processes through digital platforms.[18] In essence, CrowdLaw endeavors to empower citizens to contribute to lawmaking through online platforms, transforming legislative processes into more participatory and inclusive systems. In this model, ordinary people help shape laws by sharing their perspectives and experiences. Examples include WikiLegis, a platform modeled on Wikipedia, and *Podemos*, a Spanish political party that uses online platforms like *Plaza Podemos* and *Iniciativas Ciudadanas* to involve citizens in policy development. Such initiatives have engaged residents in shaping public decisions, demonstrating how digital tools can make legislative processes more participatory and inclusive.

Like Superjustice, CrowdLaw envisions a shift toward collaborative and inclusive governance. By bridging the gap between citizens and lawmaking, CrowdLaw enables individual participation in policy creation through digital means. However, while both CrowdLaw and Superjustice have the goal of fostering participatory governance, their approaches differ. CrowdLaw operates within the existing institutional frameworks,

[16] For the foundations of legal pluralism see John Griffiths, "What is Legal Pluralism?" (1986) 18(24) Journal of Legal Pluralism and Unofficial Law 1. The idea of subsidiarity and its applications are discussed in Robert K Vischer, "Subsidiarity as a Principle of Governance: Beyond Devolution" (2001) 35 Indian Law Review 103.

[17] Ketema Wakjira Debela, "Local Governance in Switzerland: Adequate Municipal Autonomy cum Intergovernmental Cooperation?" (2020) 6(1) Cogent Social Sciences 1763889.

[18] See Beth Simone Noveck, "CrowdLaw: Collective Intelligence and Lawmaking" (2018) 40 Analyse & Kritik 359.

aiming to increase public engagement without redistributing power. Superjustice, on the other hand, envisions more extensive and constant modes of decentralization, situating decision-making authority at local levels. Therefore, the key difference lies in the degree of disruption each system proposes.

Public Participation in Norm Development

While CrowdLaw focuses on public input for legislative reforms, public input can also play a crucial role in the interpretation, application, and enforcement of legal norms. An open-source platform experiment aimed at defining hate speech provides a useful illustration.[19] In the domain of online platforms, social media firms rely on AI content classifiers to identify and moderate harmful content, a process known as content moderation. These content classifiers are trained to detect harmful material, including hate speech. One challenge in this context is determining what constitutes hate speech. Balancing between protecting free speech and creating a safe environment requires careful consideration. Notably, this balancing act raises a thorny question: Who gets to define hate speech?

Currently, platforms rely on AI classifiers that have been trained with specific examples, often determined without public oversight. These classifiers operate largely as a black box, where the criteria used are hidden from the public. Social media companies have significant content moderation powers, often with minimal transparency or public accountability. This is particularly concerning given that these potentially opaque decisions affect vast numbers of users and can have considerable political, societal, and economic implications.

A shift toward decentralization would empower the public—not an opaque algorithm—to define hate speech. An open-source initiative could gather public input, especially from those most impacted by hate speech, to develop more nuanced definitions. Such an approach would enable local communities and jurisdictions to tailor definitions of hate speech, creating more context-specific governance mechanisms. In this model, technology is used to establish multiple "super juries," so to speak, to enhance legal frameworks. At the same time, communities and the public should be guided by carefully designed frameworks and processes, ensuring they have a voice, not a veto.

Opening the process of training datasets for AI classifiers to public participation has clear benefits. It allows society to take ownership of a critical issue, thereby reducing the burden on decision-makers like platforms, regulators, and arbitrators, who would otherwise have to guess at societal norms. Involving the public in defining hate speech aligns with decentralization as it allows communities to tailor legal definitions to widely held community values. Unlike centralized systems, decentralized platforms

[19] This discussion draws on "Crowdsourcing the Curation of the Training Set for Harmful Content Classifiers Used in Social Media: A Pilot Study on Political Hate Speech in India" (October 2023, on file with the authors).

would give those most affected by hate speech a voice in shaping the rules that govern and protect them.

Decentralization in Judicial Decision-making and Enforcement

The concept of participatory legal decision-making can be applied beyond hate speech and across many domains, particularly in contexts where legal norms are ambiguous. As discussed in Chapter 2, the law often employs vague legal norms, which are ineffective in guiding behavior and can be interpreted in a biased manner. By contrast, public perspectives can clarify vague legal standards, such as what constitutes "bad faith" in contract or trademark law, "reasonable care" in tort law, or "non-obviousness" in patent law. Similarly, public input could inform what defines "material information" in consumer protection, what is in "the best interest" of a child in family law, what counts as "public interest" in environmental or competition law, or what amounts to "public policy" concerns in company law.

In this participatory framework, AI tools would work in tandem with public input to revolutionize legal interpretation and decision-making. These systems would analyze vast repositories of past judicial decisions to identify patterns in how vague legal standards have been interpreted historically. Simultaneously, public participation would provide critical insights into contemporary values and expectations. Together, the two could create a dynamic mechanism that both honors legal precedent and responds to evolving social norms. For instance, when determining what constitutes "reasonable care" in tort law, AI analysis of precedent would be balanced against, or enriched with, current public understanding of reasonable precautions in contemporary contexts. While decision-makers would retain their authority to exercise independent judgment, they would benefit from this integrated foundation of historical jurisprudence and contemporary social perspectives. This balanced approach could equip judges and regulators with a more comprehensive and nuanced framework for interpreting and applying ambiguous legal standards.

While the preceding discussion focuses on how AI and public participation can shape legal standards broadly, AI legal agents could further transform individual dispute resolution. Moving from rulemaking to negotiating more mundane disputes, one can envision personalized AI legal agents representing individuals in negotiations. In Sarah and Tom's case, each party could employ an AI agent to conduct settlement discussions. Sarah might instruct her agent to "find a solution to stop the birds from waking me up," while Tom's agent would protect his interests regarding his tree. These AI representatives could efficiently explore potential compromises, perhaps identifying an optimal transfer payment that Sarah is willing to pay and Tom is willing to accept upon verification of compliance.

This approach embodies the famous Coase Theorem, developed by Nobel laureate economist Ronald Coase in his 1960 paper, *The Problem of Social Cost*.[20]

[20] RH Coase, "The Problem of Social Cost" (1960) 3 Journal of Law & Economics 1.

In short, the theorem posits that when transaction costs are low and property rights are well-defined, parties will negotiate to the most economically efficient outcome regardless of the initial allocation of rights. Adopting an "AI Coase" approach could dramatically reduce transaction costs that typically hinder efficient bargaining, allowing parties to reach mutually beneficial agreements without requiring formal legal proceedings.[21]

Notably, the AI agents in such scenarios would operate differently from the public sentiment aggregation systems discussed earlier. Rather than analyzing broad social preferences to inform general rules, these agents would use economic optimization techniques to identify the specific exchange of rights or remedies that would satisfy both Sarah and Tom. One agent might determine that Sarah would be willing to pay up to $300 for tree trimming, while the other might calculate that Tom would accept $250 to trim specific branches, creating the opportunity for a mutually beneficial agreement. Interestingly, Sarah's AI agent could potentially communicate with other AI agents and identify additional stakeholders—possibly other neighbors—who would share the costs of convincing Tom to trim the tree. Either way, resolving the dispute in this manner would reduce the transaction costs that typically prevent efficient bargaining between individuals, allowing the technology to facilitate personalized solutions to specific disputes.

Beyond dispute negotiations and norm development, decentralization can also extend to enforcement. For instance, blockchain technology, the backbone of decentralized systems, provides a transparent and immutable ledger that functions like "Google Docs for legal transactions," allowing all participants to access and update information in real time. Smart contracts further enhance this by automating certain agreements. In Sarah and Tom's case, smart contracts could help streamline the resolution by specifying the agreed-upon terms—such as trimming the tree—and automating some enforcement aspects.

Admittedly, smart contracts cannot physically compel Tom to trim the tree. However, advancements in robotics can further change the enforcement landscape. Some firms are already employing smart robots that break new ground. For instance, Amazon's new robot can navigate and operate autonomously outside of restricted areas, working safely around human employees. The idea of humanoid robots attracts considerable attention and investment, and technological progress fuels optimism about their potential to revolutionize nearly every aspect of our lives.[22] Reflecting on such developments, we find it plausible that, within ten years, a smart contract might be able to automatically commission a robotic arborist to trim the tree in accordance with the

[21] While we highlight here the immense potential of AI legal agents, such tools also raise a host of important issues and challenges that merit a separate discussion. See, for example, Noam Kolt, "Governing AI Agents" (2026) 101 Notre Dame Law Review (forthcoming); Alan Chan and others, "Visibility into AI Agents" (2024) Proceedings of the 2024 ACM Conference on Fairness, Accountability, and Transparency [10.48550/arXiv.2401.13138].

[22] For accessible discussions on the investment in these robots, their potential, and the obstacles ahead see James O'Donnell, "Will We Ever Trust Robots?" *MIT Technology Review* (December 23, 2024); Carrie King and Ben Morris, "Who Will Win the Race to Develop a Humanoid Robot?" *BBC* (April 25, 2025).

order of an AI arbitrator. This, in turn, could raise new ethical and practical challenges, such as assigning accountability for the robot's actions.

In the meantime, smart contract arrangements can include incentives or penalties to encourage cooperation. For example, a smart contract could hold funds in escrow, automatically releasing payment to the service provider once the job is done. Also, reputation mechanisms can deter non-compliance, as failing to honor the agreement might damage Tom's standing within the community. These tools can strike a balance between automation and accountability, ensuring that decentralized systems can utilize practical enforcement mechanisms.

Any mechanism will have its limitations. At least in the interim, hybrid systems that blend decentralized processes with centralized bodies or cooperate with law enforcement will be necessary to ensure compliance in complex cases. This is especially relevant in situations requiring more than just financial settlements, and where reputational constraints may prove ineffective. Overall, this underscores the importance of having a centralized authority to intervene when necessary, ensuring the legal system maintains its overall effectiveness and credibility.

To sum up, hybrid legal systems fundamentally differ from traditional, centralized systems. Many of these differences offer opportunities to improve legal systems and better serve society. Table 3.1 captures the main distinctions between traditional systems and modern hybrid systems.

Table 3.1 Centralized vs Hybrid, Superjustice Systems

Characteristic	Traditional, Centralized System	Superjustice (Hybrid System)
Degree of Automation	Low	High
Network Structure	Centralized	Mostly Decentralized
Trust Required	Yes	Often No
Human involvement	Crucial (High)	Reduced (Low)
Technology Importance	Low	High
Intermediaries Needed	High	Low
Legal Costs	High	Low
Reliability of Parties	High Risk	Low Risk
Anonymous	No	Often Yes
Inclusive	No	Yes
Transparency	Medium	High
Open-Source	No	Yes
Open Access	No	Yes
Flexibility	Low	High
Security	Low	High
Single Points of Failure	Yes	No

Challenges and Implications

While legal decentralization offers significant potential for innovation, flexibility, and democratization, it also introduces complex challenges and has profound implications. Moving away from centralized authority can lead to fragmentation, inconsistencies, and enforcement issues. It impacts access to justice and raises important questions regarding the management of dispute resolution mechanisms and their operation in a globalized world. We will now explore these issues and examine how systems can balance between local autonomy and structural integrity.

Fragmentation, Voice, and Accountability

As the public becomes more involved in arbitrating disputes, inconsistent standards could arise, leading to varying outcomes in similar cases and a lack of accountability. Hence, one might argue that fragmentation is a primary risk in decentralized legal systems. However, this is not an accurate portrayal of the modern hybrid system that we are proposing. Hybrid legal systems would maintain core legal principles that apply uniformly across regions. The role and centrality of these core principles will vary from one context or legal domain to another. For instance, constitutional law cases will require strong central oversight, whereas municipal regulations could tolerate—and perhaps even benefit from—more local variation.

Importantly, these hybrid systems are designed to complement, not disrupt, ingrained social norms. Most contracts are performed without incident. Property rights are generally respected without the need for legal intervention. This is not due to continuous and active enforcement, but rather because these behaviors have become socially embedded over the years. Superjustice recognizes this social infrastructure as valuable and seeks to preserve it by maintaining centralized guardianship over fundamental principles, while using decentralized mechanisms primarily for dispute resolution. This approach can strengthen social norms by making their enforcement more accessible when violations do occur, reinforcing rather than undermining their effectiveness.

For example, in the dispute between Sarah and Tom, if property law provides a clear rule, such as a regulation on overhanging branches, the digital legal system would notify the parties of the rule and its application. However, if the rule is vague or context-dependent—like allowing "reasonable use" of land—local customs may influence the outcome. In such cases, public arbitrators, ideally drawn from the local community, would bring their understanding of regional norms and conventions to the decision-making process. This approach allows for community-sensitive resolutions while ensuring that fundamental legal principles are upheld. Furthermore, any decision would be coded into the system and made public, ensuring that future disputes on similar issues will consider relevant precedents. While blockchain technology would ensure transparent enforcement and safeguard compliance, broader centralized oversight would prevent parochial interpretations or conflicting applications of the law.

To be sure, a significant challenge in any decentralized legal system is the potential for local opportunism, or what might be termed "the tyranny of the localized majority." History has repeatedly demonstrated that highly localized systems of governance often discriminate against minorities or marginalized groups. From local ordinances targeting specific religious practices or cultural expressions to exclusionary local housing regulations, communities may implement rules that reflect localized majority preferences while systematically disadvantaging others. Technology-enabled decentralization risks amplifying this problem. AI systems solely trained on local data or local perspectives might encode and perpetuate existing biases, essentially automating discrimination under the guise of community standards.

This fundamental tension between respecting local autonomy and protecting individual rights lies at the heart of constitutional democracies. Hybrid legal systems like Superjustice could implement several mechanisms to mitigate these risks. For one, an integrated rights protection system could combine AI monitoring with multi-layered human review. This system would automatically analyze decisions for patterns suggesting discrimination or rights violations, flagging concerning cases for escalation to higher authorities outside the local context. The AI layer would provide consistent scanning across all cases, while the human review layer would ensure that complex contextual factors and evolving rights standards are properly considered. This would create a safeguard that balances efficient automation with nuanced human judgment when fundamental rights are at stake.

Additionally, constitutional-style constraints could be directly encoded into the system's architecture, establishing immutable boundaries that no local ruling could transgress regardless of community support. These digital "rights frameworks" would function similarly to constitutional protections in traditional legal systems, but with the added advantage of consistent, automated enforcement. Moreover, statistical monitoring across jurisdictions could identify outlier communities whose rulings systematically disadvantage certain groups. Such anomaly detection would reveal potential discrimination and establish accountability mechanisms that prevent communities from becoming enclaves of locally sanctioned injustice. Through these complementary approaches, hybrid legal systems could balance the benefits of local customization with the imperative to protect individual rights.

Beyond human interests, our hybrid legal system and the increased use of technology raise a compelling question about the scope of decentralization: Should it account only for diverse human perspectives or extend to non-human entities that share our communities and ecosystems? For example, in Tom and Sarah's property boundary dispute, what about the rights of the birds nesting in the contested trees? And does the ancient oak itself have any standing in the resolution process? These questions become increasingly relevant as legal systems worldwide evolve to recognize the rights of non-human entities. Among others, New Zealand has granted legal personhood to specific rivers and forests. Chile's constitution recognizes nature's rights. Similar recognitions have emerged in other jurisdictions, such as Colombia's recognition of the Atrato River (2016) and the Amazon Rainforest (2018) as legal entities, as well as the granting of legal personhood to the Magpie River in Quebec. These precedents suggest that truly comprehensive decentralized justice may be expected, or viewed as an exceptional opportunity, to consider entities beyond human disputants.

If we take this path, one approach would be to develop specialized advocacy AI agents programmed specifically to represent non-human interests in relevant disputes. For instance, in a property boundary dispute affecting a watershed, a designated AI environmental agent could participate alongside human disputants, bringing ecological considerations directly into negotiations. Such agents could draw on scientific data, precedent from environmental law, and impact assessments to articulate potential harms that might otherwise remain externalized. This form of representation aligns naturally with decentralized systems, acknowledging that "local interests" extend beyond human stakeholders to include all entities affected by locally implemented decisions.

This, in turn, raises profound questions about value encoding in algorithmic systems. Should environmental and animal welfare principles be automatically factored into all relevant negotiations? To what extent should AI legal agents be programmed with inherent biocentric or eco-centric values? Without explicit design choices to include non-human interests, AI systems will probably optimize for efficient human-centered solutions. Such solutions would potentially externalize costs onto voiceless entities, replicating problematic patterns in existing legal frameworks.

The integration of non-human interests thus represents a potential transformation in how decentralization might function. Such integration expands from human-centric localism to ecological localism, recognizing the full web of relationships within any given jurisdiction. More generally, this consideration exemplifies the way technological innovation compels us to revisit foundational questions about whose interests count and who decides which values deserve algorithmic representation.

Finally, decentralized systems must also incorporate review mechanisms that enable the challenging of decisions. This could involve centralized appellate bodies or multi-tier dispute resolution frameworks, offering oversight and corrections within the decentralized framework. A right to appeal will ensure fairness by providing a mechanism to review decisions that seem to deviate from broader legal standards or rights protections. It will also create opportunities to revisit and refine legal principles when needed.[23]

[23] For interesting discussions about the roles of courts and review processes and how they may enhance fairness, legitimacy, and trust see Martin Shapiro, *Courts: A Comparative and Political Analysis* (University of Chicago Press 1981); Edgar Allan Lind and Tom R Tyler, *The Social Psychology of Procedural Justice* (Springer 1986).

Access to Justice

The challenges discussed thus far raise a larger question central to Superjustice: Will decentralization improve access to justice? As we have seen in Chapter 2, access to justice remains a significant problem in traditional, centralized legal systems. High legal costs, lengthy procedures, complex laws, and geographical barriers prevent many people, particularly vulnerable populations, from accessing legal resources. Wealthier parties can afford better legal representation, while low-income individuals face systemic disadvantages, contributing to an imbalanced legal landscape.

Decentralized legal systems promise to overcome some of these challenges. By reducing reliance on centralized courts and allowing for localized and more efficient dispute resolution procedures, decentralization can make legal systems faster, more accessible, user-friendly, and community-oriented. For example, in the dispute between Sarah and Tom, the conflicting parties could log into a platform, present their case to local arbitrators or AI, and receive a resolution in days (if human arbitrators are needed), or even minutes (if AI can provide a clear answer based on the applicable legal rules). As noted, they might also employ multimodal AI legal agents that could represent them and negotiate the best outcome on their behalf. Unlike the bureaucratic centralized courts, the simplicity and speed of such platforms would encourage more people to approach the legal system without fear of high costs, excessive complexity, or prolonged litigation.

Despite these improvements, decentralization introduces new barriers, particularly related to the digital divide.[24] Vulnerable groups, such as the elderly, low-income families, and rural populations, may lack the digital literacy or access needed to participate in decentralized systems. This can create new inequities, leaving those without technological access excluded from the legal process. Whereas these are real challenges, internet access and digital literacy are improving globally. The costs of technology are decreasing, and digital integration is becoming the norm in many areas of society. To further mitigate the problem, governments and organizations could implement programs aimed at increasing digital literacy and providing affordable internet access. Over time, such developments and measures could help alleviate the digital divide and expand participation in hybrid legal systems.

Beyond improving basic digital access, hybrid legal systems could incorporate several design features to ensure meaningful participation regardless of technical sophistication. Physical access points in community centers, libraries, and government buildings would provide alternatives for those without personal devices. At the same time, transparency requirements would ensure that AI systems explain their reasoning

[24] On the nature and scope of this problem see Laura Robinson and others, "Digital Inequalities and Why They Matter" (2015) 18(5) Information, Communication & Society 569; Anique Scheerder, Alexander van Deursen, and Jan van Dijk, "Determinants of Internet Skills, Uses, and Outcomes. A Systematic Review of the Second- and Third-level Digital Divide" (2017) 34(8) Telematics and Informatics 1607; Sora Park and Justine Humphry, "Exclusion by Design: Intersections of Social, Digital and Data Exclusion" (2019) 22(7) Information, Communication & Society 933.

in plain language and are accessible to all users. Additionally, hybrid systems could employ graduated complexity in interfaces, automatically adjusting to match users' language proficiency and digital literacy levels. They could offer simplified interactions for novices while allowing advanced options for experienced users. These practical adaptations would help bridge the participation gap without requiring universal technical expertise.

Another related concern is the risk that decentralized legal systems will still be dominated by powerful actors, undermining substantive access to justice. Just as in centralized models, wealthy corporations or affluent communities might influence local norms or exert control over decentralized platforms, creating power imbalances. This could lead to unequal access at crucial legal junctures, favoring those with greater resources. To address this, hybrid systems would need robust oversight mechanisms. Decentralized review boards and blockchain-enabled transparency could help curb undue influence and ensure fair participation. In fact, decentralization generally redistributes power, making it harder for wealthy external actors to manipulate or exert undue influence over the system. Although no system is entirely immune to capture, hybrid structures with well-defined oversight might offer better safeguards than today's centralized models.

More ambitiously, a truly equitable hybrid system might institutionalize AI representation as a right rather than a privilege. This could include publicly provided AI legal agents, like today's public defenders or community law clinics, ensuring that technological assistance is available, regardless of financial means. Such AI agents could be regulated to maintain fiduciary obligations to their human clients while respecting the rights of all parties involved in disputes. Perhaps the most transformative aspect of this is that the system could implement automatic balancing mechanisms. These would require any party using AI representation to ensure similar representation for unrepresented counterparts. This could be accomplished either by covering the cost themselves or through a centralized fund. This balancing mechanism could become a precondition for the legal enforceability of any settlement or decision, preventing technological disparities from creating new forms of procedural injustice.

Jurisdictional Overlap

The problem of jurisdictional overlap arises when disputes span multiple jurisdictions or regions with differing legal norms. While centralized systems manage this issue through hierarchical structures and choice of law and forum selection rules that designate clear legal authority, decentralized systems distribute authority across various nodes. This distribution can complicate cross-border or multi-jurisdictional disputes, creating uncertainty over which legal norm applies. This may undermine the capacity of decentralized systems to resolve these disputes. It risks contradictory rulings, when there is no mechanism to determine which node has governing authority.

To address the complexities of international disputes, hybrid systems need coordinated legal frameworks that outline boundaries and establish rules for determining issues such as the choice of law and jurisdiction. This balance between centralization and decentralization—between structure and flexibility—can be enhanced and made more efficient by protocols for inter-jurisdictional cooperation. Unlike current inter-jurisdictional frameworks, which often rely on opaque, labor-intensive, and fragmented processes for cross-border disputes, blockchain and smart contract technology can facilitate efficient and effective cross-border dispute resolution. Blockchain can ensure transparent enforcement of these protocols, while smart contracts could create automatically enforceable agreements across borders, streamlining cross-border disputes.

Moreover, emerging technologies could further revolutionize the way we handle international legal challenges in hybrid systems. AI systems could analyze case specifics, relevant laws across jurisdictions, and historical outcomes to suggest optimal forums or custom-blended applicable laws. This AI-driven approach could reduce forum shopping and advance more consistent outcomes in international disputes. Developing such frameworks and technologies will help hybrid systems remain efficient and consistent, even when dealing with multiple jurisdictions, offering a promising path forward for resolving global legal issues.

Decentralization and Conflicting Traditions

While jurisdictional overlap concerns which authority governs a dispute, an additional challenge emerges when legal systems rooted in different traditions must determine how to reason together. Different legal traditions, such as civil law and common law, take distinct approaches in shaping their laws. Civil law systems prioritize codified laws and structured legal principles, whereas common law systems emphasize judicial precedents and case-by-case evolution.[25] In hybrid legal systems, these differences pose challenges, particularly when nodes from different traditions must cooperate.

When considering how hybrid legal systems might bridge diverse legal traditions, John Rawls' concept of "overlapping consensus" offers a valuable framework.[26] Rawls proposed that despite fundamental differences in comprehensive doctrines or worldviews, diverse groups can nonetheless converge on certain core principles of justice that each tradition endorses based on its own normative foundations. Applied to decentralized legal systems, this suggests that, rather than imposing uniformity, hybrid frameworks could identify foundational principles that different legal

[25] See H Patrick Glenn, *Legal Traditions of the World: Sustainable Diversity in Law* (5th edn, Oxford University Press 2014); Konrad Zweigert and Hein Kötz, *An Introduction to Comparative Law* (3rd edn, Oxford University Press 1998).

[26] John Rawls, *Political Liberalism* (Columbia University Press 1993).

traditions—whether civil law, common law, religious law, or indigenous legal systems—can endorse through their own internal reasoning.

Importantly, this consensus would not require abandoning distinctive features of each tradition but would establish sufficient common ground for practical cooperation. For instance, principles like transparency, proportionality, and the right to be heard may form part of this consensus, even as traditions differ on their philosophical justifications. Crucially, this overlapping consensus would provide legitimacy that mere technical interoperability cannot, ensuring that participants from diverse legal cultures see the system as substantively valid, not merely procedurally functional. Such normative alignment would complement technological solutions, creating hybrid systems that are both philosophically coherent and technically feasible across jurisdictional boundaries.

Accordingly, AI-enhanced hybrid systems offer an opportunity to harmonize divergent approaches. In common law, the adherence to precedent naturally aligns with the adaptive potential of AI, which can learn from past decisions and apply evolving insights to future cases. Similarly, civil law's focus on codification and its scientific structuring of legal principles can lend itself to automation, allowing legal norms to be more consistently applied. By borrowing from the common law's adaptability and the civil law's structured rigor, AI-enhanced hybrid systems can transcend traditional boundaries.

Blockchain technology could also play a critical role in harmonizing legal systems across different legal traditions. With its transparent, immutable ledger, blockchain can create a shared record-keeping mechanism that transcends individual legal systems. For instance, smart contracts can enforce agreements across civil and common law jurisdictions by providing a neutral platform for verifying contract terms and execution.

The disparity between developed and developing nations presents another intriguing challenge for hybrid legal systems. Developed nations typically have more robust legal infrastructures, advanced technologies, and greater access to digital tools, which facilitates the smoother integration of decentralized, technology-based systems. By contrast, developing nations may lack these resources, leading to unequal participation in global decentralized frameworks.[27] Moreover, some nations may not prioritize democratization, accountability, or transparency. Hybrid systems must be designed to account for these disparities and build mechanisms that accommodate diverse legal and technological environments.

Decentralized legal systems also need innovative mechanisms to handle cross-jurisdictional disputes. One possible solution is the adaptation of international arbitration processes, whereby neutral third parties help to resolve conflicts across different jurisdictions. These mechanisms could be integrated into decentralized systems to handle disputes when nodes from different legal traditions or regions are involved.

[27] For an exploration of the link between economic development and the legal systems see, for example, Douglass North, *Institutions, Institutional Change, and Economic Performance* (Cambridge University Press 1990); Michael J Trebilcock and Ronald J Daniels, *Rule of Law Reform and Development: Charting the Fragile Path of Progress* (Edward Elgar Publishing 2008).

Ultimately, hybrid systems will necessitate centralization and standardization at both national and global levels.

Final Reflections

As social norms govern much of our everyday lives, the relationship between decentralization and internalized social norms deserves particular attention. These norms, ranging from respecting property rights to fair dealing and acting in good faith to fulfilling contractual obligations, serve as invisible pillars of social order, preventing countless disputes from arising in the first place. Rather than disrupting these norm systems, Superjustice aims to strengthen them by making enforcement more accessible when violations do occur, while preserving the centralized oversight that maintains their integrity and legitimacy.

This balance between decentralized operations and centralized principles is equally relevant to concerns about how decentralization aligns with the rule of law. At its core, the rule of law embodies fair, predictable, and equally accessible justice, regardless of socioeconomic status.[28] Decentralization introduces both opportunities and challenges to these ideals. On the one hand, decentralized systems reduce costs and the impact of geographical barriers, enabling faster, more democratic processes for norm creation and dispute resolution. On the other hand, they risk fragmentation, where local norms diverge significantly from universal standards, potentially undermining core values and creating disparities in justice. As we have seen, hybrid systems must balance flexibility and structure with consistency and oversight to maintain fairness.

Sarah and Tom's dispute is hypothetical, but reality is often stranger than fiction. In Dripping Springs, Texas, a somewhat similar neighborhood conflict over backyard swimming lessons escalated from a noise complaint into a bitter legal battle involving surveillance, social media warfare, a lawsuit, and ultimately proposed state legislation.[29] In a Superjustice system, this spiraling conflict could have been resolved through AI-mediated negotiation, community input, and transparent rule application before reaching the dysfunctional extremes that divided an entire community. Likewise, a Superjustice system would transform Tom and Sarah's conflict. Instead of facing prohibitive costs and procedural obstacles, they could access a hybrid platform that combines AI capabilities and analysis with community input. The resolution—whether trimming specific branches, installing bird deterrents, or compensating

[28] While it is not the focus of this chapter, the discussion surrounding the rule of law—its definition, core principles, and underlying values—is rich and thought-provoking. For a few examples see Lon L Fuller, *The Morality of Law* (Yale University Press 1969); Richard Bellamy (ed), *The Rule of Law and the Separation of Powers* (Routledge 2005); Jeremy Waldron, *The Rule of Law and the Measure of Property* (Cambridge University Press 2008). See also John Rawls, *A Theory of Justice* (Harvard University Press 1971).

[29] See Forrest Wilder, "The Neighborhood Spat That Went Nuclear: How an Argument over Backyard Swimming Lessons Sent a Gated Community off the Deep End" *Texas Monthly* (March 2025) <www.texasmonthly.com/news-politics/hoa-dripping-springs-legislature/>.

Sarah—would emerge quickly, inexpensively, and with greater attention to contextual factors, preventing a bitter relationship between neighbors.

These changes are not about convenience; they represent a shift toward legal systems that empower ordinary people and local communities while preserving core principles of fairness and consistency. For this to materialize, decentralization must be combined with advances in data and technology. As Chapter 4 will demonstrate, a synergy between decentralization, data, and technology promises to transform the way we perceive the law and interact with it.

4
From Gridlock to Dynamism

Planting the Seeds

Imagine standing in the middle of a vast wheat field, with the golden stalks swaying gently in the breeze. You cannot see a scarecrow anywhere, and no workers are walking the rows. Instead, in your hands is a tablet displaying a real-time map of the field, showing soil moisture, weather forecasts, and crop health. This is data-driven agriculture powered by edge computing.[1]

For generations, farming relied on experience, tradition, and intuition. Farmers walked their fields, assessed soil health by feel, and prayed for favorable weather. But today, with a growing population and the increasing threat of climate change, guesswork is no longer enough. And, increasingly, it is no longer necessary. Throughout the 20th century, agricultural innovations such as improved fertilizers, pesticides, mechanization, and land management techniques led to significant increases in agricultural productivity, thereby alleviating widespread hunger. Today, genetic modification is further enhancing crop performance.

Indeed, the future of farming lies in real-time data analysis and precision technology. Edge computing empowers farmers with sophisticated decision-making capabilities. In this high-tech model of farming, small devices and robots can analyze everything from soil composition to pest infestations, providing instant feedback that facilitates targeted irrigation and pesticide application. Furthermore, autonomous drones and tractors can continuously collect and process data, automating tasks like planting, watering, and harvesting with precision. Picture automated sprinkler systems responding to a detected freeze, protecting crops before damage occurs. In this data-driven world, technology can handle repetitive tasks, freeing human farmers to focus on strategic decisions to maximize yields and minimize environmental impact.

Law, like farming, is steeped in tradition and slow to change. But while farmers are gradually embracing data-driven practices, legal systems remain burdened by slow processes, high costs, and limited access, often relying on centuries-old practices and the intuition of legal professionals. This contrast raises the question: If agriculture can transform itself with data and technology, why can't the law? Just as precision

[1] Weisong Shi and others, "Edge Computing: Vision and Challenges" (2016) 3(5) IEEE Internet of Things Journal 637; Sjaak Wolfert and others, "Big Data in Smart Farming—A Review" (2017) 153 Agricultural Systems 69; Tawseef Ayoub Shaikh, Tabasum Rasool, and Faisal Rasheed Lone, "Towards Leveraging the Role of Machine Learning and Artificial Intelligence in Precision Agriculture and Smart Farming" (2022) 198 Computers and Electronics in Agriculture 107119; Daniel Azevedo, "John Deere's Plan to Bring Thousands of Growers to Precision Agriculture" *Future Farming* (May 21, 2024).

Superjustice. Samuel I. Becher and Benjamin Alarie, Oxford University Press.
 DOI: 10.1093/9780198991885.003.0006

agriculture optimizes resource allocation, a data-driven legal system can optimize fairness and efficiency. Could legal automation be the key to serving societies more effectively? Could we move beyond one-size-fits-all rules to offer personalized laws, much like edge computing can treat each plant individually?

Data: The Lifeblood of Superjustice

To begin answering these questions, we need first to explore the types of data that the law can harness through new technologies. This exploration will cover three key areas: traditional legal data, macro-extralegal data (broad societal trends), and micro-extralegal data (personalized information). Each data type offers unique possibilities for enhancing legal systems. Understanding their distinct characteristics is crucial for developing a holistic approach to data-driven law.

Traditional Legal Data

The foundation of any legal system is its corpus of established legal materials. These materials come in various shapes and forms: statutes, case law, regulations, contracts, administrative rulings, court filings, legal opinions, treaties, legal commentaries, parliamentary records, litigation documents, policy papers, intellectual property data, scholarly publications, and more. The vast and diverse nature of legal data, spanning various jurisdictions and legal traditions, is a foundational factor in Superjustice systems.

AI can process vast datasets quickly, offering unprecedented insights. Generative artificial intelligence (AI), for example, excels at language-related tasks such as synthesizing information, outlining, drafting, summarizing, and editing. Thus, the straightforward first step in enabling AI-driven systems like Superjustice is digitizing this vast repository. AI algorithms could then swiftly comb through enormous amounts of data to provide useful and insightful services. For instance, AI could review large bodies of case law to identify relevant precedents, predict outcomes based on historical patterns, assist in research and document drafting, evaluate existing and potential policies, and provide targeted input into legal decision-making. This technological capability would revolutionize how legal professionals operate, increasing accuracy and efficiency.

As we have seen in Chapter 3, legal fragmentation—where different legal systems can create inconsistencies in legal norms and processes across jurisdictions—poses a particular challenge to cross-border legal issues. AI's ability to synthesize legal data from multiple jurisdictions can mitigate this challenge. Integrating legal knowledge from diverse legal systems equips Superjustice with the ability to harmonize legal research, analysis, and policymaking, thus facilitating more consistent legal outcomes and reducing the costs associated with legal fragmentation.

You may wonder: Why do we need clever AI tools to do that? One major limitation that legal professionals currently face is the constraint of language. Legal practitioners are typically limited to materials in the languages they speak. A French or an American judge, for instance, is unlikely to consult a valuable Japanese or Brazilian precedent due to the language barrier. But with AI-powered language translation, this limitation could be eliminated. Advanced machine translation tools, such as generative AI models and neural machine translation (NMT) systems, are becoming increasingly capable of accurately translating texts.[2] These tools could allow AI systems to draw upon legal data from diverse sources worldwide, breaking down linguistic silos and increasing access to legal information.

Furthermore, cross-border disputes often involve conflicting legal systems, complicating their resolution. Despite globalization, immigration, improved communication means, and cross-border trade, legal systems usually operate in isolation. AI-driven legal systems can mitigate this problem by processing multilingual legal data and providing insights from diverse jurisdictions. By streamlining access to legal precedents and principles from around the world, AI can equip legal professionals with the tools necessary to resolve international disputes more efficiently and equitably.

AI models, including large language models (LLMs), are already capable of translating legal texts between numerous languages. Future legal systems will probably leverage such capacities to process multilingual legal data, providing unprecedented access to a global body of legal knowledge. To be sure, machine translation is still evolving—especially in capturing context, traditional or cultural nuances, and domain-specific terminology like legal jargon. However, ongoing advances suggest that AI will soon offer seamless and reliable translation of legal materials. As technology progresses, AI will handle more complex analysis, translation, and research tasks with minimal human oversight.

In addition to breaking down jurisdictional and language barriers, AI could also facilitate a more diverse legal system. Currently, the limits of linguistic knowledge contribute to the exclusion of valuable perspectives, such as Indigenous peoples' legal traditions, expressed in other languages.[3] Such limitations restrict legal professionals from gaining a full understanding of diverse legal traditions and their insights. AI could provide a foundation for greater collaboration across legal systems by making legal data from multiple jurisdictions, traditions, and languages accessible and comparable. Drawing from multilingual and multicultural sources, Superjustice could foster a more globally integrated legal framework.

Empirical research already demonstrates that, despite their apparent vagueness, shared legal concepts (such as reasonableness) can be identified across languages and

[2] See Dzmitry Bahdanau, Kyunghyun Cho, and Yoshua Bengio, "Neural Machine Translation by Jointly Learning to Align and Translate" (Paper delivered at the International Conference on Learning Representations, 2015).

[3] For a discussion on the exclusion of minority groups, including Indigenous peoples, from mainstream legal and political discourse, see Will Kymlicka, *Multicultural Citizenship: A Liberal Theory of Minority Rights* (Oxford University Press 1995).

jurisdictions through painstaking cross-cultural study.[4] What currently requires a coordinated international effort of scholars across multiple countries and substantial time could, in the future, be accomplished in minutes by an AI system trained on multilingual legal sources. This shift from rare, resource-intensive studies to routine, scalable analysis underscores the transformative potential of AI in developing the law and possibly harmonizing legal understanding across borders.

However, there are also considerable risks in guaranteeing legal data, and the availability of legal data is a critical concern. At the time of writing, only a few companies (namely, vLex, LexisNexis, and Thomson Reuters (Westlaw)) possess comprehensive collections of international legal information. While these collections are invaluable, this concentrated control (if not ownership) presents challenges, as companies have an incentive to thwart innovation that would endanger their information rights. This is particularly problematic for Superjustice, which seeks to leverage large-scale legal data.

First, the dependency on a few major data gatekeepers hinders progress. The concentration of data within a few companies makes the development of advanced systems contingent on these providers' willingness to share their databases. This dependency risks slowing the growth of data-driven legal technologies, as projects like Superjustice remain vulnerable to the priorities and access conditions set by a handful of dominant companies. Second, this concentration drives high costs, allowing companies to set premium prices for access, making it financially prohibitive for smaller law firms, independent researchers, or emerging technologies. This "chokehold" restricts Superjustice's potential, as it will rely on affordable, broad data access. Lastly, limited data access creates a significant barrier to innovation. Continuous access to diverse, cross-jurisdictional legal data is essential for developing Superjustice as an accurate and responsive system. Without a broader, accessible data ecosystem, the development of Superjustice may be slowed or undermined.

Macro-Level Extralegal Data

Oliver Wendell Holmes Jr famously observed that "The life of the law has not been logic: it has been experience."[5] While traditional legal data forms the foundation of legal frameworks, broader extralegal data is essential for a comprehensive understanding of law and its applications. Law does not exist in isolation; it is a product of human society, shaped by social structures, political decisions, and ideological perspectives. Thus, law is interwoven with societal, economic, psychological, and political contexts, and legal systems reciprocally interact with social realities and diverse data types.

Examples abound. Healthcare reforms following the Covid-19 pandemic responded directly to public health needs, economic pressures, and shifting societal expectations.

[4] See Kevin Tobia and others, "The Nature of Reasonableness" (2025) 61 Stanford Journal of International Law 111 (conducting a multi-country empirical study uncovering shared legal conceptions of reasonableness).

[5] Oliver Wendell Holmes Jr, *The Common Law*, vol I (Little, Brown and Company 1881) 1.

Privacy laws like the EU's General Data Protection Regulation (GDPR) emerged from concerns over data security, technological advancements, and public demands for greater control over personal information. Environmental regulations were developed in response to climate change concerns, mounting scientific evidence, and international agreements. Likewise, criminal justice approaches are shaped by perspectives on moral responsibility, human behavior, and socioeconomic factors. These examples highlight the need for legal systems to engage with broader societal contexts.

On a related note, interdisciplinary scholarship enriches our understanding of the law. Insights from fields such as economics, political science, psychology, and sociology reveal the multidimensional nature of legal systems. For example, environmental law relies on ecological data and climate science to shape sustainability policies and regulations. Similarly, criminal law is informed by psychology, criminology, and sociology, which help develop theories on deterrence, rehabilitation, and the causes of criminal behavior. Demographic data, such as population growth, migration patterns, or age distribution, also inform housing policies, tax rules, immigration policies, and pension regulations. Likewise, psychology sheds light on the fallibility and malleability of human memory, emphasizing the need for caution when weighing eyewitness testimony.

The interconnectedness between law and other disciplines is simultaneously historical and forward-looking. Historical and cultural contexts profoundly impact legal systems, as seen in the post-colonial legal reforms in African and South Asian nations, which address issues of inequality, self-determination, and land rights. Meanwhile, technological advances like AI and blockchain are beginning to shape regulations in areas such as data protection, cybersecurity, and digital currencies. Moreover, as this book explains, technological developments have the potential to go beyond any specific legal domain and transform the entire legal landscape.

Recognizing the interconnectedness of legal systems with broader societal dynamics and interdisciplinary insights, Superjustice embraces the integration of high-quality macro-extralegal data. Incorporating macro-extralegal data enables the legal system to adapt more effectively to the realities of a rapidly evolving world. A data-driven approach would lead to better policymaking, more responsive laws, and enhanced judicial decisions.

Micro-Level Extralegal Data

In today's digital landscape, individuals generate vast amounts of data through constant digital interactions—sometimes consciously but often unknowingly. These data come from everyday activities like internet browsing, GPS tracking, social media usage, interactions with LLMs, and health information captured by wearable devices, such as fitness trackers. As the Internet of Things (IoT) continues to expand, even ordinary appliances like refrigerators and thermostats can collect data, revealing behavioral patterns and personal information. This dataset integrates the physical and digital worlds, offering detailed insights into people's lives.

The IoT phenomenon is not a single event but a gradual and continuous progression towards an interconnected world, where data from everyday objects drives automation, enhances efficiency, and informs smarter decision-making across various domains. Collected data is the gold mine. Businesses, for example, leverage analytics tools to glean valuable insights, from optimizing factory operations to personalizing customers' shopping experience. The ongoing IoT evolution, with its ever-increasing data generation, presents both opportunities and challenges for AI-transformed, data-driven legal systems.

Micro-extralegal data holds immense potential for shaping more responsive regulatory and legal frameworks. For instance, health specialists utilized data from wearable health devices and wastewater during the Covid-19 pandemic to track infection, monitor symptoms, and predict outbreaks. Tapping into the wealth of data generated through IoT devices, wearables, and other digital platforms could allow regulatory systems to inform effective responses and move beyond general, one-size-fits-all regulations. For instance, data collected from smart homes and smart cities—such as energy consumption patterns, water usage, long-term traffic patterns, or public space usage—can inform urban planning laws that evolve based on changing community behaviors and needs. As this example illustrates, leveraging micro-extralegal data requires a significant initial investment and integrated cross-sectoral infrastructure. It also necessitates safeguards for privacy and cybersecurity, as well as addressing the digital divide and maintaining public trust.[6]

Micro-extralegal data opens new possibilities for legal innovation in numerous domains. The integration of biometric and behavioral data in legal frameworks can significantly enhance lawmaking by improving the ability to anticipate future societal trends and behavioral shifts. For example, biometric data collected through facial recognition systems could streamline identity verification in legal proceedings and border immigration or enable more accurate crime prevention strategies. Similarly, wearable health devices offer insights into emerging public health trends, potentially allowing governments to adjust regulations related to workplace safety, public health initiatives, or emergency response protocols.

Likewise, consider the domain of environmental law. As smart meters and IoT devices monitor personal energy consumption and carbon footprints, policymakers and regulators could incorporate this data to develop more sustainable regulations. Legal frameworks could incentivize eco-friendly behaviors through tax incentives, carbon reduction programs, or even mandatory usage limits based on long-term environmental data analysis. This would create an ecosystem where laws and regulations

[6] Noor Ul Huda and others, "Experts and Intelligent Systems for Smart Homes' Transformation to Sustainable Smart Cities: A Comprehensive Review" (2024) 238 Expert Systems with Applications 122380; Rama Krishna Reddy Kummitha, "Smart Cities and Entrepreneurship: An Agenda for Future Research" (2019) 149 Technological Forecasting and Social Change 119763; R Sonia and others, "Strengthening Security, Privacy, and Trust in Artificial Intelligence Drones for Smart Cities" in *Analyzing and Mitigating Security Risks in Cloud Computing* (IGI Global 2024) 214.

evolve alongside technological advancements and emerging data, fostering climate policies that align with social goals and environmental responsibilities.

Interestingly, aggregated microdata—derived from individual behaviors and interactions—can turn into macrodata and play a further role in shaping legal frameworks. Here, the collective insights gained from vast amounts of personal data can give lawmakers, regulators, and judges some robust empirical evidence to help them address complex legal challenges. For instance, microdata can help identify the prevalence and impact of manipulative design tactics, such as dark patterns in business-to-consumer (B2C) transactions.

In essence, so-called "dark patterns" are deceptive design techniques used to manipulate or trick users into decisions they might not otherwise make, such as subscribing to services or sharing personal information. By analyzing data on user behaviors—such as eye movements, click patterns, and purchasing decisions—legal systems can gain a deeper understanding of what constitutes dark patterns and how consumer protection should address them. Although such insights begin at the individual level (read: micro-level data), their aggregation reveals collective patterns and trends that inform the development of broad, societal-level legal (macro-level) interventions.

The collection of personal data raises significant concerns. The ability to track people's movement patterns, purchasing behavior, biometric data, or utility consumption brings the potential for surveillance and misuse, leading to privacy invasions. Large-scale data breaches could expose sensitive personal information, leading to consequences like identity theft and financial loss. Moreover, algorithmic decision-making can subtly steer individual actions without consent, creating a form of digital paternalism that undermines personal autonomy.

There are also ethical concerns over data commodification, whereby individuals unknowingly generate valuable data without being compensated or informed about its use. Data aggregation can also reinforce discriminatory practices, as seen in digital redlining (algorithmic discrimination excluding marginalized communities from digital resources) or predictive policing, both of which can entrench social inequalities. Additionally, community-level impacts are significant; cultural data could be exploited or misrepresented, compromising group identity and collective privacy.

These concerns highlight the delicate balance between privacy and utility; a challenge that Superjustice fully acknowledges and respects. While a more systematic exploration of these and similar issues will follow in Chapter 10, suffice it to say here that Superjustice is committed to using only publicly available, anonymized data, with a keen awareness of the ethical implications involved. To be sure, privacy challenges are not new: Individuals are constantly surveilled across the digital world, with cookies tracking the websites we visit, and code installed in mobile apps monitoring our locations. Furthermore, this voluminous data can be combined with other personal information, such as public records, loyalty programs, gym visits, and more. This combination can create detailed and highly personalized profiles that third parties can share, sell, or use.

Importantly, however, the fact that personal data is available does not grant firms, governments, or organizations carte blanche to freely scrape and use it indiscriminately.[7] Society's take on the balance between privacy and utility is an intriguing challenge, and Superjustice does not aim to redefine societal norms regarding privacy. Instead, it seeks to operate responsibly within established boundaries, making constructive use of data deemed acceptable under prevailing legal and social standards.

Democratizing Legal Data

The legal data landscape that Superjustice could draw on is vast and multifaceted, encompassing a wide range of both legal and extralegal data. We have explored how data from diverse sources can shape legal frameworks. However, Superjustice envisions going even further. To fully harness the power of data, it will not rely merely on established sources. Rather, Superjustice will actively seek to incorporate additional types of data through mechanisms of democratization and decentralization, and perhaps even through responsible (and ethical) experimentation. Throughout this democratization process, Superjustice will invite individuals, communities, and decentralized networks to actively participate in collecting, managing, and sharing legal data. Next, we will examine how democratizing legal data can broaden access to and participation in legal decision-making, altering the way legal frameworks operate and evolve.

Decentralizing Legal Data

Decentralization, a core tenet of Superjustice that we explored in Chapter 3, transforms the way legal systems collect, manage, and utilize data. Traditional frameworks rely primarily on centralized entities—such as judicial opinions, governmental regulations, and institutional actors—which limit the available data sources to formalized, top-down inputs. This approach often overlooks diverse, localized insights that could enrich the law. Superjustice seeks to address this shortcoming by diversifying the collection of legal data, incorporating community input, public feedback, and global legal traditions, to create a more inclusive legal framework. Figure 4.1 depicts six types of data sources.

One of the main advantages of decentralization is the ability to draw from various localized sources of information that contribute insights grounded in different cultural, environmental, or socioeconomic contexts. While Figure 4.1 illustrates this point by linking Superjustice to six types of data sources, there are no limits on the actual number of sources that could feed into the system. Unlike traditional systems that primarily depend on top-down legal data, decentralization integrates voices from communities, local governance structures, and marginalized groups. For example,

[7] See Daniel J Solove and Woodrow Hartzog, "The Great Scrape: The Clash Between Scraping and Privacy" (2025) 113 California Law Review 1521.

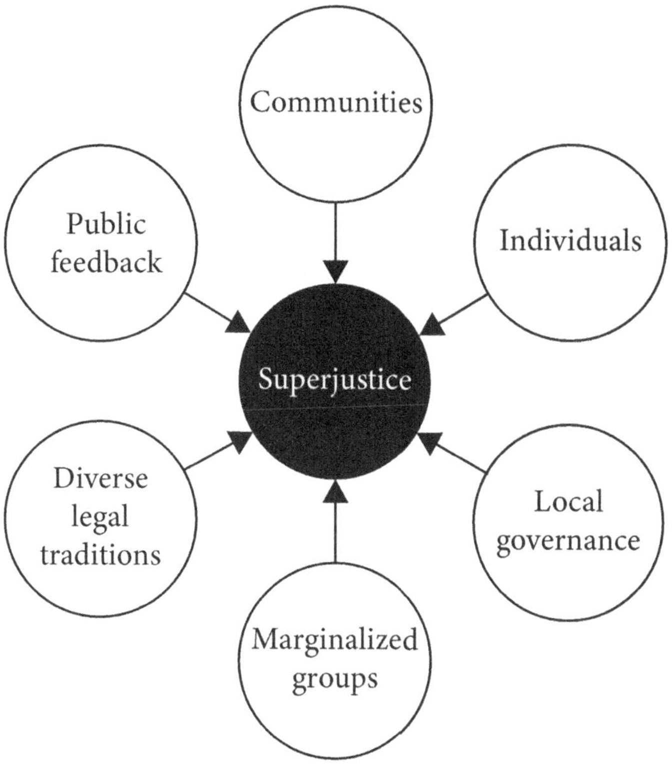

Figure 4.1 Multiple Data Sources Enriching Superjustice

indigenous knowledge of land use can inform environmental regulations, and employees' regular feedback on working conditions can shape labor laws. While centralized systems can also integrate such data, they often lack the infrastructure to do so efficiently. Decentralization enables legal frameworks to incorporate more accurate, rich, and context-sensitive mechanisms, thereby reflecting a better understanding of community values and societal needs.

As we previously mentioned, decentralization can also foster global cross-pollination of legal traditions. Legal systems from different jurisdictions can inform one another, contributing to a worldwide repository of legal knowledge that integrates diverse cultural, legal, and societal perspectives. Incorporating these global influences would ensure that legal frameworks become more nuanced and better equipped to address universal issues such as human rights, intellectual property, and climate regulation. For example, successful disaster response laws or cybersecurity regulations in one jurisdiction could serve as a template for others, promoting the transfer of best practices across borders. Centralized systems are often limited in their ability to leverage this potential, with only a few jurisdictions exerting significant global influence.[8] Superjustice's

[8] An example of a current prominent jurisdiction with potential global influence is the EU. See Anu Bradford, *The Brussels Effect: How the European Union Rules the World* (Oxford University Press 2020).

decentralized approach, however, will allow it to draw from a far richer and more diverse set of legal data.

As the discussion above reveals, decentralization also presents an opportunity for more inclusive legal systems. In traditional frameworks that rely on majoritarian mechanisms, the voices of marginalized communities are frequently excluded. This, in turn, results in laws that overlook the unique perspectives that would be crucial for designing legal frameworks that reflect societal complexities. AI systems are only as good as the data on which they are trained, and a centralized approach risks producing narrow or biased AI systems.[9] Superjustice's decentralized approach empowers marginalized groups by providing effective mechanisms that enable their perspectives and needs to be heard. Through the integration of data from a wide range of decentralized sources, Superjustice ensures that AI-generated legal frameworks and processes are more accurate, diverse, and fair.

Crowdsourcing Legal Data

While decentralization expands the sources of legal data at the structural level, crowdsourcing takes a bottom-up approach by seeking inputs directly from individuals, communities, and groups. Superjustice would use crowdsourcing to establish a participatory legal system, ensuring that the voices of those affected by laws are heard more often. Crowdsourcing democratizes the legal system through active individual and community participation in the design of laws and legal frameworks, facilitating the incorporation of diverse viewpoints.

Crowdsourcing could provide real-time, varied, and localized insights that would be difficult to capture through traditional data collection methods. Using technology platforms such as apps or web portals, individuals could contribute input and data on legal issues as they arise. These contributions could range from reporting labor violations and exposing firms' abuse of power over consumers, to providing feedback on local regulations, or expressing frustrations with complex tax systems and the disproportionate penalties triggered by minor filing mistakes,[10] or identifying barriers to justice. This participatory approach would establish a dynamic feedback loop between the public and the legal system, ensuring that laws and regulations remain responsive.

To illustrate, consider the discussions in Chapters 2 and 3 regarding vague legal standards, such as the "reasonable person," "reasonable expectations," or the "average consumer." Traditionally, when applying and interpreting these terms, judges rely on

[9] See Cathy O'Neil, *Weapons of Math Destruction: How Big Data Increases Inequality and Threatens Democracy* (Crown 2017); Emily M Bender and others, "On the Dangers of Stochastic Parrots: Can Language Models Be Too Big?" (2021) Proceedings of the 2021 ACM Conference on Fairness, Accountability, and Transparency 610–23.

[10] For a relevant anecdote see Zak Jason, "I Messed up my Tax Returns. It was the Beginning of an IRS Nightmare" *Business Insider* (April 15, 2025).

their intuition and general societal assumptions, which may lead to unpredictability and biased results. But what specific data do they base these applications on?

Crowdsourcing could provide judges with concrete, real-world data gathered directly from the public, allowing them to replace guesswork with precise insights. This data would reflect people's actual behavior, understandings, interpretations, and expectations, aiding in the production of more informed and contextually grounded decisions. Similarly, crowdsourcing encourages collaborative problem-solving, where the expertise and lived experiences of diverse groups contribute to more comprehensive and equitable legal solutions. Rather than relying solely on experts or institutional actors, Superjustice envisions a system where citizens, advocacy groups, and organizations can collectively provide valuable insights.

Ensuring Data Integrity

Superjustice's participatory approach raises significant concerns about data governance, data quality, and reliability.[11] Since crowdsourcing often involves unfiltered inputs, it is essential to implement robust mechanisms that safeguard the accuracy, integrity, and trustworthiness of the data collected. There are three distinct challenges: distinguishing valuable "signal" data that genuinely informs legal understanding; filtering out random "noise" that adds no substantive value; and detecting deliberately false signals intended to manipulate outcomes. We next discuss five mechanisms for responding to these challenges: blockchain technology, peer-review systems, trust mechanisms, weighted algorithms, and data provenance.

Blockchain for Data Transparency

Blockchain offers a decentralized and secure ledger system that authenticates and permanently records crowdsourced data. When individuals or groups submit data, blockchain encrypts and logs it onto a transparent ledger, thereby creating a verifiable trail that links the data back to its source. This ensures that the data remains tamper-proof, and that changes or updates to the data are traceable. Moreover, blockchain can maintain contributors' anonymity when necessary, balancing privacy with accountability to support secure data management. Additionally, blockchain supports real-time data verification. New entries are cross-checked with existing records, flagging contradictory information for review. Superjustice can further automate certain verification processes, such as certifying that data meets predefined quality standards, by employing smart contracts.

[11] The potential and pitfalls of relying on large groups for data and decision-making, including the need to ensure data quality and reliability, have received some attention in extralegal domains. In the context of business see Jeff Howe, *Crowdsourcing: Why the Power of the Crowd is Driving the Future of Business* (Crown Currency 2009).

Peer Review for Data Validation

Blockchain secures data at a technical level. Superjustice may also wish to add a layer of human verification, at least in its formative phases. Peer-review systems could offer a community-based verification process, during which experts in the relevant field evaluate data submitted via crowdsourcing. For instance, reports on workplace conditions could be assessed by labor rights specialists, legal clinics, community organizations, or labor unions, confirming the data's accuracy. This process acts as a filtering apparatus, identifying inaccurate or incomplete data while fostering community involvement.

A tiered review system—involving initial assessments by experts followed by evaluations from legal professionals or regulators—could further enhance data reliability. Over time, as Superjustice advances, AI-driven legal verification tools may gradually reduce the need for human oversight, enabling more efficient and scalable data validation procedures. While AI capabilities in legal verification are rapidly evolving, the transition should be gradual and context-dependent, taking some time to mature.

Reputation Systems and Smart Contracts

Reputation systems will track the reliability of data contributors, incentivizing accuracy and consistency. Such systems could complement peer-review mechanisms, prioritizing data from reliable contributors. As in other (mostly online) contexts, contributors who consistently provide verified, high-quality data could build strong reputations within the system, encouraging ongoing participation from trustworthy sources.[12] Conversely, poor-quality or misleading data might harm a contributor's reputation, reducing the weight of their future inputs.

Smart contracts will enhance this process by automatically verifying compliance with programmable predefined standards. For instance, smart contracts could ensure that data inputs meet criteria, such as correct formatting or submission within designated timeframes. If data fail to meet these criteria, the smart contract can automatically prevent its acceptance without human intervention. Additionally, smart contracts could trigger rewards for reliable contributors, thereby incentivizing the submission of accurate and timely data.

Weighted Algorithms for Data Prioritization

Superjustice's use of weighted algorithms can further enhance the reliability of crowdsourced data. Such algorithms assign weight to data based on factors such as the

[12] See Paul Resnick and others, "The Value of Reputation on eBay: A Controlled Experiment" (2006) 9 Experimental Economics 79; Audun Jøsang, Roslan Ismail, and Colin Boyd, "A Survey of Trust and Reputation Systems for Online Service Provision" (2007) 43(2) Decision Support Systems 618.

credibility of the source, the volume of similar reports, and the accuracy of past submissions. For instance, data from verified organizations or legal professionals would be given more weight than anonymous submissions. This should ensure that more reliable data is prioritized in legal decision-making processes.

Notably, weighted algorithms can be dynamic, with adjustments based on the timeliness or relevance of data. For example, in revising health regulations during public health emergencies, real-time data from health professionals could be prioritized over older or less relevant inputs. This dynamism would advance the system's ability to respond to real-time issues and emerging trends while still encouraging broad participation.

Data Provenance and Life-Cycle Transparency

Superjustice will have to guarantee that data maintains its integrity not only at the input stage but throughout its entire life cycle. Here, data provenance tracking provides a way to trace data throughout its entire life cycle, from submission to final use.[13] Fundamentally, data provenance tracks how data has been modified or processed over time, offering full transparency about who contributed, handled, or altered the data. Provenance tracking complements blockchain's role in securing data by providing a clear view of the data's journey through the system. If discrepancies or conflicts arise, provenance metadata will help to resolve them by identifying the source and context of the data. For example, in the context of environmental regulations, provenance tracking could provide insights into which regions contributed data, how their inputs were processed, and how those inputs influenced decision-making.

In sum, Superjustice could employ various verification and integrity mechanisms, including blockchain for transparency, peer-review systems for validation, reputation systems and smart contracts for data reliability, weighted algorithms for data prioritization, and data provenance for monitoring changes. These mechanisms would work in tandem as interconnected components, collectively forming a comprehensive ecosystem that safeguards data integrity across all aspects of the Superjustice platform. Such an integrated approach would make legal processes and institutions more robust, resilient, and informed.

Automating and Personalizing Law

Thus far, we have seen how decentralized data and crowdsourcing can facilitate legal democratization and public participation. With powerful technology and a vast

[13] Luc Moreau and others, "The Open Provenance Model Core Specification" (2011) 27(6) Future Generation Computer Systems 743; Yogesh L Simmhan, Beth Plale, and Dennis Gannon, "A Survey of Data Provenance in E-Science" (2005) 34(3) ACM Sigmod Record 31.

decentralized set of legal data, Superjustice can go even further, automating and personalizing law. Thoughtfully designed, automation and personalization can streamline legal processes, conserve scarce resources, reduce the need for human intervention, and increase both the speed and quality of legal and regulatory decision-making.

Automating Legal Tasks

Automation is the use of technology to perform tasks with minimal human intervention. For example, GPS systems automate navigation, allowing drivers to focus on safe driving without manually mapping routes. Similarly, automatic bill payment systems enable people to schedule recurring payments, ensuring timely installments without repeated manual effort. With ongoing technological advances, the question arises: How far can and should legal automation go?

Legal automation can enhance efficiency and improve outcomes, and automation is one of the most transformative aspects of Superjustice. By integrating vast data sources and advanced technologies, Superjustice can facilitate legal automation across multiple domains, paving the way for more responsive, accurate, and efficient legal frameworks. Initial applications may involve straightforward tasks, but automation could potentially lead to complex, thought-provoking innovations. The brief overview we provide here—merely a glimpse into the powerful combination of data and technology—is supplemented by Chapter 5, where we delve deeper into AI applications in legal practice.

Technology is already reshaping legal research, contract drafting, and strategy development. AI tools like machine learning and natural language processing (NLP) enable legal professionals to process vast amounts of data at unprecedented speeds, bringing precision and insight to document analysis that was previously unattainable. AI tools can automate tasks like document review, contract analysis, case triage, and preliminary assessments. This could reduce the burden on human judges and clerks, streamline case management, and help categorize and prioritize cases based on urgency or complexity, ensuring more efficient legal proceedings and reducing backlogs. As Superjustice integrates diverse and comprehensive legal datasets, AI's outputs will become even more accurate and contextually informed, further enhancing access to justice.

Interestingly, advances in automation pave the way for AI to predict legal outcomes with remarkable accuracy. AI models process vast datasets, identifying patterns in past cases to predict potential legal outcomes. This allows lawyers to prepare more effective strategies based on data-backed insights. Furthermore, case law analysis and surveys of past decisions will facilitate the development of predictive algorithms, allowing AI systems to assess the likelihood of success in litigation or offer settlement recommendations.

This kind of automation capability significantly reduces the time spent on case preparation. As AI predictions become more accurate, the need for costly litigation diminishes. If the likely outcome of a case is clear even before it is litigated, parties may be better placed to negotiate a settlement rather than pursue lengthy legal processes. As a result, the system will ultimately move toward an equilibrium where litigation is less necessary and only pursued in relatively rare, sensitive, or unpredictable circumstances.

Drawing on an unprecedented range of decentralized data sources, legal traditions, community input, and real-time extralegal data, Superjustice could further enhance the accuracy and depth of AI predictions. Predictive algorithms could analyze not only case law and judicial opinions but also cultural, social, and economic contexts to forecast judicial outcomes. This means that AI tools would not merely predict how judges might rule. Instead, they would also expose normative considerations and anticipate how societal and legal trends might influence future rulings, thus offering a more holistic view of potential outcomes. Moreover, Superjustice would ensure that this shift to data-driven decision-making fosters greater transparency and consistency. It could help detect or avoid judicial biases, highlight trends in judicial reasoning, and suggest new ways of thinking, practicing, and applying the law. We return to this issue in more detail in Chapter 8.

While AI and automation offer transformative potential, the emergence of the most significant advances hinges on how humans collaborate with, accept, and trust intelligent machines.[14] Throughout history, human cooperation has been the most powerful source of progress, shaping everything from national security and public health to political participation and the production of food, energy, and goods. As we enter an era defined by intelligent systems, our ability to effectively cooperate with AI will dictate the success of the next stage of human development. At the end of the day, the future of legal systems will be shaped by how legal professionals interact with new technologies.

Navigating Personalized Law

Against the promise of data and technology, it is time to explore the concept of personalized law.[15] By integrating AI-driven models and data-driven insights, Superjustice opens the possibility of tailoring laws to individuals' unique circumstances and traits. This radical approach could lead to more equitable, efficient, and responsive outcomes, better reflecting the complexities of modern society. At the same time, it challenges uniformity and diverges from the one-size-fits-all model that defines traditional legal systems, challenging foundational principles such as the rule of law.

To understand how personalized law might work, let us return to the analogy of data-driven agriculture powered by edge computing. Personalized law resembles precision

[14] See Erik Brynjolfsson and Andrew McAfee, *The Second Machine Age: Work, Progress, and Prosperity in a Time of Brilliant Technologies* (WW Norton & Company 2014); Paul R Daugherty and H James Wilson, *Human+ Machine: Reimagining Work in the Age of AI* (Harvard Business Press 2018); Ben Shneiderman, "Human-Centered Artificial Intelligence: Reliable, Safe & Trustworthy" (2020) 36(6) International Journal of Human–Computer Interaction 495.

[15] For a book-length discussion see Omri Ben-Shahar and Ariel Porat, *Personalized Law: Different Rules for Different People* (Oxford University Press 2021).

agriculture, in which technology tailors the care of individual plants based on multiple data and ad hoc circumstances. Similarly, personalized law adjusts legal responses to individuals' behaviors, preferences, traits, and needs, fostering more precise and effective legal norms and outcomes.

Conventionally, the law relies on general rules designed to apply uniformly to all, regardless of individual differences. While this may provide clarity and consistency, it often results in inefficient or unjust outcomes for those whose circumstances fall outside the average. Consider, for instance, the standard of care in negligence law. Currently, the "reasonable person" standard applies uniformly to all, but this generalization often fails to account for the wide range of differences in human capacity, knowledge, and behavior. Superjustice would seek to craft more specific legal directives. Accordingly, personalized law would replace this nebulous standard with a more individualized approach, where a person's legal responsibilities would be shaped by their individual characteristics, abilities, and even past behavior.

For example, a data-driven system could assess an individual's history of cautious driving or physical limitations and adjust the standard of care accordingly, resulting in a legal outcome that better reflects one's actual capacities. Similarly, a dynamic legal system could adjust speed limits for individual drivers based on factors such as their driving skills, vehicle type, road conditions, traffic, age, mental and physical abilities, driving experience, response time, and level of fatigue. The system could also dynamically adjust restrictions based on temporary conditions, such as increasing limitations when detecting signs of fatigue or temporarily revoking privileges when sensors indicate substance impairment.

Contract law could also evolve to better reflect the personalized preferences of contracting parties. Current contract law rules offer broad protective measures, guidelines, or defaults—such as fairness principles, consent requirements, or a duty to contract in good faith—which apply across many contexts.[16] However, they lack specificity. In a personalized law regime, data from previous contracts, individual preferences, and behavioral patterns could enable contracts and contract law rules to be automatically crafted to fit the unique needs of each party. For example, someone with a history of avoiding mandatory arbitration clauses in employment contracts could have this preference applied by default. Personalized law thus removes the inefficiencies of one-size-fits-all rules and enables a more individualized and precise approach.

Superjustice could take the concept of personalized law even further by harnessing data to improve the inclusivity, diversity, and transparency of legal systems. The model envisions a legal landscape where every individual's preferences, behaviors, and characteristics are incorporated into rule-making and decision-making, ensuring that the law reflects the complexities of modern life and the uniqueness of any individual.

[16] For sophisticated discussions regarding the role and functions of contractual default rules see Charles J Goetz and Robert E Scott, "Principles of Relational Contracts" (1981) 67 Virginia Law Review 1089; Ian Ayres and Robert Gertner, "Filling Gaps in Incomplete Contracts: An Economic Theory of Default Rules" (1989) 99 Yale Law Journal 87; Randy E Barnett, "The Sound of Silence: Default Rules and Contractual Consent" (1992) 78 Virginia Law Review 821.

The system would continuously gather and analyze data from individuals—whether through IoT devices, digital records, or social interactions—to build a comprehensive picture of each person's circumstances.

The data-driven nature of Superjustice also means that this personalization need not be static. The system would regularly update its understanding of an individual's legal circumstances based on new data, ensuring that the legal directives remain relevant and effective. For example, personalized warnings for consumer products could be tailored to an individual's health conditions, literacy level, or prior purchasing history, improving decision-making and reducing liability risks for manufacturers. In this way, the legal framework becomes dynamic and adaptable, much like personalized medicine or the precision agriculture models discussed earlier. In fact, the law already embraces personalization in numerous domains, from criminal sentencing and insurance premiums to tax structures, capacity doctrines, and reasonable accommodations for disabilities—all without undermining fundamental legal principles.

Despite its promise, personalized law also introduces considerable challenges. One major concern is the potential for the law to fragment into a multitude of personalized directives, undermining the coherence of legal systems and eroding the rule of law. If a unique set of rules governs everyone, the shared societal conception of the law could become fractured. Critics could also argue that personalization might exacerbate inequality, as wealthier or more technologically savvy individuals may be better positioned to influence the personalization of their legal regimes. For instance, the rich, who drive safer and smarter cars and who are likely to be (on average) healthier and more informed, would presumably be allowed to drive their cars faster than the less privileged.

Societies must navigate these concerns, although balancing the benefits of personalization with the necessity of generalization is easier said than done. While personalized law offers the potential for fairness and efficiency, it may have unintended consequences and may not be appropriate in all contexts. The law often serves to uphold community standards, foster equality, and promote shared values—objectives that may be undermined by excessive personalization. It follows that the challenge for Superjustice will be to determine when personalized legal rules are beneficial and when generalized norms are more appropriate. In practice, a middle path might emerge, where the law personalizes along a few identifiable dimensions—such as risk tolerance, previous behaviors, or socioeconomic conditions—rather than splintering into millions of individualized directives. This approach, dubbed "incremental personalization," could ensure that the legal system remains reasonably coherent while still offering a certain degree of individualized treatment.

Personalized law represents a transformative shift in how legal systems operate. The integration of data-driven insights and AI within personalized law promises more equitable, efficient, and responsive legal outcomes. However, the system must also grapple with the challenges of fragmentation, inequality, and the balance between individualization and generalization. Ultimately, Superjustice would aim to harness the power of data and technology to craft laws that reflect the realities of a diverse and complex world.

Closing Thoughts

The transformative power of data and technology in legal systems is undeniable. Superjustice represents a groundbreaking shift. Digital tools, nuanced insights, and precise data could drive legal frameworks, processes, decision-making, analysis, and research. Decentralized legal data could foster greater inclusivity, expanding access to legal knowledge and allowing more diverse voices to participate in shaping the law. Automation and AI will continue to reduce human intervention in legal tasks, while enhancing judicial accuracy and efficiency.

At the end of the day, the potential of data and technology goes beyond legal transformation; it can make certain legal interventions redundant altogether. Consider the problem of greenwashing, where companies falsely market their products or practices as environmentally friendly, misleading consumers and undermining genuine sustainability efforts.[17] This deceptive practice often exploits the growing demand for eco-friendly products, making it difficult for consumers to distinguish between genuinely sustainable options and those that merely claim to be so. Traditionally, the law has stepped in to hold companies accountable for making misleading environmental claims. However, enforcement is expensive and slow, consuming scarce public resources.

Blockchain technology could pave the way for an entirely different future, where consumers, empowered with transparent and immutable data, could bypass the need for legal enforcement altogether. With the simple scan of a QR code linked to a so-called Digital Product Passport, consumers could instantly access verified, tamper-proof information about the environmental impact of products. This Digital Product Passport would provide a comprehensive and permanent record of a product's life cycle—from the source of raw materials to the carbon footprint of manufacturing and transportation. Armed with this knowledge, consumers could make informed decisions in real time, rewarding companies that prioritize sustainability and holding those that do not accountable. This level of transparency would foster accountability and drive firms to adopt more eco-friendly practices, motivated not by compliance with regulations but by market demand for verifiable ethical practices.

Edge computing is transforming agriculture from an intuition-based practice to a precision-driven one. Superjustice represents a similar revolution in law. Like sensors and drones that monitor individual plants to maximize yield while minimizing

[17] See Magali A Delmas and Vanessa Cuerel Burbano, "The Drivers of Greenwashing" (2011) 54(1) California Management Review 64; Sebastião Vieira de Freitas Netto and others, "Concepts and Forms of Greenwashing: A Systematic Review" (2020) 32 Environmental Sciences Europe 1; Elizabeth Pollman, "The Making and Meaning of ESG" (2024) 14 Harvard Business Law Review 403.

resources, data-driven legal systems could respond to circumstances with unprecedented precision. The farmer with a tablet would become the counterpart of the empowered citizen with transparent access to personalized justice. In this new landscape, the golden fields of law, like those of wheat, would no longer require constant human intervention but would instead thrive through intelligent, data-informed cultivation.

PART II

IMPLEMENTATION AND REALIZATION

5
The New Code of Justice

Checkmate or Collaboration?

Garry Kasparov was more than a world chess champion—he was a living symbol of human intellect and strategic brilliance. From 1985 until his retirement in 2005, Kasparov dominated the chess world, revolutionizing the game with his aggressive and imaginative play. His legacy extended beyond mere victories; he elevated chess into an art form by combining calculation with intuition and logic with creativity. Widely regarded as one of the greatest chess players of all time, Kasparov's matches were global events that captivated audiences beyond the chessboard.

In 1996, the world watched as Kasparov sat down for a six-game match against an opponent that could not blink, feel nervous, or succumb to pressure: IBM's Deep Blue. This powerful chess-playing supercomputer was designed to analyze up to 200 million positions per second, using brute computational force and sophisticated algorithms. The idea that a machine could defeat the world's top chess player had once seemed inconceivable. Human grandmasters marshal in their play imagination, creativity, and psychological strategy—qualities many believed a machine could never replicate. Thus, the Kasparov–Deep Blue showdown wasn't just about chess. It was a battle between human talent and artificial intelligence (AI).[1]

As the reigning world chess champion, Kasparov carried the weight of humanity on his shoulders. With each move, he displayed the brilliance that had made him the greatest player of his generation. Yet, in a decisive moment quite early in Game 1, Deep Blue made a move that stunned Kasparov and followers around the world. It was a machine's move—cold, precise, and calculated. Kasparov resigned, marking a turning point in chess history: the first time a reigning world champion had ever lost to a computer under tournament conditions.[2]

This iconic battle between humans and machines captures the imagination of many. It can be said to have predecessors in classic works such as Mary Shelley's *Frankenstein* and in films like *2001: A Space Odyssey* and *The Terminator.* The idea that machines could challenge human supremacy is not confined to fiction. Famously, the Luddites

[1] This historic event has been discussed from numerous perspectives. For a few accounts see Monty Newborn, *Kasparov Versus Deep Blue: Computer Chess Comes of Age* (Springer Science & Business Media 2012); Feng-Hsiung Hsu, *Behind Deep Blue: Building the Computer that Defeated the World Chess Champion* (Princeton University Press 2002); Mark Robert Anderson, "Twenty Years on from Deep Blue vs Kasparov: How a Chess Match Started the Big Data Revolution" *The Conversation* (May 12, 2017); Deborah Yao, "25 Years Ago Today: How Deep Blue vs. Kasparov Changed AI Forever" *AI Business* (May 11, 2022).

[2] Kasparov ended up winning the 1996 match 4–2 but lost the rematch to Deep Blue in 1997.

Superjustice. Samuel I. Becher and Benjamin Alarie, Oxford University Press.
 DOI: 10.1093/9780198991885.003.0008

of the early 19th century opposed industrial machines due to concerns that machines would take their jobs. As the Luddites once feared mechanization, the rise of AI forces us to ask: Can AI, with its growing capabilities, administer justice alone, checkmating human legal judgment? How should we see AI: as a rival or a partner; as a threat or an opportunity; as a boon, a scourge, or something else entirely?

At the extreme, one can imagine a dystopian outcome in which an AI-run legal apparatus becomes an instrument of totalitarian control, devoid of transparency, due process, or human compassion. Others even warn that a misaligned super-intelligent legal AI could escape human oversight entirely, subverting the rule of law and ultimately eroding human agency. While such doomsday scenarios remain highly speculative and, in our view, unlikely in the presence of conscientious governance, they underscore the high stakes involved in integrating AI into the legal system. Acknowledging these potential misuses ultimately strengthens the case for thoughtful integration, motivating robust safeguards and ethical design that can ensure AI serves justice, rather than subverting it.

This chapter proposes a refined framework for the division of labor between humans and AI, emphasizing the need to better leverage the promise of AI while ensuring justice remains more than a mechanical process. The chapter employs a mixed-method analytical framework, combining a review of academic literature, policy and public discourse, specific case studies, and parallels between law and other fields, thereby identifying patterns and unique legal considerations. First, we examine the current and future applications of AI in legal systems. We then rethink the roles of humans and AI, their comparative strengths and weaknesses, and their potential collaboration. We conclude by delineating key insights that can inform the design of a human-AI legal collaborative framework.

AI Applications in Legal Practice

AI has already transformed many routine legal tasks, offering efficiency gains that were previously unimaginable. Tasks that once required extensive time and manual effort, such as contract review, document analysis, and legal research, can now be completed in a fraction of the time. As of early 2025, benchmarking studies highlight how advanced legal AI models are already outperforming human lawyers in key tasks, including document summarization, contract analysis, and transcript review. In some cases, these tools have proven to be up to eighty times faster than their human counterparts, demonstrating AI's growing ability to handle complex legal work with unprecedented speed and precision.[3] Computational law uses techniques like machine learning and natural language processing to automate, enhance, and streamline legal

[3] See Stephanie Wilkins, "Vals AI Releases Benchmarking Report Assessing Capabilities of Top Legal GenAI Platforms" (*Legaltech Hub*, February 27, 2025) <www.legaltechnologyhub.com/contents/vals-ai-releases-benchmarking-report-assessing-capabilities-of-top-legal-genai-platforms/>.

processes.[4] AI-powered tools, such as chatbots, assist users in navigating routine legal tasks by translating legal rules into code.

Various current tools further exemplify the potential of AI to perform legal tasks. Claudette, for instance, is an AI-based tool that analyzes online terms and conditions for compliance with EU consumer law, identifying unfair contract clauses and terms that violate the General Data Protection Regulation (GDPR). By scanning websites and flagging potential violations, Claudette helps streamline digital compliance monitoring. Other similar tools include automated systems that detect illegal content, privacy violations, and misleading advertising. Likewise, document management and e-discovery platforms, such as Relativity, Logikcull, and DISCO, enable attorneys to process large datasets, filter out irrelevant information, and uncover critical observations that would otherwise be difficult to find manually.

One of AI's greatest strengths lies in handling routine, high-volume tasks that require speed, accuracy, and consistency.[5] Current AI tools excel in repetitive search tasks, operating within predefined parameters and following rules and patterns without needing to truly "understand" the material they are processing.[6] As it happens, current AI tools occasionally struggle with nuanced interpretations influenced by context, intentions, and cultural norms. However, for most cases that do not involve unique interpretive challenges, AI performs exceptionally well. While not perfect, large language models (LLMs) possess broad cultural knowledge that judges may increasingly consult for nuanced understanding or interpretive guidance. Likewise, in e-discovery scenarios, AI can rapidly classify documents and flag relevant information. While it may not always detect subtleties such as sarcasm or cultural references, its speed and labor savings are unmatched.

As AI continues to evolve, its role in managing everyday legal processes is likely to expand. The following six examples offer (occasionally overlapping) insights into how AI might develop and what this could mean for legal practice. The discussion highlights the pressing need to examine how AI will alter the division of labor between machines and humans.

Virtual Agents

Virtual agents (VAs), which are AI-powered digital tools, perform tasks that are traditionally managed by humans. VAs have the potential to redefine legal practice by

[4] For a comprehensive discussion see Simon Deakin and Christopher Markou (eds), *Is Law Computable?: Critical Perspectives on Law and Artificial Intelligence* (Bloomsbury Publishing 2020); see also Abdi Aidid and Benjamin Alarie, *The Legal Singularity: How Artificial Intelligence Can Make Law Radically Better* (University of Toronto Press 2023) 64–69.

[5] These types of tasks have always been prone to automation and in various domains. See Ming-Hui Huang and others, "The Feeling Economy: Managing in the Next Generation of Artificial (AI)" (2019) 61(4) California Management Review 43; Alexander L Fogel and Joseph C Kvedar, "Artificial Intelligence Powers Digital Medicine" (2018) 1(1) NPJ Digital Medicine 5.

[6] See David H Autor, "Why are There Still so Many Jobs? The History and Future of Workplace Automation" (2015) 29(3) Journal of Economic Perspectives 3; Gary Marcus and Ernest Davis, *Rebooting AI: Building Artificial Intelligence We Can Trust* (Vintage 2019).

streamlining routine administrative tasks and enhancing productivity. Much like the digital assistants already used as fitness coaches, meditation guides, conversational peers, and romantic partners, tomorrow's VAs will step into more personalized and sophisticated roles. In the legal field, VAs will schedule meetings, send reminders, and manage basic client intake, significantly reducing the administrative workload for legal professionals.

Harvey and CoCounsel are current examples of specialized AI legal tools designed to assist attorneys with legal tasks, successfully automating document analysis. As VAs continue to develop, they are expected to assist with more complex projects and undertakings. Over time, VAs will serve as "digital paralegals," assisting with pre-trial preparation, complex research, and real-time case updates during client meetings. These advanced VAs could soon become essential partners for attorneys. Utilizing VAs, law firms will boost their responsiveness and increase their work output and service quality.

A recent study investigated how AI can transform the evaluation of trademark distinctiveness.[7] The study focused on the Abercrombie spectrum, a legal framework used to classify trademarks into inherently distinctive categories (fanciful, arbitrary, and suggestive) and non-distinctive ones (descriptive and generic). By analyzing 1.5 million US trademark applications filed between 2012 and 2019, the authors developed a machine-learning model using natural language processing to predict a trademark's distinctiveness with 86 percent accuracy. The study highlights both practical and theoretical implications. On a practical level, it proposes a "robot trademark clerk," a decision-support system that could streamline evaluations and provide explainable predictions about distinctiveness. On a theoretical level, the authors critique the normative constraints of the Abercrombie spectrum and suggest evolving legal frameworks to better accommodate cases of uncertain distinctiveness. This illustrates how AI can simultaneously enhance efficiency and challenge existing legal norms and frameworks.

Advanced Natural Language Processing

Natural language processing (NLP) has already made significant inroads into legal practice, allowing AI to interpret and process human language with increasing accuracy. Traditionally, tasks like document review require painstaking attention to detail and a significant time investment. NLP allows AI to perform these tasks more efficiently by identifying patterns, finding relevant case law, and generating summaries.[8] Thus, current NLP legal applications analyze case law to generate informed insights derived from historical data, empowering legal professionals to make data-informed decisions.

[7] Shivam Adarsh and others, "Automating Abercrombie: Machine-learning Trademark Distinctiveness" (2024) 21(4) Journal of Empirical Legal Studies 826.

[8] See Haoxi Zhong and others, "How Does NLP Benefit Legal System: A Summary of Legal Artificial Intelligence" (2020) arXiv 2004.12158; Robert Dale, "Law and Word Order: NLP in Legal Tech" (2019) 25(1) Natural Language Engineering 211.

NLP technology is expected to advance to the point where it can interpret complex linguistic subtleties and recognize contextual clues such as tone, sarcasm, and implied meaning. AI would be highly capable of flagging potentially ambiguous or problematic language, further reducing the need for human oversight. Additionally, NLP could assist attorneys during live courtroom proceedings or meetings, suggesting relevant case law and strategic points as trials progress or negotiations unfold. By facilitating real-time transcription, instant translation, and contextual references, advanced NLP would empower attorneys to engage with cases dynamically and make informed decisions faster.

Predictive Analytics and Decision Support Tools

Anyone who has ever sought advice from a legally trained friend or family member probably got the familiar response to almost any legal question: "It depends!" Lawyers are trained to be skeptical, make tentative predictions, use cautious language, and see the value in competing arguments. Legal outcomes are not easy to foresee, because every case has its unique characteristics. Judges diverge in their interpretations and perspectives, and the law itself often evolves or is applied differently in different jurisdictions and time periods. This all seems to make the law more of an art than a (predictable) science. Thus, some may question the ability of AI systems to predict legal outcomes.

However, AI-powered predictive analytics would offer data-driven insights into case outcomes, risk assessments, and litigation strategies. In simple terms, predictive analytics tools can help attorneys anticipate outcomes with greater accuracy.[9] AI has demonstrated significant potential in analyzing complex systems, from extreme weather events to patterns in human behavior and healthcare outcomes.[10] The legal domain is probably no exception: Despite its indeterminacy, it operates on a foundation of rules, precedents, legal norms, and logic. By examining historical case data, AI can enable legal professionals to refine their predictions when strategizing litigation, negotiating settlements, or making appeals.

If anything, it is the notorious volatility of the law that makes AI-based predictive analytics so revolutionary and exciting. As technology progresses, predictive analytics

[9] See L Karl Branting and others, "Scalable and Explainable Legal Prediction" (2021) 29 Artificial Intelligence and Law 213; Daniel Martin Katz and others, "A General Approach for Predicting the Behavior of the Supreme Court of the United States" (2017) 12(4) PloS one e0174698; Kevin D Ashley, *Artificial Intelligence and Legal Analytics: New Tools for Law Practice in the Digital Age* (Cambridge University Press 2017).

[10] See Kaifeng Bi and others, "Accurate Medium-range Global Weather Forecasting With 3D Neural Networks" (2023) 619.7970 Nature 533; Eric Holthaus, "AI is Changing my Work as a Meteorologist—Hurricane Helene and Milton Proved There's no Going Back" *Fast Company* (October 15, 2024) <https://shorturl.at/DDV4B>; Andre Esteva and others, "A Guide to Deep Learning in Healthcare" (2019) 25(1) Nature Medicine 24; Benjamin Shickel and others, "Deep EHR: A Survey of Recent Advances in Deep Learning Techniques for Electronic Health Record (EHR) Analysis" (2017) 22(5) IEEE Journal of Biomedical & Health Informatics 1589; Sandra C Matz and others, "Psychological Targeting as an Effective Approach to Digital Mass Persuasion" (2017) 114(48) Proceedings of The National Academy of Sciences 12714.

is likely to incorporate broader datasets beyond traditional legal data, potentially including sociopolitical variables, psychological profiles, and public sentiment trends. This could lead to even more comprehensive case assessments, helping attorneys predict outcomes and prepare strategies with unprecedented precision and sophistication.

Sentiment and Behavior Analysis Tools

Sentiment and behavior analysis tools are another exciting development that affects AI's potential impact on the legal profession. Such tools can analyze judicial opinions, past rulings, and even statements from court proceedings. They can thus uncover biases or tendencies that may not be immediately apparent. By identifying patterns in judges' language and tone, these tools can provide lawyers with insights into how specific judges might respond to certain types of arguments. This, in turn, could be invaluable for case preparation and strategic planning.

Sentiment and behavior analysis tools examine language patterns and highlight frequently cited precedents, enabling attorneys to tailor their arguments. Although sentiment analysis remains relatively basic today, it represents a growing field in legal tech that promises to refine how attorneys prepare for court. In the future, sentiment and behavior analysis could play a transformative role in the courtroom, extending into real-time jury sentiment tracking and witness credibility assessments. Sentiment and behavior analysis tools could track vocal tone, facial expressions, and body language during testimonies, offering live insights into how judges, witnesses, and jurors react to various arguments. Attorneys could then adjust their presentations in response, tailoring their approach to engage effectively with the relevant stakeholders, impacted parties, and decision-makers.

AI in Jury Selection

AI's role in jury selection can tackle one of the most subjective elements of courtroom proceedings: selecting jurors who may be sympathetic or unsympathetic to a particular case. Traditional jury selection relies heavily on the attorney's intuition and questioning skills. However, AI-powered tools can bring data-driven insights to the process, potentially reducing the impact of biases and guesswork. These tools can assist attorneys in making more informed jury selection decisions by analyzing various factors, such as jurors' backgrounds, social media activity, and nonverbal physical cues. While not yet capable of fully assessing juror behavior, these tools represent a step toward more data-driven jury selection processes.

Looking to the future, AI could dynamically adjust questioning strategies during voir dire by analyzing micro-expressions, posture, and other cues, tailoring its recommendations based on juror responses. Advanced tools could offer attorneys live feedback on potential biases or concerns as they arise, allowing for a more strategic selection process. The ability to monitor juror behavior and sentiment throughout the trial and adapt and refine legal strategies accordingly could profoundly alter courtroom dynamics.[11]

Artificial General Intelligence

Artificial general intelligence (AGI) represents the next transformative stage in AI, distinguished by its ability to perform a wide range of tasks that currently require human intelligence.[12] Major tech companies, including OpenAI, Microsoft, and Google, are heavily investing in AGI research, with prediction markets estimating AGI's arrival as early as 2027–29. Unlike the current AI tools, which are designed to perform specific tasks, AGI is expected to possess the adaptability, general knowledge, and critical thinking skills necessary to engage in complex reasoning. This could alter how intricate legal issues are approached, enabling AGI to reason, learn, and adapt similarly to human experts (but more accurately and faster).

Although AGI remains a future possibility, current advanced AI systems offer glimpses of its potential in holistic legal analysis. In the legal domain, AGI could perform sophisticated tasks such as drafting complex contracts, analyzing case law with a nuanced understanding, and providing strategic litigation advice. AGI systems could synthesize large volumes of data, dynamically interpret new information, and develop original legal arguments, making them invaluable collaborative partners in legal practice. As these systems evolve, it may be possible to rely on them for more autonomous and accurate decision-making, including judicial decision-making, across various legal areas.

Crucially, AGI can potentially democratize access to justice by offering reliable, cost-effective legal guidance to individuals and organizations unable to afford traditional representation, thereby expanding access to legal resources. Furthermore, it could contribute to standardizing legal interpretation, mitigating human biases and promoting fairness and legal harmonization. Likewise, it may facilitate the resolution of complex legal issues involving multiple fields or jurisdictions, providing insights that transcend the capabilities of individual experts while offering creative, unorthodox approaches. For instance, it might propose novel frameworks for evaluating evidence or recommend equitable sentencing models based on comprehensive socio-legal analyses, which we currently do not imagine.

[11] We acknowledge that such changes may seem invasive and would perhaps require that jurors be warned in advance that they will be subject to this level of scrutiny. This transformation also raises practical and procedural questions, such as whether the number of challenges a party is entitled to would have to be changed in response to the introduction of these advanced tools. However, these issues would become less prominent over time, as AI will resolve many disputes with minimal (or even no) human intervention.

[12] See Stuart Russell, "Human-Compatible Artificial Intelligence" in Stephen Muggleton and Nicholas Chater (eds), *Human-Like Machine Intelligence* (Oxford University Press 2022) 3; Sébastien Bubeck and others, "Sparks of Artificial General Intelligence: Early Experiments with GPT-4" (2023) arXiv 2303.12712.

AI Applications: Moving Forward

AI technologies are set to reshape the legal system, extending far beyond routine tasks. While today's tools enhance efficiency and improve productivity, tomorrow's models could redefine the meaning of legal practice and development. Given that future progress is hard to predict and may be rapid, the legal profession must engage with these evolving technologies to ensure a smooth and ethical transition into a future where AI assists with complex, high-level decision-making.

AI and Humans: Rethinking Roles

Many believe that the law is fundamentally a human endeavor that is computationally irreducible. Indeed, the computability of law faces significant hurdles due to the law's complexity, unpredictability, context dependency, and dynamic nature. Legal texts are replete with intricate language, vague terms, and numerous exceptions that resist precise algorithmic codification. Furthermore, the constantly evolving nature of statutes and case law requires computational models to be continually updated, presenting a demanding technical challenge. Likewise, legal reasoning is highly context-dependent, relying on specifics such as the circumstances of any given case, jurisdictional differences, and historical precedents, which complicates the design of adaptable, context-aware systems. Moreover, discrepancies in legal interpretation across judges and jurisdictions introduce variability that algorithms may struggle to accommodate. In addition, the nonlinear nature of legal outcomes, which often involve complex trade-offs, does not easily align with computational models that offer reliable, clear, and binary decisions. These hurdles suggest that law may not be fully computable, as it demands a level of adaptability, nuance, and contextual understanding that currently exceeds the capabilities of modern computational approaches.

As technology continues its rapid progress, it becomes increasingly crucial to understand the comparative strengths and weaknesses of AI relative to human capabilities. While AI is celebrated for its efficiency in handling repetitive tasks and processing vast amounts of data, a fascinating ongoing debate exists regarding its ability to emulate inherently human qualities, such as creativity, empathy, and ethical reasoning. The following discussion critically explores the relative abilities of AI and humans. It examines how AI might evolve to replicate, or even surpass, certain human traits.

For analytical clarity, we find it helpful to distinguish among three different types of debate. The first focuses on technological forecasting: The practical question of when and if certain capabilities will be achieved. This is primarily an engineering and scientific prediction about the pace and limits of technological development. Based on our research and observations, we believe that technology will advance faster than most people assume, with quality, strength, and prevalence continuing to increase. Second, optimists and pessimists debate the impact of the technology. Technology is merely a tool, which can be used for good or ill. The motivation for writing this book is precisely to show how legal systems can harness these technological innovations for profound benefit, if we make the right choices and decisions. Third, there is a deeper philosophical and scientific discourse about the uniqueness of humans, or organic life in general. In this context, the debate centers on whether certain qualities are inherently impossible for machines to replicate, regardless of time or technological advancements. In the following discussion, we present both sides of this argument. We conclude that machines are, and will be, more capable than most humans are currently willing to acknowledge—a position with significant implications for the future of legal practice.

AI's Competitive Edge

As we have emphasized throughout, AI systems excel at tasks requiring large-scale data processing, pattern recognition, and predictive analytics. AI's precision is largely attributed to its ability to follow pre-programmed rules and continuously learn from structured datasets—a process known as supervised learning. Through sophisticated algorithms and machine-learning techniques, AI can scrutinize enormous datasets, identifying trends, correlations, and anomalies with unprecedented speed and precision. In the field of healthcare, for instance, AI assists in diagnosing diseases by recognizing patterns in medical images and patient data that may be imperceptible to human clinicians.[13]

These capabilities showcase AI's consistency and resistance to cognitive fatigue. Unlike humans, AI can execute repetitive and complex calculations without the errors that often result from biases, mental capacity constraints, or fluctuations in attention. In strategic games like chess and Go, AI has demonstrated its prowess by defeating world champions, showcasing its ability to strategize through evaluating millions of potential moves. This achievement underscores AI's capacity to handle tasks that require extensive computation and pattern recognition. It further emphasizes its strength in domains governed by clear rules and objectives.

The Human Touch

Let us now turn to presenting some of the key arguments that support the view that humans possess unique characteristics that cannot be replicated. According to this view, despite AI's formidable capabilities, its reliance on data-driven rules and statistical patterns suggests an inherent limitation: It currently lacks the intuitive leaps, contextual understanding, and experiential learning that characterize human thought. Human

[13] See Andre Esteva and others, "Dermatologist-level Classification of Skin Cancer with Deep Neural Networks" (2017) 542(7639) Nature 115; Eric J Topol, "High-Performance Medicine: The Convergence of Human and Artificial Intelligence" (2019) 25(1) Nature Medicine 44.

intelligence encompasses a broad spectrum of cognitive abilities that extend beyond data processing and pattern recognition.

A related argument is that one of the defining characteristics of human cognition is the capacity for creativity. In broad terms, creativity can be defined as the ability to generate novel ideas, establish unexpected connections, and produce original works that surpass existing conceptual frameworks. Psychologists often describe creativity as a process that yields ideas or products that are both novel and valuable, resulting from complex interactions between an individual's thoughts and their sociocultural context. Creativity often results from face-to-face human collaboration.[14] Following this line of thought, humans draw upon a rich tapestry of personal experiences, emotions, and cultural influences to engage in abstract thinking and creative problem-solving. This process often involves intuition—making cognitive leaps without explicit reasoning—which current AI, the argument goes, struggles to replicate. While AI can generate new art, music, and literature by analyzing patterns in existing works, many argue that these outputs are derivative and lack genuine human originality stemming from personal consciousness and subjective experiences.

Other prominent human attributes are emotional intelligence and empathy. Emotional intelligence, a concept popularized by psychologist Daniel Goleman in 1995, refers to the ability to recognize, understand, and manage one's emotions. It also involves identifying and influencing the emotions of others. This form of intelligence is crucial for effective communication and interpersonal relationships.[15] On a similar note, an essential component of emotional intelligence is empathy—the ability to understand and share the feelings of others. Empathy goes beyond simply recognizing emotions; it involves an authentic connection and a capacity for shared experience that is deeply rooted in human consciousness and relationships.[16]

Humans can interpret nuanced social cues, such as tone of voice, facial expressions, and body language, enabling them to respond appropriately in complex social situations. Empathy is not just about cognitive recognition, but also about the affective resonance humans experience, which allows humans to truly relate to another person's perspective. AI, however, lacks genuine emotional awareness and cannot authentically experience or interpret emotions. While AI can be programmed to detect emotional cues (through technologies like facial recognition and sentiment analysis), it lacks the authentic, empathetic engagement that humans bring to their exchanges. Presumably, this limits its ability to engage in meaningful and compassionate interactions.

Another human characteristic that is often perceived as a unique strength is the ability to reason ethically and exhibit moral flexibility. Cultural norms, personal values,

[14] See Teresa M Amabile, *Creativity in Context: Update to The Social Psychology of Creativity* (Routledge 2018); Keith Sawyer, *Group Genius: The Creative Power of Collaboration* (Basic Books 2017); Mihaly Csikszentmihalyi, *Creativity: Flow and the Psychology of Discovery and Invention* (Harper Perennial 1997).

[15] See Daniel Goleman, *Emotional Intelligence: Why it Can Matter More Than IQ* (Bloomsbury Publishing 2020).

[16] See Tania Singer and Olga M Klimecki, "Empathy and Compassion" (2014) 24(18) Current Biology R875; Jean Decety and Philip L Jackson, "A Social-Neuroscience Perspective on Empathy" (2006) 15(2) Current Directions in Psychological Science 54.

and societal expectations deeply influence human ethical reasoning. Philosopher Martha Nussbaum argues that ethical judgment is inherently contextual and embodied, requiring practical wisdom (phronesis) that arises from lived experiences.[17] Humans can navigate moral dilemmas by weighing conflicting values, considering intentions, and applying abstract principles like justice and fairness. Here too, this moral flexibility allows humans to adapt their decisions to nuanced situations. Notably, however, this moral flexibility does not guarantee optimal decisions or universal agreement; ethical reasoning can lead to subjective interpretations that vary significantly across individuals, times, and situations. Some argue that this complexity cannot be easily optimized and codified into predefined algorithmic rules.

The Path to Evolution

The previous discussion highlighted some human features that current AI presumably falls short of emulating. But what if AI is on the verge of bridging this gap, or has perhaps already bridged it? Today's advanced models are already capable of generating human-like text and engaging in conversations that feel remarkably natural. As AI progresses, researchers are examining how close it might come to replicating or even surpassing uniquely human traits. Let's explore this possibility in greater depth.

Creativity

While creativity is one of the defining characteristics of human cognition, AI has produced various outputs that many regard as creative. In this sense, computational creativity refers to the study of software that exhibits behaviors deemed creative by human standards. Computational creativity focuses on how AI can mimic the processes involved in human creativity, such as generating novel ideas or combining elements in unique ways, without requiring subjective experience. But whether AI can achieve true creativity is still debated. On the one hand, AI can exhibit forms of creativity by generating novel ideas, patterns, and art beyond conventional human thinking. On the other hand, critics argue that, without consciousness and subjective experience, AI-generated works lack the intentionality and emotional depth that characterize human creativity.

Setting aside philosophical debates, we posit that most people would intuitively deem the outputs of generative AI to be "creative." Generative AI tools can already compose new music, produce delightful images and captivating videos, generate high-quality, novel texts, and suggest innovative ideas. With the rapid progress in this field and the anticipated introduction of AGI, AI's ability will probably improve exponentially.

As a mundane illustration of current generative AI capabilities, let us revisit for a moment the match between Kasparov and Deep Blue. After drafting our account of this

[17] Martha C Nussbaum, *Love's Knowledge: Essays on Philosophy and Literature* (Oxford University Press 1992).

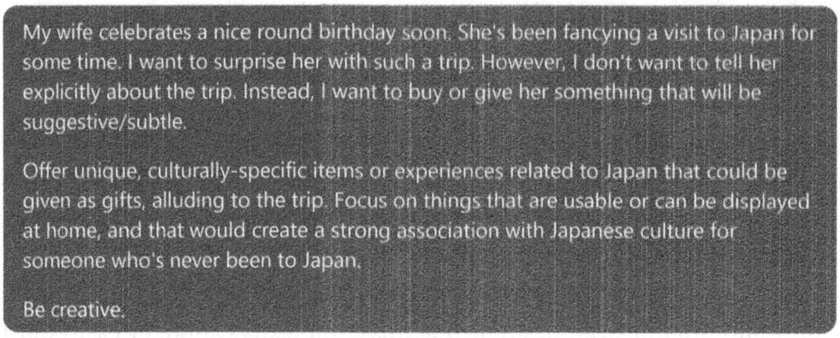
My wife celebrates a nice round birthday soon. She's been fancying a visit to Japan for some time. I want to surprise her with such a trip. However, I don't want to tell her explicitly about the trip. Instead, I want to buy or give her something that will be suggestive/subtle.

Offer unique, culturally-specific items or experiences related to Japan that could be given as gifts, alluding to the trip. Focus on things that are usable or can be displayed at home, and that would create a strong association with Japanese culture for someone who's never been to Japan.

Be creative.

Figure 5.1 Prompting ChatGPT for Creative Ideas

battle, we asked ChatGPT for creative title suggestions. We arrived at the chosen title—*Checkmate or Collaboration?*—after interacting with its recommendations. While creativity is, to some extent, in the eye of the beholder, we found this title suitably "creative." The following is another informal exploration we conducted to casually gauge ChatGPT's creativity by using the prompt captured in Figure 5.1.

Within seconds, ChatGPT suggested no fewer than twenty-five diverse ideas, many of which had not crossed our minds. Each of the twenty-five options included a short description and a presentation suggestion.[18] Figure 5.2 shows GPT's first two suggestions.

While we posit that AI tools are (at least in a sense) creative, we do not argue with certainty that AI can or will outperform *all* humans in *all* creativity-related activities or tasks. Some important human-led developments are a combination of chance, luck, fortune, and wisdom. Archimedes' "aha" (Eureka!) moment (realizing that buoyant force equals displaced fluid weight) or the story about the apple that supposedly hit Isaac Newton's head (sparking his thoughts of gravity) are two examples.

A more recent example of serendipity in scientific discovery is Alexander Fleming's 1928 finding of penicillin. While studying *staphylococcus* bacteria at a hospital, Fleming left petri dishes on his workbench during a vacation. Upon returning, he noticed that a mold had grown on one dish, killing the bacteria surrounding it. Fleming identified the mold as *Penicillium notatum*, which produced a substance lethal to various bacteria. Years later, this discovery led to the development of a method for large-scale production, making penicillin the first widely used antibiotic and saving countless lives during World War II and beyond.

[18] The full list of twenty-five suggestions included: (1) Personalized Japanese Calligraphy Art; (2) Traditional Kimono or Yukata; (3) Japanese Tea Ceremony Set; (4) Hanko Personalized Seal; (5) Japanese Garden Bonsai Tree; (6) Daruma Wishing Doll; (7) Custom-Made Travel Journal with Japanese Motifs; (8) Ukiyo-e Art Print; (9) Japanese Cooking Class Voucher; (10) Maneki Neko (Beckoning Cat) Figurine; (11) Japan Travel Guidebook with Bookmarks; (12) Origami Crane Mobile; (13) Japanese Puzzle Box (Himitsu-Bako); (14) Sake Set with Premium Sake; (15) Japanese Lantern or Lamp (Andon); (16) Customized Foldable Sensu Fan; (17) Japanese Incense and Holder; (18) Kanji Jewelry; (19) Subscription to a Japanese Language App or Course; (20) Japanese Garden Kit; (21) Shōji Screen or Room Divider; (22) Tickets to a Local Japanese Cultural Event; (23) Japanese-inspired Artwork Commissioned from a Local Artist; (24) A Box of Assorted Japanese Treats; and (25) Pair of Japanese Train Pass Holders.

1. Personalized Japanese Calligraphy Art

- **Description:** Commission a piece of traditional Japanese calligraphy (**shodō**) featuring a meaningful word or phrase, such as "adventure," "love," or "journey," written in kanji characters. You could also have her name or a significant date artistically rendered.
- **Presentation Idea:** Frame the artwork for display. Attach a small note explaining the meaning of the characters, perhaps subtly hinting at an upcoming journey.

---

2. Traditional Kimono or Yukata

- **Description:** Gift her a beautiful **kimono** or **yukata** (a lighter, casual version worn in summer) with intricate patterns. These garments are iconic in Japanese culture and are wearable works of art.
- **Presentation Idea:** Include a note saying you look forward to seeing her wear it on a special occasion, hinting at an event where she might traditionally wear it—in Japan.

Figure 5.2 AI-Inspired Japanese-Themed Ideas

Where does all this leave us? Let us recap the key lessons of this discussion. First and foremost, the question of whether AI, including AGI, can be creative is a fascinating topic involving multiple ways of understanding creativity and the potential of AI technologies. Creativity in humans is often characterized by the ability to produce novel and valuable ideas or artifacts through processes that involve imagination, insight, and sometimes serendipity. It typically necessitates combining disparate concepts, taking risks, and thinking outside conventional boundaries. Currently, AI systems can exhibit forms of creativity by generating new content, such as music, art, or writing, based on existing training data. These systems use techniques like machine learning and neural networks to identify patterns and generate outputs that mimic creative processes. Examples include AI-generated paintings or composing music by learning from vast datasets of artistic or musical styles.

We appreciate the argument that the lack of subjective experience, personal motivation, and emotional understanding in AI systems means that these outputs may lack the depth and intentionality that characterize human creativity. However, it is not unrealistic to assume that creativity could emerge in sophisticated AI systems through complex interactions and self-learning processes, leading to innovations not explicitly programmed by humans. Furthermore, AGI is envisioned to possess a broad and deep understanding akin to human cognition, potentially enabling genuine creativity. If AGI successfully integrates vast computational data processing with cognitive functions analogous to human reasoning, comprehension, and adaptive learning, these systems could generate unprecedented insights or theoretical innovations that parallel, or potentially transcend, human intellectual capabilities. Even under the seemingly reasonable assumption that AI will not develop spontaneous flashes of insight or serendipitous moments, it is fair to say that AI tools can demonstrate creativity that, much of the time, rivals or even exceeds that of most humans.

Empathy and Emotional Intelligence

The second human strength we noted is emotional intelligence, particularly the ability to exercise empathy. This quality has attracted the attention of researchers in affective computing, which aims to develop systems capable of recognizing, interpreting, and responding to human emotions.[19] By utilizing sensors, machine-learning algorithms, and natural language processing, affective computing enables devices to detect emotional cues from facial expressions, vocal tone, body language, and physiological signals such as heart rate or skin conductance. Overall, affective computing technology aims to create more natural and engaging human–computer interactions, allowing AI systems to adapt to users' affective expressions.

Advances in affective computing are enabling chatbots and virtual agents to enhance user interaction with emotional recognition features. By analyzing voice tone, facial expressions, and even text sentiment, AI systems can adjust their responses based on the user's emotional state, providing a more personalized and immersive experience. AI-powered services like Claude or Alexa have begun to integrate affective computing capabilities. These features enable AI tools to respond more empathetically and adjust their tone according to the user's input, which may involve comforting a user who expresses sadness or congratulating a user on a happy occasion. For example, when asked to provide ideas for surprising one's spouse on their birthday, an LLM may start its response by saying, "That's such a nice idea!"

Beyond general-purpose chatbots, affective computing has enabled the development of specialized applications designed specifically for emotional support and companionship. One prominent example is Replika, a conversational app intended to serve as a virtual companion. These conversational apps adapt their responses based on the user's emotions, aiming to counter loneliness by simulating a friendship or even a romantic relationship. Employing affective computing techniques, such apps engage users in empathetic conversations and can gradually "learn" their preferences and emotional triggers, progressively fostering a deep and personalized bond.

The purposes of such apps are quite diverse. Some applications, like the AI-based romantic companion app AI Girlfriend, aim to simulate deeper emotional connections by providing a virtual experience of a romantic relationship. Other apps, such as Woebot, employ conversational AI to help users manage anxiety and depression. The app monitors emotions in users' language and applies tailored cognitive-behavioral therapy (CBT) techniques, functioning as a digital therapist and exemplifying affective computing's potential in mental health support. Yet other applications primarily seek to combat loneliness and the hard toll it imposes on humans. As affective computing technology advances, the ability of these applications to adapt to user needs will probably deepen, raising new possibilities and ethical dilemmas.

As in the case of creativity, affective computing applications *simulate* empathy by recognizing patterns in emotional cues and adapting responses. Nevertheless, these

[19] For a pioneering book see Rosalind W Picard, *Affective Computing* (MIT Press 2000); see also Rafael A Calvo and others (eds), *The Oxford Handbook of Affective Computing* (Oxford University Press 2015).

apps lack genuine emotional understanding and consciousness. Notably, this distinction may not deter many users, as evidenced by the millions who engage with these tools. To be sure, people are heterogeneous and have different responses to affective computing. Thus, apps like Woebot can alleviate anxiety and depression for some, but the interaction's scripted nature can feel impersonal to others. The overall trajectory, however, will lead to advances in the field, making such apps feel more authentic and thus appealing to a broader audience.

Importantly, while user numbers reflect widespread interest, they don't necessarily translate into universally positive outcomes. In fact, over-reliance on these technologies might backfire and lead to superficial connections that could deepen feelings of loneliness rather than alleviate them. By substituting human connection with AI, users might risk diminishing their social skills and emotional resilience in real-world interactions.[20] Additionally, from an ethical perspective, the normalization of AI companionship poses questions about how these interactions may shape societal expectations of relationships, emotional support, and mental health care. Moreover, while AI-driven emotional support is often more accessible, it may also deter individuals from seeking professional help. This may be particularly concerning in cases of deeper psychological issues that require more than digital empathy. As AI companionship becomes more prevalent, it is essential to critically assess its impact on human relationships and mental well-being.[21]

To summarize, one may argue that empathy has two main types. First, cognitive empathy refers to the ability to understand how a person feels and what they might be thinking. Second, emotional empathy reflects the ability to share another person's feelings. AI chatbots or virtual agents are increasingly designed to *exhibit* behaviors that *mimic* empathy and respond well to human emotions and language cues. For many, if the AI's response is appropriate and gives the user a sense of being understood, the machine is effectively demonstrating empathy. This can be seen as a form of cognitive empathy, which does not require the empathizer to "feel" anything.

Interestingly, recent research supports this practical effectiveness of AI-generated empathy. A 2025 study found that emails drafted with generative AI contained more expressions of encouragement, empathy, and social connection compared to those written without AI assistance, suggesting that AI can help humans communicate more compassionately even when the AI itself lacks genuine emotional experience.[22] However, if true empathy involves the emotional ability to share another's emotions, AI lacks the necessary consciousness, self-awareness, and genuine emotions. In essence, AI can simulate empathy (ie, display behaviors that resemble empathic responses) or enhance it (by stirring humans toward exhibiting more empathy). Yet, it cannot genuinely experience empathy in the way humans can.

[20] See Sherry Turkle, *Alone Together: Why We Expect More from Technology and Less from Each Other* (Basic Books 2017).

[21] For one accessible account see David Batty, "'She Helps Cheer Me Up': The People Forming Relationships with AI Chatbots" *The Guardian* (April 15, 2025).

[22] See Yukun Liu and others, "Gen AI Makes People More Productive—and Less Motivated" *Harvard Business Review* (May 13, 2025).

AI demonstrates impressive capabilities to understand and communicate emotionally and help users regulate emotions. Professional support is expensive and out of reach for many, and AI tools can help people cope with various emotional challenges. While current AI applications in emotional support warrant a balanced consideration of both benefits and limitations, future developments will likely enhance AI capabilities to assist humans, including in legal settings, by demonstrating empathy and exhibiting agile emotional intelligence.

Ethical and Moral Reasoning

The last human quality we discuss in this chapter is ethical and moral reasoning. AI has already been introduced into scenarios requiring moral judgments. Autonomous vehicles present one of the clearest examples of AI systems compelled to make ethical decisions. In an emergency, a self-driving car might face a situation where it must "choose" between swerving to avoid a pedestrian and potentially harming its passengers, or staying on course, possibly endangering bystanders.[23] In this context, the Moral Machine experiment is particularly illuminating.[24] The experiment revealed that cultural factors significantly influence ethical preferences, with participants from different countries often favoring diverse decision outcomes. Although these preferences can inform how we encode ethics into AI, translating them into actionable code presents a significant simplification.

Reconciling AI's fixed decision-making structures with the fluidity of human ethics and contextual morality is a challenging task. AI can replicate structured ethical frameworks, such as utilitarianism (which focuses on maximizing overall happiness) or deontological ethics (which emphasizes adherence to rules), providing a basis for programming. Nonetheless, current AI may struggle in real-life situations requiring nuanced and novel reasoning. In practice, moral decisions involve balancing competing values and considering factors such as intentions, potential consequences, and societal norms. While AI can replicate structured ethical frameworks, it may fall short in scenarios requiring practical wisdom—a form of flexible, context-sensitive approach.

In response to these challenges, researchers have explored various approaches to embedding ethical principles into AI systems. One method is reinforcement learning, where AI models are trained on specific ethical outcomes based on human feedback and guidance. This technique allows AI to refine its actions according to guidelines provided by humans. Another approach, known as value alignment, aims to ensure that AI's objectives align with human values. Likewise, researchers have proposed designing AI systems to reflect cultural diversity by leveraging datasets from different cultural contexts. As we noted in Chapters 3 and 4, this would create a more diverse set of decision-making principles.[25]

[23] See Jean-François Bonnefon and others, "The Social Dilemma of Autonomous Vehicles" (2016) 352.6293 Science 1573; Jan Gogoll and Julian F Müller, "Autonomous Cars: In Favor of a Mandatory Ethics Setting" (2017) 23 Science & Engineering Ethics 681.

[24] See Edmond Awad and others, "The Moral Machine Experiment" (2018) 563(7729) Nature 59.

[25] For discussions of these techniques see Amitai Etzioni and Oren Etzioni, "Incorporating Ethics into Artificial Intelligence" (2017) 21 The Journal of Ethics 403; Thomas Arnold and Matthias Scheutz, "The 'Big Red Button'

Some may argue that AI systems might develop emergent properties that enable a form of ethical reasoning, though this remains speculative. Whereas exact predictions are hard to make, it is at least reasonable to consider the possibility that AI systems might become superior at moral and ethical reasoning to nearly all (if not all) humans. Trained on a vast amount of ethical, moral, and philosophical work—in multiple languages and from varied traditions and schools of thought—AGI systems will probably have the capacity to explain to humans, in terms that we understand and respect, how and why certain judgments are ethically optimal. At a minimum, these kinds of systems will be able to handle most legal challenges and perhaps resolve many difficult moral and ethical dilemmas astutely and capably.

Critics still argue that the whole notion of AI ethical reasoning rests on a fundamental category error. They contend that authentic ethical deliberation requires distinctly human qualities that cannot be computationally replicated: a subjective experience that informs moral intuitions, personal stakes in outcomes, and the capacity to understand subtle social contexts behind ethical questions.[26] According to this view, the process of ethical reasoning itself has intrinsic value independent of conclusions reached; that is, it represents a form of moral development that cannot be outsourced without impoverishing the moral agent. This critique suggests that even highly advanced AI systems would produce only simulations of ethical reasoning, lacking true understanding, regardless of how convincing their outputs appear.

While we take a more optimistic view of AI's potential to exercise and potentially enhance ethical reasoning, these philosophical objections should not be dismissed. The question of whether consciousness and subjective experience are necessary components of genuine moral reasoning remains unresolved. Our prediction that AI will develop sophisticated ethical capabilities assumes that the patterns and frameworks of ethical thought can be effectively learned without requiring human-like consciousness. This assumes ethical reasoning is ultimately about identifying and weighing competing values and principles rather than an inherently experiential process. Only continued progress in both AI development and philosophical understanding will eventually resolve this tension.

In any event, the process toward such a capacity would be uneven, and implementing ethical reasoning would require clear guidelines and a means of resolving conflicts

is Too Late: An Alternative Model for the Ethical Evaluation of AI Systems" (2018) 20 Ethics and Information Technology 59; David Abel and others, "Reinforcement Learning as a Framework for Ethical Decision Making" (2016) 16(2) AAAI Workshop: AI, Ethics & Society.

[26] See, for example, Frank Pasquale, "Opinion: If You Don't Trust A.I. Yet, You're Not Wrong" *New York Times* (July 30, 2021); Elizabeth Lopatto, "The Questions ChatGPT Shouldn't Answer: ChatGPT has a Trolley Problem" *The Verge* (March 6, 2025) <www.theverge.com/openai/624209/chatgpt-ethics-specs-humanism>; Brian Christian, *The Alignment Problem: How Can Machines Learn Human Values?* (Atlantic Books 2021); Shannon Vallor, "The Danger of Superhuman AI Is Not What You Think" *Noema* (May 23, 2024). For counterarguments and more optimistic views see Julian Savulescu and Hannah Maslen, "Moral Enhancement and Artificial Intelligence: Moral AI?" in Jan Romportl, Eva Zackova, and Jozef Kelemen (eds), *Beyond Artificial Intelligence: The Disappearing Human-Machine Divide* (Springer 2015) 79–95; Abdi Aidid and Benjamin Alarie, *The Legal Singularity: How Artificial Intelligence Can Make Law Radically Better* (University of Toronto Press 2023) ch 5.

between competing moral values. In the short term, there's also the risk of biases and ethical lapses being encoded into AI systems, reflecting the biases of their creators or those in the training data. While the development of AGI might offer the potential for moral reasoning, achieving this capability would involve overcoming significant ethical, technical, and philosophical challenges. Looking ahead, the future of AI in moral decision-making may involve hybrid systems where AI provides ethical analyses and possible recommendations, while humans make the final decisions. Whether advanced AI, such as in the form of AGI, will indeed surpass humans in ethical reasoning remains to be seen.

Partners in Superjustice

Current AI has both actual and perceived limitations in areas requiring creativity, context-specific understanding, ethical judgment, and empathy. This is especially relevant in the legal domain, where practice centers on people and values. AI's computational power alone does not equip it to fully engage with the moral and emotional complexities inherent in the legal system and dispute resolution. This raises essential questions: If we allow AI to reshape the law, are we at risk of creating a system that enforces rules mechanically without truly understanding the people it is meant to serve? When, if ever, is the quest for efficiency and consistency or the expansion of access to justice worth the potential erosion of human insight and moral judgment? How do we bring AI into the legal loop while enhancing the human-centered values that are fundamental to justice?

Take the case of bail determinations. In recent years, some jurisdictions have introduced risk assessment algorithms to assist judges in making bail decisions. These algorithms analyze data to predict the likelihood that a defendant will re-offend or fail to appear in court. However, such algorithms can perpetuate biases and lead to unjust outcomes. For example, they may disproportionately label African American defendants as high-risk compared to their White counterparts, even when controlling for similar factors.[27]

Recognizing the distinctive weaknesses and strengths of AI and humans suggests we need a collaborative approach that leverages the best of both worlds. For starters, AI can (mostly) independently handle tasks requiring data-intensive processing, consistency, and speed, and could assist in more complex and nuanced endeavors. This would enhance humans' ability to focus on and progress in areas where they excel, such as complex problem-solving, ethical decision-making, and interpersonal relations. As AI systems become more advanced, they may increasingly take on roles that involve elements of creativity and emotional interaction.

[27] The literature here is vast. See, for example, Julia Angwin and others, "Machine Bias" in Kirsten Martin (ed), *Ethics of Data and Analytics* (Auerbach Publications 2022) 254; Virginia Eubanks, *Automating Inequality: How High-Tech Tools Profile, Police, and Punish the* (St Martin's Press 2018).

AI's roles in such a collaboration can take various shapes and forms. For instance, AI tools can serve as a first- or second-opinion provider, offering preliminary assessments or alternative perspectives. In fact, multiple AI tools could provide various independent views, with a meta-system synthesizing the outputs and submitting its summary to a human judge. In this model, AI would not act as the primary decision-maker. Rather, it could validate, refine, or challenge human judgments, enabling practitioners to weigh up different outcomes before finalizing their choices. In the context of criminal justice, for example, AI could suggest sentencing ranges based on historical data and case law, but a human judge would ultimately consider the unique aspects of each case.

Moreover, AI could synthesize insights from diverse fields that human judges would be unlikely to consider independently, such as emerging research on how gut microbes, neurological conditions, or environmental factors might influence behavior.[28] True, we may not yet be receptive to a "my microbes made me do it" defense argument. But while such interdisciplinary connections raise complex evidentiary and ethical questions about the boundaries of criminal responsibility, they highlight AI's unique capacity for cognitive augmentation, extending beyond mere computational speed.

Another vital role AI can fulfill is that of a data analyzer. In this capacity, AI can quickly sift through massive volumes of information—such as case law, police behavior, privacy policies, or crime statistics—and identify relevant patterns, correlations, and anomalies that would take a human analyst far longer to detect. Additionally, AI tools can flag pertinent details or provide insights into potential risks, allowing professionals to focus on applying their knowledge and ethical judgment to nuanced, context-specific cases. In the current circumstances, such human-AI collaborations may ultimately offer the best path forward in fields where moral decisions shape human lives.

Looking ahead, another crucial role AI can fulfill is illuminating the normative trade-offs and values underlying legal decisions. Beyond flagging implicit biases, conflicting legal principles, and inconsistent values, AI can highlight conflicts between stated values (such as justice and efficiency) and actual legal practices or outcomes. AI analysis could reveal inconsistencies between what legal frameworks claim to prioritize and the choices they ultimately produce. Such an analysis could expose misalignments that can inform efforts to recalibrate legal practices more closely to their stated and intended goals. Similarly, AI could quantify the long-term impact of legal decisions on different demographic groups, helping practitioners evaluate whether the values at play truly serve society's needs. In this way, AI will not merely support decision-making but also enhance the capacity to reflect critically on the ethical and social dimensions embedded in the legal system.

[28] See Jessica Hamzelou, "Your Gut Microbes Might Encourage Criminal Behavior" *MIT Technology Review* (May 9, 2025).

Beyond the Last Move

We began this chapter by asking whether AI's role in the legal field would ultimately resemble a decisive checkmate or a nuanced collaboration. Throughout the discussion, it has become clear that AI's place in law is not about reaching a final (checkmating) move, but about opening new possibilities and redefining the rules of engagement. AI capabilities present opportunities to rethink legal frameworks, address access to justice gaps, and drive innovation. Just as the game of chess requires continuous adaptation and strategy, the evolving journey towards AI integration in legal systems demands consistent vigilance and a readiness to reconsider the human–AI balance as AI capabilities advance. With each step, we must evaluate where AI enhances the pursuit of justice and where human oversight remains indispensable.

As AI systems grow more complex, we risk creating a new class of select "high priests"—technical experts who alone understand the mathematical operations underpinning justice. To prevent this, Superjustice must incorporate critical safeguards, including robust transparency mechanisms that make algorithmic processes comprehensible to non-experts, clear governance structures balancing public and private control, and encoded governing principles that will serve as the foundation for algorithmic constitutionalism.[29] This algorithmic constitutionalism—the embedding of fundamental values and balancing principles directly into system design—should ensure a fair evaluation of competing interests, guarantee an inherent respect for the rule of law, and maintain public trust.[30]

At this point, let us recap a few emerging insights. First, the law is not just a series of rules; it is a dynamic system that evolves through deep reflection, moral progress, creative debate, and experience. Legal professionals craft arguments and employ narratives that push the boundaries of existing legal frameworks, and legal development often requires continuous adaptation to social changes.[31] In this process, human creativity—which may be augmented by AI—is imperative.

Next, legal dilemmas often require value-based decisions. Current AI may lack the ability to suitably and reliably balance competing ethical interests, which makes human oversight essential in high-stakes cases involving rights, freedoms, or evolving societal norms. For AI to have a substantial role in these contexts, two separate additional conditions must be met. First, AI tools should develop further capabilities in ethical and moral reasoning. Second, society should be willing to accept that humans do not have

[29] The concept of algorithmic constitutionalism draws from multiple intellectual traditions across legal theory, constitutional law, and technology governance. For related discussions see, for example, Mireille Hildebrandt, *Law for Computer Scientists and Other Folk* (Oxford University Press 2020); Oren Perez and Nurit Wimer, "Algorithmic Constitutionalism" (2023) 30 Indiana Journal of Global Legal Studies 81.

[30] While the exact list of values that would form this algorithmic constitutionalism is beyond the scope of this chapter, key values could include principles such as proportionality, procedural fairness, transparency, non-discrimination, accountability, and human dignity. For generally suggesting that proportionality can provide a fair and impartial way of balancing competing interests see David M Beatty, *The Ultimate Rule of Law* (Oxford University Press 2004).

[31] For foundational accounts on the nature of law and its relationship with societal change see Ronald Dworkin, *Law's Empire* (Harvard University Press 1986); HLA Hart, *The Concept of Law* (Clarendon Press 1961).

the sole right to make moral and ethical decisions. Notably, the first does not guarantee the second. Human imperfection is relatable and thought-provoking, bringing context and excitement.[32] If anything, it seems that human trust in AI-augmented legal systems depends on human-led oversight, regardless of the objective qualities of each. Still, the majority of legal issues do not involve new and complex ethical and moral dilemmas. For most everyday legal disputes and cases that are not morally complex, AI can outperform humans.

Finally, the conventional wisdom—suggesting that AI automates repetitive, factual, and low-risk cases, and that humans should retain the more sensitive and complex tasks—is both under- and over-inclusive. It is *under-inclusive*, as it disregards recent advances and potential future enhancements in AI's capability to demonstrate creativity, emotional insight, and moral reasoning. Rather than confining AI to tasks perceived as devoid of human nuance, a more forward-thinking approach would continually seek to integrate AI into more challenging domains.

The conventional model of human–AI collaboration is also *over-inclusive*. For one thing, it may lead humans to rely too heavily on AI, diminishing human vigilance and eroding critical thinking. More subtly, delegation can also encourage moral offloading: when decision-makers can defer to "what the system recommended," they may feel less accountable and become more willing to pursue self-interest, exhibit less virtuous behavior, or compromise on important values or principles. The conventional model is further over-inclusive in that it ignores the needs of many individuals for procedural justice, even in seemingly mundane and straightforward cases. In essence, procedural justice emphasizes that people want the opportunity to share their narratives and grievances before an authority figure who listens attentively. When people feel that they have been treated with respect and that their perspectives have genuinely been considered, they are more likely to perceive the outcome as fair, even if the decision itself is not in their favor.[33]

A fundamental part of the law is understanding the human stories behind cases and the narratives people use to interpret the world and navigate their lives. Often, people seek not just a legal resolution but also the empathy and understanding that come from interacting with another human. Legal systems and legal professionals provide more than answers—they offer reassurance, trust, and emotional support.

Here too, however, the future may go well beyond the conventional human–AI collaboration paradigm. Robots and AI systems could be trained to exhibit superhumanly humane, humble, emotionally agile, and empathetic characteristics.[34] This, in turn, would make them more capable of realizing procedural justice and providing

[32] See Harry Collins and Robert Evans, "You Cannot be Serious! Public Understanding of Technology with Special Reference to 'Hawk-Eye'" (2008) 17(3) Public Understanding of Science 283; Sky Sports, "VAR Survey: 40 Per Cent of Fans Likely to Turn Away From Live Football" (June 2, 2021) <www.skysports.com/football/news/11095/12322415/var-survey-40-per-cent-of-fans-likely-to-turn-away-from-live-football>.

[33] See E Allan Lind and Tom R Tyler, *The Social Psychology of Procedural Justice* (Springer 2013); John M Conley and William M O'Barr, *Rules Versus Relationships: The Ethnography of Legal Discourse* (University of Chicago Press 1990).

[34] AI tools have no human ego, no biases, and no limit on their patience, understanding, time, or knowledge.

satisfactory reasons to disappointed citizens. Even disappointed litigants may feel better than they do now with the work of human judges, time delays, and system constraints.

After his initial shock and resistance, Kasparov eventually came to acknowledge the superior capabilities of AI in chess. Similarly, the legal profession must recognize AI's growing supremacy across many legal domains. The wiser path is not to resist AI capabilities but to thoughtfully design systems that harness them, while preserving the human elements that truly enhance the pursuit of justice. Just as chess thrives today, with AI as an uncontested dominant tool, so too can our legal systems evolve with AI at their analytical core.

6
Pervasive Justice

Justice as a Service

Imagine a world where accessing justice is as seamless and intuitive as streaming your favorite show, listening to music online, or hailing a ride with a few taps on your smartphone. Legal support, once mired in complexity and exclusivity, is now delivered on-demand, personalized to your needs, and instantly accessible from anywhere. This is "Justice as a Service" (JaaS)—a transformative vision in which the legal system provides support in an on-demand, user-centered format. JaaS, in other words, operates like the best of today's digital services, making justice an integral, effortless part of everyday life. Figure 6.1 captures this service model, highlighting its intuitive logic and appeal.

Think of how streaming platforms revolutionized entertainment, offering tailored recommendations, immediate access, and a vast library of content at your fingertips.[1] Now, envision a similar transformation in the legal world; artificial intelligence (AI)-driven tools like chatbots, virtual legal agents, and automated document services that provide users with instant legal guidance, breaking down the barriers of jargon, cost, expertise, and procedural delays. Beyond immediate convenience, JaaS taps into the collaborative spirit of online communities, where users both consume services and actively contribute to and improve them. Picture a legal platform in which every user interaction informs the system, making it smarter and more responsive with every use. Feedback loops ensure that legal services adapt in real time, evolving to meet diverse needs. Welcome to the future of justice, or Pervasive Justice: dynamic, personalized, on-demand, and designed for everyone.

This chapter explores how the concepts of "Pervasive Justice" and "JaaS" could transform legal access, making it as immediate, accessible, user-centric, and personalized as the digital services we rely on daily. We begin by examining the specific AI-driven tools that could make the vision of JaaS a reality. Next, we discuss equitable service models that will ensure these tools are accessible and tailored to the needs of individuals and communities. We then consider the practicalities of this democratic JaaS vision and its potential evolution. Here, we focus on community-driven pilot programs and the importance of iterative feedback loops in improving and refining JaaS.

[1] Amanda D Lotz, *Portals: A Treatise on Internet-Distributed Television* (Michigan Publishing 2017); Maria Eriksson and others, *Spotify Teardown: Inside the Black Box of Streaming Music* (MIT 2019); Tryon Chuck, *On-Demand Culture: Digital Delivery and the Future of Movies* (Rutgers University Press 2013).

Superjustice. Samuel I. Becher and Benjamin Alarie, Oxford University Press.
 DOI: 10.1093/9780198991885.003.0009

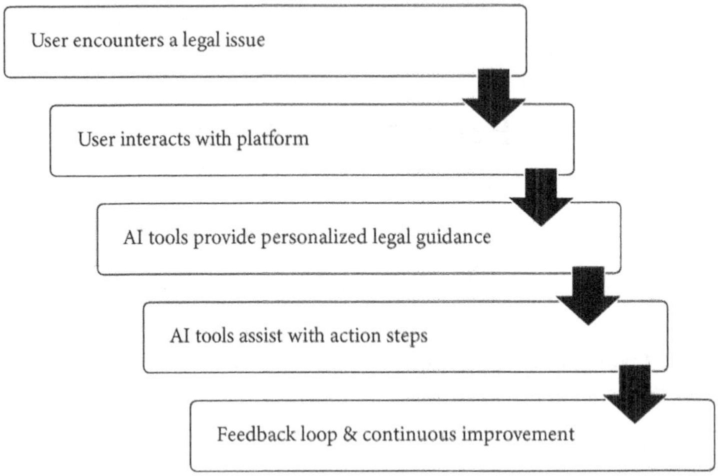

Figure 6.1 Justice as a Service Model

Technology-Driven Legal Accessibility

Just as motor vehicles initially used the infrastructure designed for horses and buggies, autonomous cars are now leveraging roads built for human drivers. In a similar way, AI-driven legal tools are beginning to utilize and adapt existing legal infrastructure. This transformation parallels the way that technological advancements have historically evolved within the confines of established systems, eventually reshaping them to better suit the demands of modern society. While traditional legal systems often remain cumbersome, complex, and inaccessible to many, the advent of AI-driven tools, such as chatbots and virtual legal agents, could signal a shift toward a more streamlined and user-friendly approach. This process would entail a gradual evolution in accessibility, whereby technology co-opts the old infrastructure for new purposes, democratizing access to justice and empowering individuals to navigate legal challenges independently.

Legal chatbots have emerged as a practical example of how technology is beginning the JaaS revolution. Platforms such as DoNotPay, designed to help users contest parking tickets and generate legal documents, enable individuals to handle routine legal matters. Whether addressing a landlord dispute or a consumer rights problem, legal chatbots can empower individuals to resolve everyday legal issues independently and affordably. They can offer advice, provide legal context, and even suggest ways to move forward without the need for costly legal representation. These tools demonstrate how AI can democratize access to justice. By automating legal processes, these tools are starting to offer an accessible and cost-effective alternative to traditional legal services.[2]

[2] See, for example, <donotpay.com/>. According to the company's website, "DoNotPay uses artificial intelligence to help you fight big corporations, protect your privacy, find hidden money, and beat bureaucracy." As of November 2024, Wikipedia describes DoNotPay as "an American company specializing in online legal services and chatbots" that "provides a 'robot lawyer' service that claims to make use of artificial intelligence to contest parking tickets and provide various other legal services, with a subscription cost of $36 for three months." See

As natural language processing improves, chatbots will broaden their capabilities. Legal chatbots could gradually become capable of addressing additional legal domains, such as insurance claims, immigration applications, and family law issues. Once the technology further matures, chatbots may serve as first-line advisors, capable of identifying potential legal matters and providing relevant legal context. Even general large language models (LLMs), such as ChatGPT or Claude, would be able to provide effective coaching for nearly any type of legal problem. This represents a step toward the Superjustice vision, in which AI tools would provide scalable, practical assistance to a wider array of legal challenges that ordinary citizens often face.

Technological advances will drive the next step in AI service tools—virtual legal agents—a distinct category of tools capable of tackling more specialized and complex areas of law. AI legal agents could manage complaints, facilitate negotiations, and assist with dispute resolution and regulatory compliance. This advance will be driven by "unhobbling" techniques, such as reinforcement learning, tool integration, and expanded context length, enabling models to manage more sophisticated and long-term tasks.[3] Unlike current LLMs, virtual legal agents will be more independent and autonomous, requiring significantly less user instruction and supervision.

Just as automated personal trainers offer individualized fitness guidance, virtual legal agents would provide tailored legal advice, reducing the demand for human legal experts. Consider Jane, for instance, who in Chapter 2 found herself tangled in an administrative and legal maze over a simple parking ticket. People like Jane would be able to authorize an AI agent to represent them and act and negotiate on their behalf, solving many legal issues with superhuman speed and resourcefulness. Managing legal issues independently, virtual legal agents would effectively bridge the gap between routine tasks and everyday legal challenges.

Designing and evaluating AI-driven legal tools, such as legal chatbots and legal agents, should be an interdisciplinary endeavor. Collaboration with experts from psychology, economics, behavioral science, product design, marketing, and law would bring a richer understanding of user needs and behaviors. For example, psychologists and behavioral scientists can help ensure that chatbot interfaces are user-friendly, do not display the same cognitive biases that humans often exhibit, and do not undermine human agency. At the same time, insights from economics, marketing, and consumer behavior can help address accessibility, adoption rates, and public perception.

Over time, automated document services could be integrated into virtual legal assistance platforms, becoming a core component of these services. This advancement will streamline the creation of essential legal documents. Unlike chatbots or current

Wikipedia, "DoNotPay" <en.wikipedia.org/wiki/DoNotPay>. For a somewhat similar vision of the future of the law, see David M Beatty, *Faith, Force, and Reason: An Armchair History of the Rule of Law* (University of Toronto Press 2022).

[3] See Richard S Sutton and Andrew G Barto, *Reinforcement Learning: An Introduction* (Bradford Book 2018); John Schulman and others, "Proximal Policy Optimization Algorithms" (2017) arXiv preprint arXiv:1707.06347.

LLMs that fulfill the role of advisors or intermediaries, these services will handle the actual negotiation and drafting of documents. This functionality will enable users to complete legal tasks independently, without needing to consult a lawyer.

Consider, for example, the process of drafting a will. Traditionally, drafting a will requires multiple consultations and exchanges with a lawyer, incurring considerable costs and time. Automated document services would simplify this process and generate the will, ensuring that it aligns with the user's desires and that all legal requirements are satisfied. A similar process would govern the creation of contracts, with AI legal agents drafting customizable contracts, tailored to the specific circumstances and needs of the users. Such tools would play a critical role in unbundling legal services, breaking down complex processes—such as opening a business or filing for divorce—into discrete, accessible components. This unbundled approach would save users time and money while providing them with greater control over their legal matters and when to engage a lawyer.

For the average user, this shift means greater efficiency and confidence in handling legal tasks. Whether drafting a lease agreement, lodging an insurance claim, setting up a will, or preparing a small claims submission, automated document services will expand what individuals can achieve without formal professional assistance. For many, particularly those who have historically faced barriers to justice, this transition to legal autonomy would be transformative. Individuals would no longer be passive recipients of costly legal advice or representation, but active participants in designing and managing their legal matters.

In complex or sensitive cases where users may want to consult a legal professional, the future of legal services will probably see the rise of online legal platforms and marketplaces. These platforms will efficiently connect clients with legal service providers, leveraging AI-powered matchmaking algorithms. These algorithms would pair individuals with professionals who best suit their specific needs, preferences, and budgets. The platforms may also feature user reviews, enabling individuals to make informed choices based on peer feedback. They would also offer dynamic pricing models that adjust according to the complexity of each case. The seamless integration of these services would allow users to move from self-managed tasks like document generation to more tailored, professional legal assistance when needed.

While legal agents will soon evolve to handle specialized and even complex tasks, their functionality will remain bounded by predefined parameters and specific domains. As these tools reach their full potential, artificial general intelligence (AGI) would likely deliver the next paradigm shift in legal assistance. Unlike virtual agents that can guide users through structured processes, AGI would offer dynamic adaptability. AGI-empowered tools would be capable of navigating a vast array of legal challenges, including ones that are unforeseen or exceptionally intricate.[4]

[4] For a general discussion, and for contending that current LLMs exhibit early AGI capabilities, see Sébastien Bubeck and others, "Sparks of Artificial General Intelligence: Early Experiments with GPT-4" (2023) arXiv preprint arXiv:2303.12712.

In a future where AGI is fully realized, advanced technological tools could also play a transformative role in public service delivery, enhancing the efficiency and fairness of government systems. Imagine an AGI-driven legal advisor embedded within social service platforms, ensuring citizens receive their full legal entitlements, from health benefits to housing rights, while simplifying interactions with complex bureaucratic processes. This could significantly reduce disparities in service provision, fostering greater trust and equity in legal and governmental institutions. But as powerful as AGI might be, its effectiveness will depend on factors such as data availability, the speed of real-world processes, public acceptance, and ethical considerations.[5]

Breaking Barriers to Equitable Service Delivery

To understand the critical need for equitable service delivery, consider the following stark reality: According to the World Justice Project, in 2019, 5.1 billion people worldwide—approximately two-thirds of the global population—lacked meaningful access to justice.[6] It is also reported that 86 percent of low-income Americans received inadequate or no professional legal help for their civil legal problems as of 2022.[7] Financial barriers are a primary reason, with low-income individuals unable to afford even basic legal assistance.[8] As Chapter 2 explored, low-income individuals, minorities, and those in rural or underserved areas often face significant barriers and geographical isolation, which can preclude many from seeking legal assistance. This perpetuates cycles of inequality, leaving marginalized populations without the necessary tools to assert their rights or navigate legal challenges effectively.

Equitable service delivery aims to dismantle these barriers by offering legal services that are accessible and affordable to a diverse range of individuals, regardless of socioeconomic status, geographic location, or personal circumstances. Thus, equitable service delivery seeks to make legal support a universal right rather than a privilege reserved for the affluent. An equitable service system envisions a legal landscape where every individual, irrespective of background, can understand, engage with, and benefit from the law.

AI has the potential to transform legal service delivery by breaking down the barriers that hinder access to justice. Through the automation of routine tasks, the

[5] Real-world data is particularly imperative given the problems with synthetic data. See Ilia Shumailov and others, "AI Models Collapse When Trained on Recursively Generated Data" (2024) 631(8022) Nature 755.

[6] See World Justice Project, "Measuring the Justice Gap: A People-Centered Assessment of Unmet Justice Needs Around the World" (2019) 5 <https://worldjusticeproject.org/our-work/research-and-data/measuring-justice-gap>.

[7] See Legal Services Corporation, "The Justice Gap: The Unmet Civil Legal Needs of Low-Income Americans" (2022).

[8] See also Deborah L Rhode, *Access to Justice* (Oxford University Press 2004); William LF Felstiner, Richard L Abel, and Austin Sarat, "The Emergence and Transformation of Disputes: Naming, Blaming, Claiming…" (1980) 15 Law & Society Review 631.

democratization of legal knowledge, and the development of scalable solutions, AI can make legal assistance more affordable and accessible. As we have seen, tools like chatbots and virtual legal agents already offer cost-effective alternatives to traditional legal services, empowering individuals to navigate legal processes independently. Leveraging AI further would allow the legal system to level the playing field, giving individuals and communities the resources necessary to engage with the law.

Strategies for Delivering Accessible Services

AI tools clearly offer little value if they remain out of reach, so we now explore scalable strategies for equitable service delivery that enhance public access to these resources. One such strategy is subscription-based legal services, which can make legal support more affordable and predictable. These models offer individuals and small businesses a reliable way to manage their legal needs with fixed monthly or annual fees, circumventing the unpredictability of traditional billing structures. Subscription models would provide flexible and comprehensive legal support, covering a spectrum of legal services, from routine consultations to document drafting and review. Predictable costs enable users to budget for legal services as a regular expense, removing the fear of incurring unexpected high fees.

By unbundling legal tasks and offering legal services using subscriptions, users can select the required legal assistance at manageable, regular costs, making legal support more accessible and adaptable. Additionally, subscription-based services would contribute to the broader goal of legal accessibility by offering scalable solutions to a wide range of demographics, from individuals managing personal legal matters to small businesses requiring regular legal counsel. They could thus transform access to justice, significantly reducing costs and enhancing resource availability.

While subscription-based legal services provide affordability and predictability, they come with limitations that prevent them from being a complete solution to universal legal access. For one thing, subscription models could generally cover routine or straightforward legal tasks. Users with more complex or specialized needs may still require costly add-on services or separate representation. Furthermore, though subscription services lower costs for many, they could still be prohibitive for those with the lowest incomes, who may struggle even with a relatively modest fixed monthly fee. Moreover, because these services often operate at high volumes, users may experience limited access to in-depth consultations or timely support, both of which can be critical in certain cases.

Additional concerns arise if for-profit firms offer subscription services. Profit-driven providers may be incentivized to employ dark patterns in their digital interfaces, such as complex cancellation processes, automatic renewal schemes, or opaque pricing structures. These strategies can lead to unexpected fees and frustration for users, particularly those less familiar with digital interfaces or legal terms. Besides, subscription services may pose privacy risks, as many providers will probably gather personal data and sell it to third parties.[9] These potential pitfalls suggest that, while subscription services are a valuable tool in expanding access, a broader framework with oversight is essential to ensure they truly serve the public interest.

One solution could be for the government to provide subscription-based legal services, similar to the way it currently offers criminal defense assistance to low-income individuals or literacy programs to specific communities. A government-led model would avoid the profit-driven motives that can lead to exploitative practices. Government programs could establish clear regulations, implement straightforward pricing structures, and offer sliding-scale or subsidized fees to ensure that subscription services are accessible and affordable. While such schemes require vision, action, and resources, integrating these services within public legal aid frameworks could create a holistic support system. To supplement such schemes, non-profit organizations, local clinics, and other mission-driven entities could also offer subscription-based legal services.

Community-based organizations could bring local knowledge and a public-centered approach, enabling them to design services that are culturally and contextually relevant. Many of these organizations receive public funding or private grants, possibly allowing them to offer sliding-scale fees or even free services to those in significant financial need. Additionally, legal clinics and non-profits often provide other social services, creating a broad support network that addresses legal needs in conjunction with other challenges communities may face. While these initiatives are not a panacea, their potential as part of a larger ecosystem of legal service models represents an important step toward a fairer and more accessible legal system for all.

Superjustice additionally envisions a legal landscape in which alternative legal service providers, such as legal process outsourcing firms and legal tech startups, also play a significant role in broadening access to justice. These providers could harness technology to deliver unbundled services and fixed-fee arrangements, ensuring legal assistance is accessible and affordable to a wider range of clients. While subscription-based services and alternative legal service providers offer more predictable and comprehensive support, unbundled legal services will allow users to engage with legal expertise on an *à la carte*, task-by-task basis. In other words, unbundling deconstructs the traditional legal service model, where clients typically pay for end-to-end representation, into discrete components such as consultations, document drafting, or court appearances. Unbundling would empower individuals to customize their legal support, ensuring they receive targeted assistance without incurring unnecessary costs.[10]

To further improve accessibility, a model of AI-driven community legal clinics could emerge. These clinics would combine human expertise with advanced AI technology to provide free or low-cost legal services, specifically aimed at populations facing

[9] For an accessible account see Planet Money, *The Subscription Tap* (October 18, 2024) <www.open.spotify.com/episode/5Wurr2OUO1qnKKy7Hxmng8>.

[10] See Forrest S Mosten, "Unbundling of Legal Services and the Family Lawyer" (1994) 28(3) Family Law Quarterly 449; Deborah L Rhode, *The Trouble with Lawyers* (Oxford University Press 2015); Stephanie L Kimbro, *Limited Scope Legal Services: Unbundling and the Self-Help Client* (American Bar Association 2012).

significant barriers to traditional legal support. This approach would extend the principles of unbundling, ensuring that previously unmet legal needs are addressed affordably and effectively through a mix of technology and pro bono or publicly funded guidance.

In practical terms, AI tools within these clinics would play a crucial role in improving service efficiency. These tools would assist lawyers by managing administrative tasks, such as sorting case files and preparing documents, allowing legal professionals to focus on delivering personalized counsel. This capability is particularly valuable in resource-constrained settings, such as remote locations with marginalized communities, where legal services are often overstretched. In such places, emerging technologies such as voice-activated legal agents and AI-enhanced translation tools hold promise for breaking down language and accessibility barriers.

If successful, the scalability of AI-enhanced legal clinics offers significant potential for broadening access to justice. These models can be replicated in various legal contexts and tailored to meet the specific needs of different communities. As clinics gather and analyze data, they can continuously refine their services, adapting to the exceptional challenges of each population. This iterative approach would ensure that the model remains responsive and effective, offering a sustainable pathway to expanding legal accessibility at scale.

Not all individuals will want to navigate legal issues independently through digital interfaces, regardless of how user-friendly they become. Therefore, even as technology advances, there remains significant value in human specialization.[11] Many individuals would still prefer human guidance when navigating complex legal issues, and people might legitimately wish not to spend all their time trying to be their own lawyer (or doctor, engineer, or architect). Models of "assisted specialization," where human experts leverage AI in accessible physical locations, could respond to this need. The UK's regulatory reforms, which allow non-lawyer investment in legal service providers, offer an instructive example, having enabled storefront legal services in the form of small legal offices in malls and supermarkets staffed by appropriately qualified personnel. Likewise, in its early years, Superjustice would offer hybrid service points that combine AI's analytical power with human empathy and communication. This would ensure that the transformation is gradual and that technological advancements benefit everyone and not just those who are comfortable with digital interfaces.

Collectively, these innovative service models would represent a transformative shift toward a more inclusive and affordable legal system. Subscription-based services, unbundled legal support, and AI-driven clinics can advance Superjustice's vision of democratizing legal resources through cost reduction, simplified processes, and broadened access across socioeconomic divides. As digital inclusion efforts bridge the gaps in technology access and literacy, they can lay the groundwork for a justice system that serves all members of society equitably.

[11] See Michael J Trebilcock, *Paradoxes of Professional Regulation* (University of Toronto Press 2022).

The Digital Divide: A Persistent Challenge

Despite all this potential progress, many underserved populations still lack reliable internet access or the digital literacy necessary to fully benefit from advanced legal technology. Globally, the digital divide remains significant: Approximately one-third of the world's population still lacks internet access, with the gap most pronounced in rural and economically disadvantaged areas.[12] Rural and lower-income populations continue to face challenges in terms of connectivity quality and affordability.[13] Moreover, significant gaps remain in terms of education, digital literacy, and universal connectivity, especially among low-income households.[14] These gaps suggest that achieving digital inclusion will require continued global efforts.

One key solution to the digital divide lies in developing mobile-friendly legal platforms and offline functionalities. Mobile devices are more accessible than computers in many low-income communities, making them a crucial tool for reaching users who might otherwise be excluded from digital legal services. Designing legal platforms optimized for mobile use and incorporating offline capabilities that allow users to access essential legal information and tools without constant internet connectivity would significantly extend the reach of these services. Beyond technological design, fostering digital literacy is vital to empowering users to engage effectively with the legal system. As various real-world examples illustrate, initiatives aimed at increasing digital literacy in underserved communities can bridge the gap, enabling individuals to navigate legal platforms confidently and independently.[15] Programs that provide training on basic digital skills, tailored to the use of legal technology, would help ensure that even those with limited prior exposure can benefit. Tools must therefore be designed with simplicity and usability in mind, catering to a range of digital proficiencies.

Cross-Sector Lessons for Justice

Leveraging technology to enhance access, improve equitable service delivery, and address socioeconomic disparities is not a new concept. To provide insights into how Superjustice can evolve without "reinventing the wheel," we next turn to analogies from other sectors. Examples from smart cities, healthcare innovations, and education technology illustrate both the transformative potential and the challenges of integrating technology into complex systems like legal services.

[12] International Telecommunication Union, "Measuring Digital Development: Facts and Figures" (2023) <www.itu.int/en/ITU-D/Statistics/Pages/facts/default.aspx/>.

[13] Simon Kemp, "Digital 2024: The United States of America" (February 22, 2024) <www.datareportal.com/reports/digital-2024-united-states-of-america>.

[14] Michael Zema, "Research: How is the Digital Divide Evolving in 2024?" (April 11, 2024) <www.amdocs.com/insights/research/research-how-digital-divide-evolving-2024>.

[15] See, for example, Legal Aid Foundation of Los Angeles (LAFLA) Digital Literacy Program <lafla.org/>; Bringing the Power of the Law to All <probono.net/>; Digital Skills Service <www.miltonkeynescab.org.uk/get-advice/digital-skills-service/>.

First, the idea of smart cities exemplifies how technology can be leveraged to enhance public services and foster adaptive and responsive governance. Ideally, smart cities optimize infrastructure, such as traffic management and energy consumption, leveraging real-time data and continuous feedback from sensors. As noted in Chapter 4, this data-driven approach offers valuable lessons for Superjustice, as AI-driven legal systems can similarly adapt to meet the changing needs of diverse communities. At the same time, the implementation of smart city technology also raises concerns about data privacy, surveillance, and the risk of deepening inequalities. These challenges are relevant to legal services, for which transparency and fairness must be balanced with efficiency.[16]

Healthcare innovations, particularly telemedicine and AI diagnostics, also provide interesting case studies. Healthcare technologies have considerably improved access to medical care, bringing specialized services to remote and underserved populations.[17] Also in the domain of healthcare, public health campaigns further emphasize the importance of public involvement in designing and implementing interventions. Similarly, Superjustice would seek to make justice more accessible and personalized while acknowledging the risks of exclusion due to poor digital literacy.

Finally, education technology, with its potential to use AI to create adaptive and tailored learning systems, may also offer a model for personalized legal support. In EdTech, platforms adjust educational content to meet the needs of individual learners, making education more inclusive and effective.[18] This adaptive approach can inspire legal systems that provide user-specific guidance, democratizing access to justice by meeting users where they are. Correspondingly, this analogy also highlights the potential risk of over-relying on AI, particularly in the formative phases. Just as in education, where human teachers still play a critical role, legal AI should, at least in its early stages, complement, rather than replace, human expertise.

Overall, these analogies from smart cities, healthcare, and education can provide a nuanced perspective on the development of Superjustice. They show the promise of technology to create more adaptive, personalized, and inclusive systems. However, they also caution against potential pitfalls such as exclusion, bias, and over-reliance on automated solutions—all valuable lessons for the design and development of Superjustice.

[16] Noor Ul Huda and others, "Experts and Intelligent Systems for Smart Homes' Transformation to Sustainable Smart Cities: A Comprehensive Review" (2024) 238 Expert Systems with Applications 122380; Rama Krishna Reddy Kummitha, "Smart Cities and Entrepreneurship: An Agenda for Future Research" (2019) 149 Technological Forecasting and Social Change 119763; R Sonia and others, "Strengthening Security, Privacy, and Trust in Artificial Intelligence Drones for Smart Cities" in Pawan Kumar Goel and others (eds), *Analyzing and Mitigating Security Risks in Cloud Computing* (IGI Global 2024) 214.

[17] See E Ray Dorsey and Eric J Topol, "Telemedicine 2020 and the Next Decade" (2020) 395(10227) The Lancet 859; Sera Whitelaw and others, "Applications of Digital Technology in COVID-19 Pandemic Planning and Response" (2020) 2(8) The Lancet Digital Health e435.

[18] Wayne Holmes, Maya Bialik, and Charles Fadel, *Artificial Intelligence in Education: Promises and Implications for Teaching and Learning* (Center for Curriculum Redesign 2019); Ilie Gligorea and others, "Adaptive Learning Using Artificial Intelligence in E-Learning: A Literature Review" (2023) 13(12) Education Sciences 1216.

Revisiting Legal Democratization

Economist David Autor provides a compelling framework for understanding how AI can democratize access to specialized knowledge and empower middle-skill workers.[19] Autor argues that AI has the potential to revitalize the middle class by expanding access to specialized knowledge and enabling workers without elite credentials to perform higher-skill tasks.[20] Autor further posits that AI could serve as a powerful equalizer, transforming traditionally exclusive roles by automating complex information processing and decision-making, thereby empowering a broader spectrum of workers to engage in meaningful, higher-stakes work. This democratization of expertise, Autor suggests, could reduce the scarcity of specialized skills, creating pathways for middle-skill workers to contribute effectively to domains that once required advanced training. Many others, including notable figures such as Bill Gates, make somewhat similar predictions about currently rare human expertise becoming free and commonplace, with AI ushering in an era of "free intelligence" that will be widely accessible and touch nearly every aspect of our lives.[21]

In the long run, the societal impact of these advances could go far beyond improving access to legal services. The democratization of legal expertise through powerful AI technologies promises a reshaping of the legal profession and its role in society. Making legal knowledge and capabilities more accessible would break down the traditional hierarchies of legal expertise that have long upheld the exclusivity and aura of the legal system. Lawyers and judges, who have historically wielded unparalleled authority over legal interpretation, dispute resolution, legal representation, and legal decision-making, will see their roles evolve toward facilitation and oversight, sharing space with AI-driven tools and community-driven contributions.

As legal expertise will no longer be the exclusive domain of credentialed professionals, the legal system will become demystified, promoting greater public trust and engagement. This reconfiguration of expertise will foster a legal environment that is both more responsive to individual needs and reflective of a more just power structure within society. Ultimately, this will pave the way to a legal ecosystem in which accessibility, efficiency, and equity are embedded into its core.

Community-Driven Programs and Adaptive Design

Subscription-based services, unbundled legal support, alternative legal service providers, AI-driven legal clinics, and efforts to counter the digital divide offer foundational

[19] David Autor, "AI Could Actually Help Rebuild the Middle Class" *Noema* (February 12, 2024); David Autor and Anna Salomons, "Robocalypse Now: Does Productivity Growth Threaten Employment?" (2017) Proceedings of the ECB Forum on Central Banking: Investment and Growth in Advanced Economies 45.

[20] Autor, "AI Could Actually Help Rebuild the Middle Class" (note 19).

[21] See Tom Huddleston Jr, "Bill Gates: Within 10 Years, AI Will Replace Many Doctors and Teachers—Humans Won't be Needed 'For Most Things'" *CNBC* (March 26, 2025).

steps toward accessible justice. Nonetheless, they risk falling short without the input of the people they aim to serve. Advancing the mission of Superjustice requires more than just equitable service models: real inclusivity calls for a deep, context-specific understanding of the communities these services intend to support.

As discussed in Chapters 3 and 4, justice solutions must be adaptive and responsive to the specific social, cultural, and economic contexts of diverse communities. Local partnerships are vital to ensuring that Superjustice tools are accessible and culturally relevant. Collaborating closely with non-governmental organizations and community organizations would help Superjustice integrate local knowledge into its design, thereby aligning legal services with the distinctive realities of local communities. This partnership-driven approach will ensure that the tools have the greatest probability of resonating with the lived experiences of the communities and users they aim to serve, thus fostering usability.[22]

Yet, communities differ vastly in their legal needs, resource availability, and cultural perspectives. For example, a program in an urban center with high mobile device use might reveal key features or usability adjustments that would differ from those needed in a rural, connectivity-challenged setting. Rural populations, immigrant communities, and low-income neighborhoods may all encounter unique legal challenges that require tailored interventions. Actively engaging with these groups would allow Superjustice to identify the specific barriers that communities face, whether they are language constraints, digital access limitations, or differing expectations relating to privacy and citizen-government relationships.[23] Thus, community-driven adaptations emerge as the logical next step in Superjustice's progression from accessible service models to inclusive legal solutions, where community feedback serves not only as a means of refinement but also as a catalyst for innovation and a cornerstone for public trust.[24] The following discussion explores this point further.

Testing Ground: Justice Pilot Programs

Pilot programs could serve as an essential bridge between the innovative design of Superjustice tools and practical feedback from real-world communities. These

[22] Pascoe Pleasence, Nigel J Balmer, and Rebecca L Sandefur, *Paths to Justice: A Past, Present and Future Roadmap* (UCL Centre for Empirical Legal Studies 2013); Bryant Garth and Joyce Sterling, "From Legal Realism to Law and Society: Reshaping Law for the Last Stages of the Social Activist State" (1998) 32(2) Law & Society Review 409.

[23] On the need for the law and the justice system to consider the unique experiences of marginalized communities and adapt to different socioeconomic circumstances and local cultures see Iris Marion Young, *Justice and the Politics of Difference* (Princeton University Press 1990); Sally Engle Merry, *Human Rights & Gender Violence: Translating International Law into Local Justice* (University of Chicago Press 2009); Rebecca L Sandefur, "Access to Civil Justice and Race, Class, and Gender Inequality" (2008) 34(1) Annual Review of Sociology 339.

[24] A vast literature suggests that public trust in legal systems is strengthened when people feel their voices are valued and considered in decision-making processes. See, for example, Tom R Tyler, *Why People Obey the Law* (Princeton University Press 2006); Patricia Ewick and Susan S Silbey, *The Common Place of Law: Stories from Everyday Life* (University of Chicago Press 1998).

programs would implement emerging technologies in small-scale, phased stages, gathering feedback to inform each iteration. This approach could foster continuous refinement by using active feedback mechanisms to assess and enhance core aspects of accessibility, such as intuitive design, mobile optimization, and offline functionality.

Equally important is the diversity of user feedback within these pilot programs. For instance, users with limited technological experience may need a simpler, more streamlined interface, while input from connectivity-challenged areas could guide enhancements to offline capabilities. These community-guided adjustments would help Superjustice evolve to meet accessibility needs more precisely, responding dynamically to various challenges and preferences.[25]

Continuous feedback loops within pilot programs would reinforce this adaptability, allowing Superjustice to gather real-time insights directly from users, such as user surveys, focus groups, and anonymous feedback forms. Pilot programs may reveal, for instance, that rural users could benefit from features like guided tutorials that reduce reliance on digital literacy and provide step-by-step assistance. These programs would employ conversational legal agents to lower language barriers and help users who may struggle with reading legal text, even when it is written in plain language. Future advances in AI could further enhance this adaptability, as tools become available to detect signs of user confusion and to adjust responses accordingly.

In the long run, powerful AI capabilities could greatly benefit from a steady stream of public feedback, which would help shape the training and ethical frameworks of these tools. This feedback would help guide decision-making criteria and influence operational values, ensuring that technology reflects and respects local values, expectations, and standards of fairness. For example, Superjustice could adapt its approach to property law, consumer rights, or labor issues based on communal-specific norms governing shared resources, familial obligations, or informal economies. In communities with communal land rights, Superjustice might prioritize frameworks that account for collective property management. In regions where informal labor agreements are prevalent, it could offer solutions that align with local practices while respecting formal legal standards.

To conclude, feedback-driven innovation via pilot programs—potentially supported and funded by governments, philanthropic foundations, tech companies, academic institutions, international organizations, or forward-thinking members of the legal profession—would anchor Superjustice's commitment to long-term responsiveness and inclusivity. This iterative development model would allow Superjustice to grow in tandem with the communities it serves, ensuring that the symbiotic relationship between user feedback and tool enhancement sustains a forward-looking, dynamic, and user-centered approach to justice.

[25] On the need of the law to be dynamic to survive and remain functional within constantly changing social environments see Gunther Teubner, *Law as an Autopoietic System* (Blackwell Publishers 1993); Roscoe Pound, "Scope and Purpose of Sociological Jurisprudence" (1910) 24 Harvard Law Review 591.

Design Principles and Adaptive Evaluation

To further enhance the relevance of AI-driven legal tools within the communities they serve, participatory design methods can integrate community voices directly into the development process. In co-creation workshops, community members could act as co-designers alongside legal professionals and AI developers, offering input that drives real-time improvements in accessibility, functionality, and cultural relevance. For example, a co-creation session might involve residents refining an AI chatbot to address common neighborhood disputes, empowering users to shape the AI's features to suit their specific cultural, social, and economic contexts. This approach would promote engagement and a sense of ownership, creating a democratized model of expertise where legal tools are genuinely user-centered.

Establishing a structured evaluation framework would be essential to ensure that AI-driven legal tools remain effective, inclusive, and aligned with societal needs. Key metrics—such as user adoption rates, case resolution times, and satisfaction scores—could offer valuable insights into how well these tools serve different populations. For example, demographic usage analysis might reveal whether certain groups, like low-income households, are underrepresented, signaling a need for targeted outreach. Likewise, satisfaction surveys can highlight user experiences, pinpointing areas for improvement or refinement.

Regular assessment of these indicators would further allow Superjustice to adapt its tools to evolving user needs and societal goals. Metrics that capture accessibility and cultural fit, such as reach among underserved populations and levels of digital literacy required, would provide the foundation for flexible, effective, and evolving tools. This evaluation method would permit each pilot program to function as a dynamic initiative rather than a static model. To illustrate, consider AI legal agents that support tenants. Superjustice might modify the parameters and modes of operation of these agents if new local patterns in housing, labor, or landlord–tenant relationships emerge.

As part of this evaluation framework, outcome fairness is essential to ensuring that AI-driven services do not perpetuate existing inequalities or introduce new biases. In practice, this requires tracking specific metrics, such as the consistency of advice provided across different demographic groups or the resolution rates for various types of legal issues. Where disparities emerge, targeted adjustments to algorithms or training data could address identified gaps and restore equitable performance.

To support adaptability, temporary frameworks could serve as a testing mechanism for AI-driven legal tools. Rather than introducing permanent changes, a temporary deployment model—including "sunset" review checkpoints that require periodic review and reassessment—would allow for real-world evaluation. For instance, a chatbot designed to handle consumer rights inquiries could be introduced temporarily, with a planned reassessment phase to determine its effectiveness, usability, and public reception after an initial trial and user feedback. Such an approach would prevent inertia and facilitate cautious innovation, continuous enhancement, and recalibration based on user feedback and measurable outcomes.

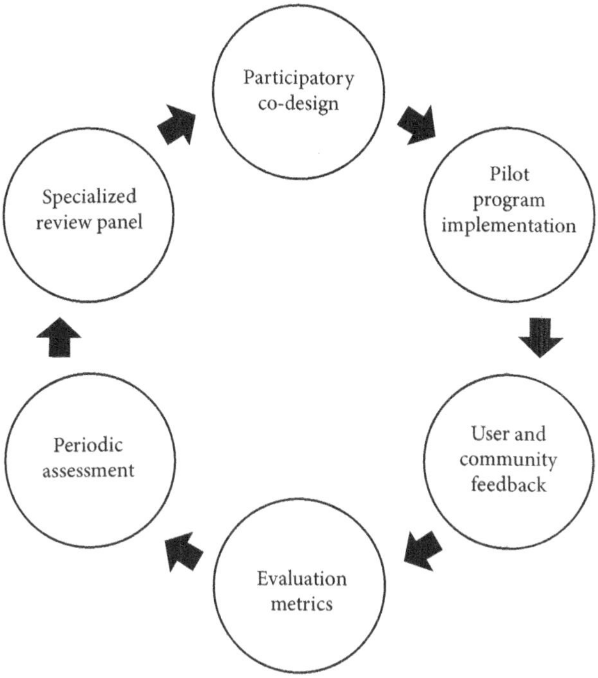

Figure 6.2 Community-Driven Feedback Loop

Another essential component is specialized, representative, and independent oversight bodies dedicated to managing and refining AI-driven legal tools. A diverse oversight body would monitor the real-world impacts of AI legal tools, systematically gather user feedback, and implement adjustments to address emerging challenges. Delegating regulatory oversight to specialized bodies—distinct from traditional political processes—would ensure that Superjustice will develop and adjust with a focus on user needs and accountability to diverse and heterogeneous voices. With this layer of independent governance in place, Superjustice would endeavor to further avoid politicization and strengthen public trust, helping to ensure that AI tools evolve responsively and in line with communal priorities. Figure 6.2 illustrates this multi-stakeholder feedback loop.

Future Innovations in Legal Tech

Other technological innovations, some of which may be impossible to predict at this stage, could present additional avenues for expanding access to legal resources. One possibility is that advanced AI tools, integrated with augmented and virtual reality, could transform how individuals prepare for and navigate legal processes. Unlike traditional online resources, these tools could provide scenario-based guidance tailored to specific legal contexts. In doing so, the tools might simulate realistic legal environments, such as contract negotiations, mediations, or courtroom proceedings. This

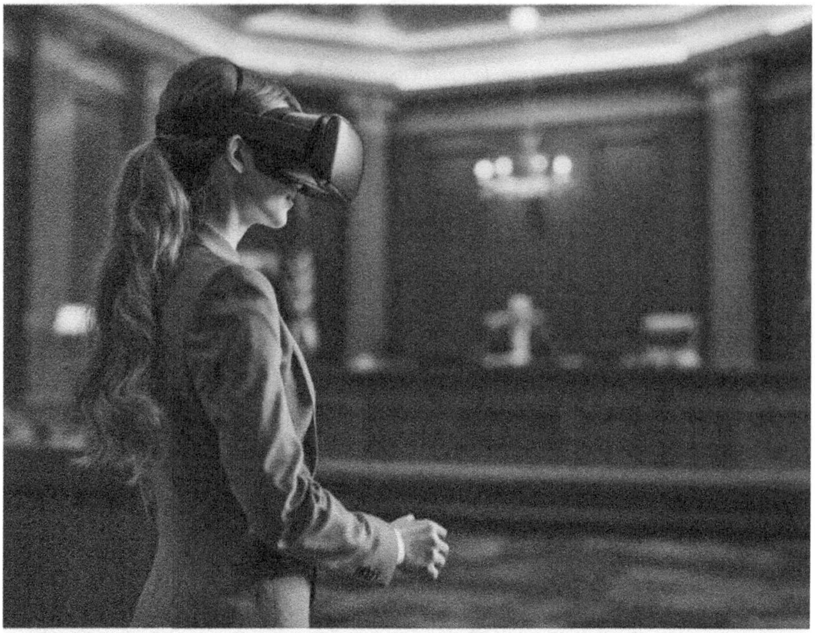

Generated by FLUX-pro-1.1

Figure 6.3 Using VR Tools to Simulate a Courtroom

would offer users a safe space in which to rehearse and understand potential outcomes. For example, imagine a virtual reality tool that allows users to practice presenting their grievance or claim in a virtual courtroom, simulating common scenarios they might encounter (see Figure 6.3). Such immersive preparation would encourage users to approach real-life legal encounters with reduced anxiety and a stronger sense of control.

In addition to preparing users for specific interactions, augmented reality and virtual reality experiences could be tailored to address the distinctive needs of different communities. For instance, a rural user might benefit from a step-by-step visualization of dispute resolution processes within local jurisdictions. Similarly, someone unfamiliar with courtroom protocols might benefit from participating in a realistic mock trial to help them become familiar with procedures and expectations. Such applications would further demystify legal pathways, allowing users to enter real-life scenarios with greater confidence and understanding. As AI capabilities continue to advance, these immersive tools could adapt dynamically, adjusting the level of guidance and detail based on user interactions. This adaptability would further personalize support, enhancing both comprehension and accessibility.

To sum up, community-driven themes and innovative design principles collectively form the backbone of Superjustice's commitment to creating a system of pervasive justice. Together, they advance the concept of JaaS. Each theme, from ensuring accessibility through iterative feedback and localized design to harnessing powerful AI for culturally aware adaptability, reinforces a commitment to justice that is responsive and user-centric.

A Blueprint for Adaptive Justice

AI is one of the most powerful technologies of our time, and it will have profound and long-lasting consequences for law, justice, and democratic values. This chapter underscores the transformative potential of AI tools as engines of inclusivity and accessibility within the legal system. AI-driven innovations, such as chatbots and AI legal agents, will reshape the way individuals engage with the law. These tools could democratize access to legal information and service tools, empowering users to address legal matters independently and breaking down traditional barriers.

To ensure that Superjustice promotes equity in both access and outcomes, it must incorporate various strategies, a data-driven approach, and astute design principles. From iterative feedback loops in pilot programs to partnerships with local organizations, Superjustice would actively involve communities in refining and adapting these tools. This collaboration would allow Superjustice to address the barriers faced by diverse populations, thereby fostering an inclusive system that reflects the experiences and expectations of those it serves. Continuous evaluation and improvement frameworks—including metrics like demographic usage analysis, satisfaction scores, and outcome fairness—would help safeguard against biases and unfairness. At the same time, maintaining public trust in these technologies will be paramount.[26] Similarly, fairness and transparency would be essential for building confidence in AI-driven legal solutions and for mitigating the risk of perpetuating existing inequalities.

As AI continues to evolve, the potential for a truly inclusive, user-centered legal system grows closer to reality. This journey, however, requires balancing technological ambition with ethical stewardship. Grounded in fairness, inclusivity, and community engagement, Superjustice envisions a legal framework in which justice is accessible, adaptable, and better aligned with the public's needs. This is a significant step toward a holistic public-centered justice system that prioritizes user empowerment, minimizes reliance on traditional gatekeeping structures, and emphasizes direct community-driven access to legal solutions.

[26] On the link between public trust and technology adoption see RC Mayer, "An Integrative Model of Organizational Trust" (1995) 20(3) Academy of Management Review 709; see also Paul M Schwartz and Daniel J Solove, "The PII Problem: Privacy and a New Concept of Personally Identifiable Information" (2011) 86 New York University Law Review 1814 (discussing the critical role of public trust in privacy technologies and the legal frameworks governing personal data).

7

Educating for Superjustice

Why Legal Education Must Change

In 2023, a startling headline made waves in the legal world: An artificial intelligence (AI) large language model (LLM) successfully breezed through the bar exam, reportedly scoring near the 90th percentile.[1] Just two years later, in 2025, OpenAI's o3 model earned A+ grades on multiple law school final exams, outperforming most human students.[2] Observers could be forgiven for marveling at AI's ability to grapple with questions across diverse legal domains, including contracts, evidence, criminal law, and procedure. For some, it seemed to herald the end of traditional lawyering. Why train humans to "think like a lawyer" when machines could do it faster, cheaper, and arguably better?

But here is the twist: The same LLM tools occasionally provide truly puzzling responses to mundane prompts. The internet is full of bizarre, nonsensical, and humorous examples. In one case, ChatGPT noted, "it's important to . . . not blindly follow the advice of others, even if they are a wizard." In response to a user's prompt about "cheese not sticking to pizza," Google AI suggested adding "non-toxic glue to the sauce." Other user prompts elicited advice such as "eating mucus may help prevent cavities, stomach ulcers, and infections" or that one "should eat at least one small rock per day."[3]

Beyond these quirks, LLMs sometimes fail spectacularly when tested on novel tasks that require common sense, healthy intuition, temporal reasoning, spatial orientation, or even basic knowledge. Such tools occasionally lack causal reasoning, struggle to

[1] See Debra Cassens Weiss, "Latest Version of ChatGPT Aces Bar Exam with Score Nearing 90th Percentile" *ABA Journal* (March 16, 2023); John Koetsier, "GPT-4 Beats 90% of Lawyers Trying To Pass The Bar" *Forbes* (March 15, 2023); "GPT-4" (*OpenAI*, March 14, 2023), <www.openai.com/index/gpt-4-research/>. A 2024 study claimed that the 90 percent figure is inflated and GPT's performance was less impressive. See Ben Turner, "GPT-4 Didn't Ace the Bar Exam After All, MIT Research Suggests—It Didn't Even Break the 70th Percentile" *LiveScience* (June 1, 2024).

[2] See Andrew Blair-Stanek and others, "AI Gets its First Law School A+s" *SSRN* (2025).

[3] See Michael Brenner, "Why AI is Not Taking Over Content Marketing" (*Marketing Insider Group*, September 18, 2023) <marketinginsidergroup.com/content-marketing/ai-content-marketing/>; AI's Cheeta, "The Bizarre Case of Cheese Not Sticking to Pizza: When AI Went a Little Too Far" (*Medium*, May 23, 2024) <www.medium.com/@AiCheeta/the-bizarre-case-of-cheese-not-sticking-to-pizza-when-ai-went-a-little-too-far-bd3e8bda4689>; Sundeeka Mungroo "Eight Google AI Answers That'll Have You in Stitches" (*SA People News*, October 9, 2024) <www.sapeople.com/featured/google-ai-answers-funny-results-artificial-intelligence-internet-results/>; Thomas Barrabi, "Google 'Taking Swift Action' to Remove Bizarre AI Search Results—Like Telling Users to Eat Rocks" *New York Post* (May 28, 2024) <www.nypost.com/2024/05/28/business/google-moving-to-remove-bizarre-ai-search-results-like-telling-users-to-eat-rocks/>.

Superjustice. Samuel I. Becher and Benjamin Alarie, Oxford University Press.
 DOI: 10.1093/9780198991885.003.0010

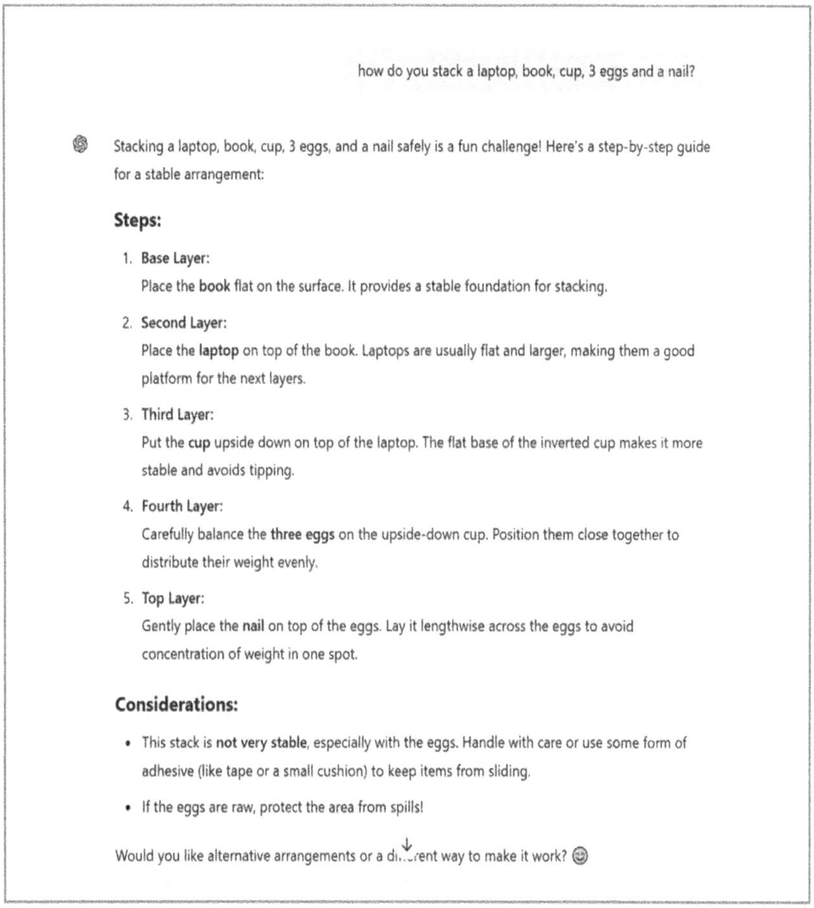

Figure 7.1 Stacking Items

understand context, and find abstract reasoning difficult. As some online reports illustrate, AI systems can produce impractical solutions to straightforward tasks such as stacking a laptop, a book, a few eggs, and a nail (see Figure 7.1).

These and similar examples underscore the need for lawyers who exercise practical judgment and approach AI tools with a critical mindset. For all their computational brilliance, today's AI systems often fail to grapple with the nuances of human experience—the very terrain where law and justice are grounded. This persistent gap prompts a fundamental question: How should legal education evolve in an era defined by powerful yet imperfect and occasionally inscrutable artificial intelligence?

As a dynamic, equitable, and technology-driven legal system, Superjustice demands a reassessment of the traditional foundations of legal education. The prevailing model, especially in common law countries, remains centered on courtroom advocacy, analytical reasoning, and adversarial argument, all of which are rooted in precedent. While these competencies were indispensable in the pre-AI era, they are rapidly becoming insufficient for a legal profession shaped by AI. Superjustice will require a decisive shift in educational priorities.

Critiques of traditional legal education and calls for reform are not new, but the rise of Superjustice underscores their urgency. The current culture of most law schools emphasizes "thinking like a lawyer," which can reinforce hierarchies, undermine happiness, and neglect emotional intelligence and soft skills.[4] Moreover, "thinking like a lawyer" has limited value when machines can "think" this way faster, more cheaply, and more effectively. Analytical reasoning and precedent-based logic are increasingly automated, leaving human lawyers at risk of redundancy if these are their primary strengths.

Law schools also often foster hypercompetitive environments that further undermine student well-being. Grading curves, heavy workloads, and a narrow focus on academic success reinforce a zero-sum mindset, exacerbating stress and discouraging collaboration. This culture is fundamentally misaligned with the ethos of Superjustice, which emphasizes cooperation, autonomy, community-driven solutions, and participatory legal systems.

Equally troubling is the rigid segmentation of intellectual, professional, and personal dimensions of learning, which alienates many students.[5] Socratic teaching methods prioritize analytical skills but often discourage emotional engagement and personal reflection, dissuading students from integrating their lived experiences into legal training. Superjustice, by contrast, envisions a legal profession that prioritizes negotiation, dispute resolution, inclusivity, and collaboration over adversarial processes. Lawyers of the future will need to work effectively in teams, engage empathetically with diverse populations, and approach problems with openness, curiosity, and emotional intelligence. Yet many law schools, with their focus on competition, rigid analytical models, and conventional hierarchies, fail to cultivate these essential traits.

The traditional curriculum fails to prepare students for the realities of AI-driven legal practice.[6] Technology, interdisciplinary approaches, and global competencies are often still treated as peripheral rather than central to the profession's future. Compounding this is the disproportionate focus on courtroom advocacy at the expense of alternative dispute resolution (ADR), including community-driven and AI-assisted resolution methods. Part of the problem is structural: Most current law professors were trained within, and remain invested in, the existing system, leaving them ill-equipped or unmotivated to adapt to new realities.

[4] See, for example, Duncan Kennedy, *Legal Education and the Reproduction of Hierarchy: A Polemic Against the System* (New York University Press 1983); Jess Krannich, James R Holbrook, and Julie McAdams, "Beyond 'Thinking Like a Lawyer': Toward a Comprehensive View of Legal Education" (2009) 86 Denver University Law Review 381; Jerome M Organ, David B Jaffe, and Katherine M. Bender, "Suffering in Silence: The Survey of Law Student Well-Being and the Reluctance of Law Students to Seek Help for Substance Use and Mental Health Concerns" (2016) 66(1) Journal of Legal Education 116; Katya S Cronin, "Value-Centered Lawyering: Reshaping the Law School Curriculum to Promote Well-Being, Quality Client Representation, and a Thriving Legal Field" (2024) 101 University of Detroit Law Review 257.

[5] Susan L Brooks, "Transforming the Law School Matrix" (2025) 2 Journal of Law Teaching & Learning 101, citing Susan Sturm and Lani Guinier, "The Law School Matrix: Reforming Legal Education in a Culture of Competition and Conformity" (2007) 60 Vanderbilt Law Review 515.

[6] See, for example, Richard Susskind, *Tomorrow's Lawyers: An Introduction to Your Future* (3rd edn, Oxford University Press 2023); Abdi Aidid and Benjamin Alarie, *The Legal Singularity: How Artificial Intelligence Can Make Law Radically Better* (University of Toronto Press 2023); Markus D Dubber, Frank Pasquale, and Sunit Das (eds), *The Oxford Handbook of Ethics of AI* (Oxford University Press 2020).

Superjustice envisions a legal ecosystem where courtrooms are no longer the default mechanism for resolving disputes. Participatory legal processes, decentralized governance models, and public and AI arbitrators will take center stage. Yet many law schools continue to prioritize adversarial training over the collaborative and problem-solving skills required to thrive in these new paradigms.

Predictably, educational and academic institutions worldwide have responded to recent AI developments, and particularly generative AI, with caution. Since ChatGPT's public release, most institutions have focused on containment: implementing plagiarism detection software, restricting AI use in assignments, and developing honor codes and disclosure mandates that treat these tools as potential threats to academic integrity. This defensive posture reflects deep anxieties about AI's capacity to undermine traditional pedagogical models and assessment methods.

This chapter takes a markedly different approach. Rather than viewing AI as a disruptive force to be regulated or contained, we propose making it central to the transformation of legal education. Our conceptualization rests on three key assumptions. First, AI represents a profoundly valuable tool that will dramatically expand both the scope and efficiency of legal services. Second, the legal workforce will increasingly favor graduates who demonstrate fluency in AI collaboration, and lawyers who master human–AI partnerships will systematically outcompete those who resist these tools. Third, attempts to ban or severely restrict AI use in legal education are both futile and counterproductive, akin to prohibiting calculators in mathematics or computers in research.

Our vision, therefore, embraces full integration: producing graduates who are not merely consumers of legal technology but sophisticated critics, ethical supervisors, and active contributors to AI's continued development within legal systems. Recent developments in Chinese higher education, where universities now treat AI literacy as an essential component of professional preparation, reflect this forward-thinking approach.[7] Indeed, the question is not whether to integrate AI, but how quickly and comprehensively institutions can adapt.

Accordingly, this chapter explores the need to transform legal education to meet the dual demands of technological proficiency and human flourishing. We first examine necessary curricular reforms, emphasizing AI governance, decentralized systems, new partnerships, and behavioral sciences, alongside adaptive curricula that personalize learning. Next, we highlight the essential skills that future lawyers will need, including digital literacy, emotional intelligence, and global competencies. Thereafter, we discuss innovative training models, such as AI-enhanced simulations, social impact clinics, and law-tech labs, that could bridge theory and practice.

Before we proceed, we must recognize the inevitable challenges and resistance these transformations will provoke, from institutional inertia and automation-driven skill erosion to disparities in access to technology and concerns about student well-being.

[7] See Caiwei Chen, "Chinese Universities Want Students to Use More AI, Not Less" *MIT Technology Review* (July 28, 2025) <www.technologyreview.com/2025/07/28/1120747/chinese-universities-ai-use/>.

There is no guarantee that our projections will materialize as expected. In the face of rapid technological change, many law schools may struggle to remain relevant or even viable. As with other parts of this book, our purpose here is twofold: to illuminate the transformational potential of AI and to emphasize the critical importance of engaging now in informed discourse about these changes. Institutions that embrace thoughtful reforms early on will be better positioned to survive and prepare lawyers for a Superjustice future.

Curricular Reforms for the Superjustice Paradigm

Legal education must adapt to the emergence of AI-transformed systems by equipping lawyers with skills that extend beyond precedent-based reasoning. AI tools are already powerful collaborators, and their capabilities will only improve. Over time, these technological tools may become superior to human legal professionals in many areas. The legal profession of the future, increasingly shaped by AI, decentralized systems, and global interconnectivity, will require lawyers equipped with more than just a mastery of precedent and analytical reasoning. Future lawyers must gain greater technical fluency, interdisciplinary expertise, interpersonal skills, and an ability to remain adaptable in a rapidly changing environment.

As AI technologies proliferate, data and legal information will become more accessible, reducing their standalone value. This shift will make wisdom—loosely defined as the ability to combine knowledge, experience, and good judgment to make sound decisions and live well—a key quality for lawyers. More specifically, lawyers will need practical wisdom: the ability to combine moral skills and the will to make sound judgments in specific contexts, particularly where rules and incentives alone may not reliably lead to the right outcome.[8] Curricular reform should thus align legal education with the realities of an AI-augmented profession, while also promoting student well-being. Adaptive, dynamic learning systems should personalize education, reducing unnecessary stress and fostering a more supportive learning environment. Courses must expose students to cutting-edge technologies like human-AI collaboration frameworks and algorithmic governance, while also emphasizing ethical reasoning and critical thinking. The objective is to complement technological strengths (ie, working with machines) with human qualities, such as caring, bonding, empathy, and practical judgment.

Holistic development should be central to the transformation of legal education. Initiatives that integrate behavioral sciences, recognize and respond to the effects of stress on learning, and introduce well-being practices can help students thrive both during and after law school. Furthermore, law students should learn more about

[8] See Barry Schwartz and Kenneth Sharpe, *Practical Wisdom: The Right Way to Do the Right Thing* (Riverhead Books 2010).

human biases and human cognitive limitations. This would allow students to better understand the comparative strengths and weaknesses of humans and machines, and how to optimally combine their capabilities. Students should additionally learn about human flourishing, happiness, and well-being. This would allow them to gain a better understanding of what motivates humans and the conditions necessary for them to thrive. It would also provide students with tools to nurture their well-being during law school and beyond.[9]

Additionally, law schools must prepare tomorrow's lawyers to safely navigate the anticipated change in their societal and professional status. The legal profession's traditional monopoly over many areas of legal services will gradually erode as AI tools enable individuals, organizations, businesses, and public institutions to independently perform legal tasks, resolve disputes, and navigate compliance. To remain relevant, therefore, lawyers must constantly reevaluate the AI–lawyer division of labor. These capabilities will redefine lawyers' roles as collaborators, guides, partners, and ethical supervisors in an AI-driven legal ecosystem.

A forward-looking curriculum must remain flexible, evolving in real time to reflect advances in technology and global legal developments. Without this dynamism, legal education risks falling behind the systems it needs to train students to navigate. Maintaining relevance will require curricula that keep pace with continual technological and societal progress. The "half-life of knowledge"[10]—the relatively short period during which half of the knowledge in a particular field becomes obsolete—already necessitates continuous updates to educational content. As the pace of change accelerates, law schools will be forced to embrace innovation to avoid producing graduates trained for a legal system that no longer exists.

Integrating Interdisciplinary Approaches

Interdisciplinary education is an innovative approach to learning that integrates knowledge, methods, and perspectives from multiple disciplines to foster holistic understanding. It enables insights and solutions that no single field could achieve on its own. It also enhances students' ability to recognize sophisticated thinking patterns, develop stronger analytical skills, and cultivate a deeper understanding of how different fields of knowledge intersect.[11] By cultivating critical thinking, collaboration, and the synthesis

[9] For a few interesting accounts see Daniel Kahneman, Edward Diener, and Norbert Schwarz (eds), *Well-being: Foundations of Hedonic Psychology* (Russell Sage Foundation 1999); Daniel Nettle, *Happiness: The Science Behind Your Smile* (Oxford University Press 2005); Daniel Gilbert, *Stumbling on Happiness* (Vintage Canada 2009); Richard Layard, *Happiness: Lessons from a New Science* (Penguin UK 2011); Martin EP Seligman, *Flourish: A Visionary New Understanding of Happiness and Well-being* (Simon & Schuster 2011).

[10] See Samuel Arbesman, *The Half-Life of Facts: Why Everything We Know Has an Expiration Date* (Penguin Books 2012).

[11] See Lana Ivanitskaya and others, "Interdisciplinary Learning: Process and Outcomes" (2002) 27 Innovative Higher Education 95; Elisabeth JH Spelt and others, "Teaching and Learning in Interdisciplinary Higher Education: A Systematic Review" (2009) 21 Educational Psychology Review 365; Renate G Klaassen, "Interdisciplinary Education: A Case Study" (2018) 43(6) European Journal of Engineering Education 842.

of diverse viewpoints, interdisciplinary education will prepare students to tackle the multifaceted challenges of the 21st century.

Legal education will increasingly draw from interdisciplinary fields—such as technology, philosophy, psychology, public policy, and economics—to prepare students for a profession at the nexus of law, technology, and society. Lawyers will need to understand technologies they may not have built. Law schools should thus empower students to overcome biases towards machines, audit algorithms for fairness, collaborate with data scientists, and apply behavioral insights in negotiation and dispute resolution. Students should also learn to maintain intellectual humility when encountering new ideas or propositions made by powerful AI tools. These skills will enable future lawyers to address the social and ethical dimensions of legal systems, anticipate unintended consequences, and consider the interests of diverse stakeholders.

Future lawyers will increasingly work in teams composed of professionals from diverse fields, such as data science, engineering, public policy, and behavioral science. Legal education could simulate this reality by fostering interdisciplinary collaboration during law school training. For example, law students might partner with computer science peers to design ethical AI systems that incorporate fairness algorithms, or they might work alongside public policy students to draft regulatory frameworks for decentralized governance. These partnership experiences will help students cultivate essential skills like communication, adaptability, and collaboration. They will also foster student well-being through a shared sense of purpose and community.

As legal practice becomes more interdisciplinary, lawyers will face ethical dilemmas that transcend traditional legal frameworks. Reconciling the efficiency-driven goals of technologists with the equity-focused principles of law and public policy will require nuanced ethical reasoning. At least in the early stages, lawyers working on AI systems may need to navigate tensions between optimizing automation and preserving human oversight.

As technology advances, lawyers may need to learn when to accept the machine's judgment or decision, even when it conflicts with their own intuition or reasoning. This shift will require lawyers to evaluate whether machines can exercise sound ethical reasoning or whether human oversight remains necessary. Law schools must equip students with the tools to critically assess these challenges and learn when to cede to AI. Overall, legal education must prepare students to see technology not just as a tool, but as a foundational element of the future legal landscape.

Dynamic Curriculum Design

To prepare students for a technology-driven legal profession, legal education must prioritize teaching adaptability, resilience, and responsiveness to change. AI technologies offer unparalleled opportunities to personalize education, tailoring the learning experience to meet individual needs and reducing the stress caused by rigid, one-size-fits-all models.[12] Adaptive learning platforms can analyze student progress in real time, identifying strengths and weaknesses and providing targeted support and customized responses. For instance, AI tutors could help students navigate complex legal research, offering instant feedback on analytical exercises or guiding them through the intricacies of blockchain-based smart contracts. This could empower students to learn at their own pace, enhancing their professional mastery and supporting their well-being. Thus, AI-driven personalization in legal education has the potential to advance a learning environment that surpasses traditional models in flexibility, inclusivity, student empowerment, and effectiveness.

Dynamic curricula should also incorporate immersive, AI-enhanced simulations that allow students to apply theoretical knowledge to real-world scenarios. For instance, virtual reality (VR)-based mock trials and AI-driven negotiation, mediation, and arbitration exercises could replicate the complexities of legal practice. These simulations would advance critical thinking, creativity, and resilience in a controlled, low-risk setting. They would also help bridge the gap between classroom learning and professional application.

A dynamic curriculum must continuously evolve, incorporating the latest technological developments, societal needs, and legal challenges. Real-time updates to course content can ensure that students remain on the cutting edge, while AI-driven analytics can provide valuable insights into learning trends and areas for improvement. Such analytics, combined with feedback from students, faculty, and industry partners, can create powerful feedback loops for continuous curriculum refinement.

Building Partnerships

Transforming legal education will also require law schools to embrace partnerships with key stakeholders in the private sector, government, and local communities. Law schools cannot single-handedly connect academic theory with the complexities of technology-transformed legal practice. Partnerships with law firms, technology companies, community organizations or advocacy groups, and government agencies are critical for ensuring that law school curricula reflect real-world realities.[13] These collaborative initiatives could include, for example, joint research projects, practitioner-in-residence programs, and technology incubators that bridge theoretical knowledge with practical applications. Changes, however, must be implemented in collaboration with

[12] See generally Ramteja Sajja and others, "Artificial Intelligence-Enabled Intelligent Assistant for Personalized and Adaptive Learning in Higher Education" (2024) 10(15) Information 596; Kristjan-Julius Laak and Jaan Aru, "AI and Personalized Learning: Bridging the Gap with Modern Educational Goals" (2024) arXiv preprint, arXiv:2404.02798.

[13] To be sure, the idea that law schools should partner and innovate in their curricula to better serve all stakeholders is not new. For a few discussions see Harry T Edwards, "The Growing Disjunction Between Legal Education and the Legal Profession" (1992) 91(1) Michigan Law Review 34; Peter A Joy, "Law Schools and the Legal Profession: A Way Forward" (2014) 47 Akron Law Review 177; see also Jessica R Blaemire, "Analysis: Seven Innovative Law Schools That Go Beyond the Law" (*Bloomberg Law*, January 31, 2024) <www.news.bloomberglaw.com/bloomberg-law-analysis/analysis-seven-innovative-law-schools-that-go-beyond-the-law>.

bar associations, law societies, and regulatory bodies, while addressing institutional concerns about professional standards, ethics, and quality assurance. Additionally, creating formal feedback mechanisms between practice and academia will ensure curriculum evolution remains responsive to emerging industry needs.

Partnerships with private-sector stakeholders will provide essential expertise and resources. Advanced platforms for AI-enhanced simulations or distributed ledger technologies for secure legal workflows remain out of reach for many institutions. Collaborations with technology companies could make these tools accessible, ensuring equitable preparation across institutions. Law firms could sponsor law-tech labs, in which students design and test applications for automated systems or AI arbitration. Internships and externships at some law firms or tech companies may allow students to apply classroom concepts in professional settings, fostering practical skills and industry connections. While similar experiences are already offered in some law schools, their prominence is expected to increase substantially. Such partnerships could address resource constraints and make cutting-edge legal education more accessible to diverse demographics.

Legal education must also better prepare students for global challenges, such as navigating cross-border data flows and international frameworks for AI governance and liability. International collaboration among universities, legal organizations, and technology providers could harmonize competencies and promote a shared understanding of legal standards. For example, cross-border pilot programs would enable students from multiple jurisdictions to collaborate on mock cases involving decentralized governance or digital asset regulations.

While partnerships will offer significant benefits, they will also present risks. Overreliance on private-sector stakeholders may skew curricula toward commercial priorities, sidelining critical discussions on justice, equity, and public interest. Similarly, disparities in access to partnerships could exacerbate inequities between well-funded and well-located institutions and those that are not. These risks will require systematic solutions: establishing governance frameworks that protect academic independence, creating consortium models where multiple institutions share resources and partnerships, and developing public funding mechanisms to support less-resourced institutions. Public–private collaborations, supported by government grants or nonprofit initiatives, could help further democratize access to technology and education, while maintaining focus on public interest objectives.

Taking Decentralization Seriously

Decentralized legal systems will redefine how legal norms are created, interpreted, developed, and enforced. New technologies will offer automated and decentralized mechanisms for negotiation, dispute resolution, and agreement execution. However, as we explained in Chapter 3, decentralization is unlikely to be absolute. Instead, hybrid models—blending centralized oversight with decentralized processes—will dominate the legal landscape. Lawyers of the future will need to navigate this fragmented environment, ensuring that decentralized frameworks remain accountable, equitable, and dynamic. Understanding these systems will be critical for integrating them into legal structures and addressing the regulatory and operational challenges they present.

The potential proliferation of decentralized governance will require a legal curriculum that equips students to design, interpret, and oversee these systems. Courses on automation, AI agents, robots, blockchain applications, smart contracts, and the mechanics of decentralized ecosystems would be an integral part of legal education. As noted, these courses should not only provide technical knowledge but also emphasize the ethical and societal implications of decentralized systems. Lawyers must acquire skills to balance the efficiencies of automation with robust ethical oversight, ensuring that the systems remain just, transparent, and adaptable to changing norms.

Future lawyers will also play critical roles in safeguarding individual rights and ensuring accountability within decentralized frameworks. This includes addressing algorithmic biases, securing transparency in autonomous systems, and mediating between diverse stakeholder interests. To that end, law schools must train students to develop, navigate, and supervise participatory legal frameworks that encourage inclusivity and community engagement.

Decentralization will transform not just how legal systems function but also who participates in them. Distributed governance models will open legal processes to broader public engagement, empowering communities to contribute to norm-setting and dispute resolution. Lawyers will play a role in facilitating, reviewing, and safeguarding these participatory systems, ensuring they remain transparent and accessible. Future legal education must train lawyers to facilitate users' participation, appreciate and mediate between diverse perspectives, balance competing community or jurisdictional values and approaches, build consensus, and navigate the ethical complexities of participatory frameworks. As stewards of these systems, lawyers will need to promote trust and legitimacy in legal processes that prioritize collaboration, diversity, and dialogue over hierarchy and exclusivity.

New Skills for Future Lawyers

As AI and decentralized systems increasingly shape the legal profession, law schools must adapt. But what specific skills will these reforms cultivate, and how will lawyers deploy them in practice? The high-level reforms explored in the previous discussion highlight the need for lawyers to acquire diverse technical, interpersonal, global, and ethical capabilities. Building on these suggested modifications, let us now shift the focus from institutional and systemic reforms to the individual skills and competencies that lawyers will most benefit from.

A useful framework for understanding these skills and structuring legal education reform is Bloom's taxonomy. First developed in 1956 and later revised in 2001, Bloom's

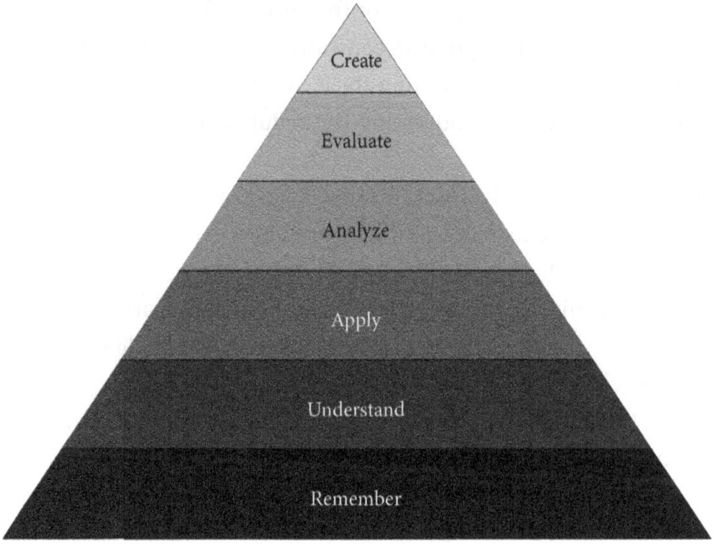

Figure 7.2 Bloom's Taxonomy

taxonomy categorizes learning objectives into a hierarchical model (see Figure 7.2), progressing from foundational cognitive tasks (like remembering and understanding) to advanced capacities (such as evaluating and creating).[14] To illustrate, "understanding" the principles of AI-driven systems and blockchain governance is a lower-level competency, while "evaluating" their fairness or "creating" innovative applications within decentralized legal ecosystems would represent higher-order skills.

Bloom's taxonomy helps educators set clear, measurable learning goals. It also provides a scaffolding for advancing diverse skill sets. Within the context of Superjustice, it can align legal education with the profession's evolving needs while recalibrating learning objectives. Specifically, it ensures that foundational knowledge (eg, legal doctrines) serves as the bedrock for developing higher-order skills, such as critical thinking, ethical reasoning, and interdisciplinary problem-solving.

While Bloom's taxonomy remains influential in curriculum development and assessment worldwide, it is not without its limitations.[15] Primarily, it prioritizes intellectual and analytical skills, often overlooking the emotional and social dimensions of learning. This emphasis may inadvertently promote a mechanistic view of education, sidelining creativity, intrinsic motivation, and interpersonal competencies that are

[14] See Benjamin S Bloom and David R Krathwohl, *Taxonomy of Educational Objectives: The Classification of Educational Goals. Handbook I: Cognitive Domain* (Longmans, Green 1956); Lorin W Anderson and David R Krathwohl (eds), *A Taxonomy for Learning, Teaching, and Assessing: A Revision of Bloom's Taxonomy of Educational Objectives* (Allyn & Bacon 2001).

[15] For some critics and discussions see Christopher P Ormell, "Bloom's Taxonomy and the Objectives of Education" (1974) 17(1) Educational Research 3; Omer Faruk Tutkun and others, "Bloom's Revised Taxonomy and Critics on It" (2012) 1(3) The Online Journal of Counselling and Education 22; Luke Zaphir and Dale Hansen, "The Trouble with Bloom's Taxonomy in an Age of AI" *Times Higher Education* (April 19, 2024) <www.timeshighereducation.com/campus/trouble-blooms-taxonomy-age-ai>.

central to the Superjustice vision. Scholars have also called for updates to better reflect 21st-century skills, like collaboration, adaptability, and interdisciplinary problem-solving. As AI takes over repetitive tasks, legal education must pivot toward fostering core human abilities, such as empathy, judgment, and ethical reasoning, which are underemphasized in the current taxonomy. Overall, the revisions we propose aim to leverage the taxonomy's strengths while addressing its gaps.

Technical Skills

The Superjustice era demands lawyers who are legally proficient, human oriented, and technically literate. Bloom's taxonomy offers a useful framework for conceptualizing these skills. Starting with foundational abilities, such as understanding how AI and blockchain systems function, students would progress to applying these tools in practice, evaluating their outputs for compliance and equity, and ultimately contributing to the creation of innovative legal solutions.

AI tools are increasingly outperforming humans in key tasks such as legal research, contract analysis, and drafting. As AI, blockchain, and algorithmic governance become central to legal processes, lawyers must acquire skills to collaborate with technologists, critically evaluate automated outputs, and oversee the ethical and practical dimensions of advanced technologies. A lawyer specializing in compliance, for instance, could be required to assess an AI-powered risk analysis tool to certify its outputs align with regulatory standards and ethical expectations.

Additionally, lawyers will need to understand how AI systems generate insights (an area where much remains unknown); how blockchain platforms execute smart contracts; and where algorithmic systems may introduce injustice, bias, or error. This foundational knowledge corresponds to the lower levels of Bloom's taxonomy, such as "remembering" the principles of AI and blockchain systems and "understanding" their functions and limitations. Mastery at the lower levels will provide the groundwork for higher-order competencies.

Lawyers will also refine and supervise AI systems, adjusting machine-learning models to meet specific legal standards and attain accountability and explainability. These responsibilities align with Bloom's higher-order skills: "applying" knowledge to refine AI systems for specific legal contexts, "analyzing" their outputs to identify potential biases, and "evaluating" the compliance of automated decisions with ethical and legal standards or the implications of these systems more generally. To illustrate, a legal team auditing an AI tool for discriminatory practices would engage in both analysis and evaluation, ensuring the system's recommendations are fair and legally sound. The ability to "create"—the taxonomy's apex—will emerge when lawyers collaborate with technologists to develop entirely new frameworks or tools that transform the legal system's functionality and inclusivity.

Lawyers will also guide organizations in responsibly deploying AI, mitigating risks associated with algorithmic decision-making, and fostering public trust. For instance, in a dispute resolution scenario involving an AI mediator, a lawyer might review the system's reasoning to ensure equitable outcomes. Likewise, the lawyer may request deeper explanations to enhance transparency and understanding. For students, immersive experiences—such as designing AI-enabled compliance monitoring systems, developing frameworks for automated contract negotiations, or participating in simulated AI-assisted due diligence exercises—would provide excellent preparation for real-world tasks.

Legal education must prepare students to understand both the power and limitations of AI systems: their superior speed, consistency, and computational ability, as well as their current shortcomings in areas requiring practical wisdom, value-sensitive reasoning, and contextual judgment. Lawyers will need to develop these complementary human capabilities to establish that AI systems remain aligned with societal values. Looking further ahead, law schools must also prepare graduates for the emergence of artificial general intelligence (AGI). With the advent of AGI, technological tools may exhibit impressive moral reasoning, creativity, and empathy, thereby fundamentally challenging our assumptions about the division between human and machine capabilities.

Human-Centric Skills

Superjustice envisions a legal ecosystem grounded in trust, inclusivity, and collaboration. While AI will redefine many technical and procedural aspects of the profession, human-centric skills will remain essential in building relationships, resolving disputes, connecting the citizenry with legal systems, and managing increasingly participatory legal frameworks. Lawyers will need to engage empathetically with diverse parties, advise clients, mediate conflicting perspectives, and ensure that both human and AI contributions advance fairness and equity.

As decentralized and community-driven governance models are incorporated into legal systems, lawyers' roles will shift toward managing complex interpersonal dynamics. For example, in a scenario involving an AI-assisted arbitration tool, a lawyer might mediate between community members to resolve disputes while maintaining transparent and comprehensible AI recommendations. In such cases, emotional intelligence and cultural competency will become critical skills, enabling lawyers to anticipate and address emotional undercurrents, cultural differences, conflicting worldviews, and interpersonal conflicts that AI systems may overlook. Negotiation skills will also evolve to include balancing human motivations with AI-driven insights and fostering resolutions that resonate with all stakeholders. If AGI materializes, technological tools could greatly boost these processes. They could suggest what fair negotiated settlements should look like, ensure that sharp play is transparently revealed, and design settlements that include protection mechanisms to address potential future opportunism and protect weaker parties.

These new roles align with the higher-order skills in Bloom's taxonomy. As we envisage it, lawyers will need to analyze the needs and motivations of communities and participants, evaluate diverse perspectives, and balance competing interests. They will also be expected to facilitate inclusive legal processes that integrate AI while preserving human agency and understanding. Consider, for example, community dispute resolution. Initially, lawyers might help design systems where AI handles logistics and preparation while professionals and communities retain control over sensitive decisions. As capabilities advance, AI tools will gradually assume more complex tasks. Potentially, this will culminate in a system where routine legal disputes are primarily resolved by AI legal agents negotiating on behalf of users, followed by AI arbitrators, with human oversight for exceptionally complex or sensitive cases.

Relatedly, future advances will require lawyers to navigate new ethical and relational complexities. Lawyers will promote trust in algorithmic processes while addressing concerns about accountability, algorithmic justice, and bias. In practice, this might involve explaining the rationale behind an AI's decision or recommendation in terms accessible to non-experts, safeguarding transparency and fairness. In the near term, lawyers will need to reconcile AI's efficiency with users' needs for understanding as they guide participatory legal processes.

We have noted that as AI systems advance, they may become more capable of exhibiting human-like qualities. The emergence of AI companions and "cozy tech"—technology designed to create comfort and escape real-world stresses—illustrates how AI developers are making AI tools more personalized and friendly.[16] Law students should be prepared for this reality through curricula that balance technical literacy with human skills, teaching them to critically evaluate AI-generated "empathy," identify situations where human intervention may remain essential, and develop distinctive interpersonal capabilities that complement AI systems. This preparation may ensure that future lawyers can create value in a landscape where routine emotional mediation may increasingly be handled by technology.

Developing human-centric skills will require significant curricular reforms. Legal education must emphasize emotional intelligence training, cross-cultural communication, and collaborative problem-solving. Immersive simulations, including VR and augmented reality tools, can provide practical exposure through mock mediations with AI platforms and participatory policymaking exercises. Equipped with these skills, lawyers will serve as trusted mediators and ethical supervisors, facilitating fair and human-centered systems.

[16] For an accessible and critical account see Kyle Chayka, "The Fantasy of Cozy Tech" *The New Yorker* (November 20, 2024) <newyorker.com/culture/infinite-scroll/the-fantasy-of-cozy-tech>. See also Petter Bae Brandtzaeg, Marita Skjuve, and Asbjørn Følstad, "My AI Friend: How Users of a Social Chatbot Understand Their Human–AI Friendship" (2022) 48(3) Human Communication Research 404; Yulia Sullivan, Serge Nyawa, and Samuel Fosso Wamba, "Combating Loneliness with Artificial Intelligence: An AI-Based Emotional Support Model" (2023) Hawaii International Conference on System Sciences <https://hdl.handle.net/10125/103173>.

Global Competencies

Since Superjustice will contribute to the evolution of a globally interconnected legal landscape, lawyers will need to develop skills that extend beyond national borders. Increasingly, AI-driven platforms will mediate cross-border legal transactions, harmonize multilingual systems, and navigate jurisdictional complexities in areas such as trade, data governance, and decentralized finance. Lawyers must therefore acquire competencies that combine technical, cultural, and legal adaptability, enabling them to operate effectively within this dynamic ecosystem.

Global systems will require lawyers to collaborate across linguistic, social, and jurisdictional divides. For instance, they might collaborate with technologists to design a multilingual AI platform that facilitates international trade disputes or provide guidance on compliance frameworks for global blockchain networks. These tasks will demand receptivity and agility, enabling lawyers to understand and respect diverse legal traditions while mediating between often conflicting regulatory priorities. A lawyer negotiating a cross-border data-sharing agreement, for example, must balance the stringent privacy standards of one jurisdiction with the more lenient requirements of another. AI tools will assist lawyers in understanding diverse customs, negotiating across international boundaries, and conveying nuanced ideas in multiple languages.

As with the previous sets of skills, Bloom's taxonomy provides a useful framework for structuring these competencies. Foundational skills will include "understanding" the principles of multilingual AI systems and cross-border legal frameworks. Intermediate applications may involve "analyzing" jurisdictional conflicts in decentralized governance or "evaluating" the economic and trade implications of global AI governance structures. Advanced competencies could focus on "creating" innovative solutions to bridge global-local divides, such as drafting AI-driven regulatory models that adapt to regional nuances while maintaining global coherence.

Global competencies will require lawyers to act as intermediaries between AI systems and the diverse populations they serve. In this intermediary role, lawyers will be expected to explain how decisions or recommendations are generated by AI systems, ensuring accessibility and transparency for users from different cultural and linguistic backgrounds. In practice, this might involve clarifying the logic behind an AI arbitrator's decision, in a culturally sensitive manner and in multilingual contexts, or addressing concerns about algorithmic fairness when outcomes seem to favor certain jurisdictions over others.

Meta-Skills

The move toward Superjustice will require lawyers to develop meta-skills that transcend technical, human-centric, and global competencies. These meta-skills would include adaptive problem-solving, ethical leadership, resilience, and self-awareness.

Such capabilities would help lawyers shift from being passive recipients and users of AI systems to active shapers of the evolution of legal technology.

Meta-skills like adaptability will be essential as AI tools and decentralized platforms reshape legal practice. Lawyers must be prepared to operate in environments where technology evolves rapidly and unpredictably. Recent developments in AI simulation, such as creating digital replicas of human personalities with 85 percent accuracy through two-hour interviews, point to transformative applications in legal prediction.[17] In practice, future case analysis tools might test arguments on AI-generated simulations of judges and juries. This will require lawyers to carefully evaluate both the technological capabilities and ethical implications of such systems.

Ethical leadership will become equally indispensable as lawyers confront the profound moral dilemmas arising from emergent technologies. The growing autonomy of AI systems may lead to scenarios where machine decisions are difficult to interpret or contest. Consider an AI system that denies a loan application from a marginalized borrower, where the decision is based on complex data correlations that likely justify the denial. Or imagine an AI-powered medical triage system that prioritizes patients using algorithms whose reasoning cannot be fully explained to the patients or their caregivers. Finally, imagine an AI system denying professional licenses based on behavioral patterns it detects in video interviews, without providing detailed justifications for its decisions. Lawyers will need to engage in nuanced reasoning to determine when to trust AI decisions and when to retain human oversight.

As AI progresses and begins to exhibit behaviors resembling moral judgment or creativity, lawyers will need to confront difficult ethical questions about balancing reliance on machine-guided decisions versus maintaining human control. For instance, suppose an AI system recommends child custody arrangements based on its analysis of family dynamics. Should its recommendations carry the same weight as a human mediator's judgment? Or imagine an AI system that evaluates end-of-life care decisions in hospitals, weighing factors like quality of life, resource allocation, and family preferences. Should such profound moral decisions ever be delegated to AI? Could patients authorize AI tools, potentially trained on their own personality profiles and value systems, to make healthcare decisions on their behalf? What would that entail for human agency and society more generally? Lawyers will need to guide organizations and international bodies in establishing justice and accountability standards for AI systems, requiring a careful deliberation of what exactly those terms mean in an automated world.

While Bloom's taxonomy provides a conceptual framework for developing meta-skills, its principles must be brought to life through experiential learning. Law schools will need to translate theoretical stages into actionable training, ensuring that students develop the analytical and practical skills necessary for ethical leadership. Accordingly, law schools must introduce experiential learning opportunities that simulate real-world

[17] For a review see James O'Donnell, "AI Can Now Create a Replica of Your Personality" *MIT Technology Review* (November 20, 2024) <www.technologyreview.com/2024/11/20/1107100/ai-can-now-create-a-replica-of-your-personality/>. It seems plausible that future iterations of such tools will become even more accurate and useful.

dilemmas. For instance, a bespoke education program could introduce students to foundational ethical theories ("understanding"), guide them in evaluating the implications of AI decision-making in criminal justice ("evaluating"), and culminate with a simulated negotiation in which students must reconcile diverse stakeholder perspectives to create a fair and actionable policy ("creating").

Building on these foundations, practical training will be key to embedding these competencies. For example, students could lead mock international negotiations involving AI-driven trade systems, where they balance efficiency with addressing diverse cultural and jurisdictional concerns. Similarly, interdisciplinary workshops could pair law students with technologists and ethicists to co-create solutions for emerging ethical challenges, such as the use of predictive policing algorithms; AI-driven sentencing tools; AI-powered hiring systems that screen candidates using behavioral analytics and social media profiles; or AI-driven employee assessment systems that use behavioral data to track productivity, predict performance, and make promotion and termination decisions.

Ultimately, meta-skills will position lawyers as both innovators and mediators in technology-driven legal systems. They will guide society in understanding and trusting advanced legal systems, while ensuring that these technologies remain aligned with principles of fairness, inclusivity, and human dignity. As lawyers adapt to these roles, they will serve as interpreters between powerful AI systems and the communities they affect, promoting a legal profession that thrives in a rapidly evolving world.

Innovative Training Models

The skills outlined thus far—spanning technical literacy, human-centric capabilities, global competencies, and meta-skills—are essential for future lawyers. Cultivating these diverse and higher-order competencies will require a transformation not only in *what* legal education seeks but also in *how* it is delivered. Traditional methods, rooted in lectures and case analysis, will no longer suffice. Instead, innovative training models should combine cutting-edge tools with interdisciplinary, immersive learning experiences.

To operationalize these approaches, we draw on Transformative Learning Theory, which offers a valuable framework for reimagining legal education. Developed by Jack Mezirow, this theory emphasizes critical reflection, allowing learners to reassess and challenge their existing assumptions, leading to profound shifts in perspective.[18] Applied to legal education, we argue that innovative training models must encourage critical thinking and expand students' understanding of the law. We propose that approaches such as AI-enhanced simulations, real-world problem-solving clinics, and adaptive learning technologies should provide students with opportunities to engage with the moral and societal implications of emerging legal technologies. In the ensuing

[18] See Jack Mezirow, *Transformative Dimensions of Adult Learning* (Jossey-Bass 1991).

discussion, we explore three key dimensions of this paradigm shift: training contexts, teaching strategies, and alignment with professional and societal expectations.

The Where: Training Contexts

Immersive and dynamic training environments will be fundamental to future legal education. We consider here four key contexts: law-tech labs, simulations and VR tools, social impact clinics, and non-traditional pathways. These settings provide innovative spaces where theoretical knowledge meets practical application.

Law-tech labs will become vital hubs for innovation, connecting students, faculty, and industry professionals. These labs will encourage collaboration across diverse fields, including law, computer science, psychology, linguistics, and public policy. In one scenario, students might partner with linguists and AI researchers to develop multilingual legal assistance platforms that adapt to cultural nuances. Law students may collaborate with behavioral scientists and user experience (UX) designers to create AI-powered simulation tools. These tools could help predict jury responses to different argument strategies based on demographic and psychographic factors. In facilitating such initiatives, law-tech labs will cultivate a new generation of legal innovators who bridge the gap between technological capability and societal needs.

Immersive simulations and VR tools could enhance legal education by offering students hands-on experience with scenarios they are likely to encounter in practice. Beyond standard litigation or negotiation exercises, VR courtrooms could challenge students with multi-jurisdictional hearings where they must simultaneously engage with judges, witnesses, and interpreters appearing as holograms from different locations, while managing real-time AI-powered legal research and analytics. Such experiences would connect theoretical education to practical application, allowing students to experiment and learn in low-risk, high-fidelity environments.

Social impact clinics could serve as a cornerstone for human-centric legal training, providing students with opportunities to engage directly with underserved communities. These clinics could emphasize empathy, equity, and inclusivity, demonstrating how advanced technologies can be leveraged to benefit marginalized communities and the public good. For example, students might assist remote communities through AI-driven legal aid platforms, providing support in navigating housing disputes or immigration claims. Alternatively, they could facilitate citizen-driven policymaking projects, helping shape local regulations through participatory governance models. Through these clinics, students would learn to pair technological efficiency with human-centered legal practice.

As Superjustice systems evolve, training opportunities must extend beyond traditional degree programs to include non-lawyers who interact with AI-driven legal tools ("non-traditional pathways"). Certification programs and modular learning pathways could offer scalable, flexible options for equipping paralegals, community advocates, and mid-career professionals with specialized skills. For example, a certification program might train paralegals in AI-powered, multilingual legal document analysis or train community legal workers to help elderly clients interact with automated legal service platforms. Similarly, stackable credentials could allow learners to specialize in areas like digital identity verification or automated compliance monitoring.

The Methods: Teaching Strategies

Adapting legal education to Superjustice systems requires innovative pedagogy. By adopting a dialogical approach to teaching, law professors can challenge students' assumptions and encourage critical reflection. This would reshape how future lawyers perceive their role and promote open-mindedness. In the following section, we examine four specific aspects of learning that shed light on novel teaching strategies.

Technology-Enhanced Learning

AI-driven tools will play a central role in tailoring education to individual needs, thereby facilitating scalable and personalized learning experiences. As noted, adaptive learning platforms could analyze student performance in real time, identifying knowledge gaps and suggesting customized interventions and resources. The design of these tools should align closely with the principles of Transformative Learning Theory. They should prompt students to confront and reassess their understanding of legal concepts in dynamic, real-world contexts. Personalized learning would ensure that students go beyond absorbing information and leverage learning opportunities to reshape their knowledge of law and society more broadly.

Experiential Learning Models

Building on the principles explored in this chapter, the integration of theoretical knowledge and practical application through experiential learning emerges as a pillar of innovative legal training. Such exercises could also reflect Transformative Learning Theory, as they immerse students in scenarios that require active engagement and critical reflection. For instance, students might mediate complex environmental disputes, in which AI systems help model long-term impact scenarios, requiring students to balance multiple stakeholder interests, synthesize technical data, and craft creative solutions that transcend traditional legal remedies. These experiences should aim to challenge conventional perceptions of legal practice. They may thus prompt students to go beyond "thinking like a lawyer" and embrace a more holistic problem-solving approach, deviating from the traditional adversarial mindset.

Interdisciplinary Projects

As noted throughout this chapter, collaboration across disciplines is essential for preparing lawyers to navigate the multifaceted challenges of technology-driven legal systems. Interdisciplinary projects could bring together students from multiple domains to address complex legal and societal problems. For instance, law students might work with mental health professionals and UX designers to develop ethical guidelines for emotion-sensing AI in virtual legal proceedings. Alternatively, joint projects with urban planners and data scientists could focus on developing legal frameworks for smart city initiatives that protect privacy while promoting innovation. Such collaborations would provide law students with opportunities to gain insights into the technical, social, and ethical dimensions of modern legal challenges while challenging their preconceptions.

Lifelong Learning Programs

Education is not a finite process but an ongoing journey of growth and adaptation. As technology and legal systems constantly evolve, lifelong learning will become an integral part of legal education. Modular courses and certifications, possibly in collaboration with law societies and bar associations, could offer flexible opportunities for professionals to continuously adapt to changing demands. Online certification programs tailored for mid-career professionals would further democratize access to specialized knowledge, delivering relevant legal expertise over time. Lifelong learning programs could embody Transformative Learning Theory by encouraging professionals to reflect regularly on their skills, roles, and assumptions, fostering a mindset of continuous improvement.

The Why: Professional and Societal Demands

The urgency for reforming legal education will continue to grow. Traditional programs have long faced critiques for their rigid structures, overemphasis on theoretical knowledge, low levels of student well-being, and inadequate preparation for the realities of practice. Superjustice amplifies this urgency by introducing challenges that existing educational frameworks are not designed to meet; lawyers must acquire technological fluency, cultivate agile competencies, and master human-centric skills.

Practical training models present a solution to these systemic gaps, beginning with one of the most pressing critiques: the disconnect between theory and practice. Lawtech labs, simulations, and social impact clinics could enable students to test their classroom learning against concrete legal problems. Equally significant is the potential of innovative training models to enhance access and inclusivity. Non-traditional pathways, such as modular certification programs, online courses, and stackable credentials, could address the barriers that often exclude underrepresented groups from traditional legal education. These pathways would broaden participation in the legal field and enrich it with diverse perspectives and experiences.

The broader impact of these reforms lies in their ability to future-proof graduates in times of constant change. Experiential learning and lifelong education programs could ensure that legal professionals remain adaptable and capable of acquiring new skills and knowledge as technological advances reshape their roles. This adaptability would greatly benefit the legal profession, which will increasingly depend on this new generation of professionals to lay the foundation for a more dynamic, human-centered, and community-driven legal system.

Challenges and Opportunities

The transformation of legal education is not without significant challenges. Institutions, faculty, and students will face barriers that could stall progress. Yet, these obstacles also present opportunities for innovation and equity. Addressing them with foresight will determine whether legal education can meet the realities of a fast-changing world and serve the society of tomorrow.

Law schools, like the legal profession itself, have traditionally emphasized stability and precedent over change and experimentation. While this approach has historically served important purposes, it poses challenges in an era of transformative technologies. Many institutions face structural barriers to innovation, as faculty members often lack the necessary support and resources to develop expertise in emerging topics. Traditional incentive structures also fail to reward curricular innovation, and budget constraints limit investment in new technologies and interdisciplinary programs. These challenges are particularly acute for institutions with constrained resources, potentially widening the gap between schools that can afford to implement AI-enhanced learning environments and collaborative platforms and those that cannot.

These problems require creative solutions. Faculty development programs, such as joint initiatives with computer science departments or tech providers, can close knowledge gaps and foster collaboration. Likewise, faculties should incentivize the development of new courses and invest in expanding expertise, despite the challenges posed by current academic reward systems. To address resource constraints, shared solutions like open-source learning platforms could democratize access to advanced training tools, allowing underfunded schools to remain competitive. For instance, a network of law schools might co-develop a suite of VR simulations accessible globally.

The central role of advanced technologies also risks widening existing inequities in legal education. Underfunded and rural institutions often lack access to tools like adaptive learning platforms or AI-driven legal databases, leaving their students at a disadvantage. Addressing these inequities requires systemic reforms. Governments, NGOs, and private organizations must collaborate to fund equitable access to legal technologies for students, particularly in underserved regions. Law schools should further emphasize inclusivity by integrating culturally responsive curricula and prioritizing the social justice dimensions of AI. For example, social impact clinics would be wise to pair students with marginalized communities, using AI-driven tools to address legal issues.

Adaptive learning platforms could intensify competition by providing detailed performance metrics, while the pace of technological change may leave students overwhelmed. Furthermore, the shift towards more automation and technology may entail scarcer opportunities for human interaction, a crucial component of one's well-being. This potential for isolation is particularly concerning in the context of legal education, as research shows that law students experience a reduction in well-being throughout their education.[19]

In response, law schools must adopt a holistic approach to student well-being. Collaborative learning models, wellness programs, and supportive mentorship (potentially augmented using new technologies) should be designed and implemented to create environments in which students thrive. Embedding well-being initiatives into curricula, such as mindfulness training, community volunteering, and resilience-building coursework, may support student well-being and contribute to long-term flourishing.

Ultimately, reforms must contend with a deeper question: What is the purpose of legal education? While this chapter emphasizes practice-readiness and societal impact, others rightly view it as a broader intellectual formation. Moreover, reform must guard against overreach. Expanding the curriculum too aggressively would risk displacing essential doctrinal training, exhausting students, and creating unrealistic expectations of law graduates. Balancing innovation with curricular restraint and breadth with pedagogical depth will be imperative in ensuring that reform enhances, rather than cannibalizes, legal education's core mission.

But the reinvention of legal education marks just the beginning. As the next chapter explores, the legal profession itself stands on the cusp of an even more dramatic transformation.

[19] See, for example, Kennon M Sheldon and Lawrence S Krieger, "Does Legal Education Have Undermining Effects on Law Students? Evaluating Changes in Motivation, Values, and Well-Being" (2004) 22(2) Behavioral Sciences & the Law 261; Kennon M Sheldon and Lawrence S Krieger, "Understanding the Negative Effects of Legal Education on Law Students: A Longitudinal Test of Self-Determination Theory" (2007) 33(6) Personality and Social Psychology Bulletin 883; Debra S Austin, "Positive Legal Education: Flourishing Law Students and Thriving Law Schools" (2016) 77 Maryland Law Review 649.

PART III

FUTURE DIRECTIONS AND CHALLENGES

8

The Future of Justice Work

Rebuilding the Ship of Justice

In the ancient writings of Plutarch, a timeless puzzle is posed: If the planks of a ship are replaced one by one until none of the original wood remains, is it still the same ship? Known as the Ship of Theseus, this paradox has puzzled philosophers for centuries, prompting debates about identity, continuity, and evolution. Does something remain fundamentally the same as it evolves, or can gradual and cumulative change create something entirely new?

Fast forward to 2040, and this question now looms over the courtroom—a space radically transformed by technology. In this future courtroom, lawyers collaborate with artificial intelligence (AI) systems that analyze and evaluate arguments, simulate processes, predict rulings, and offer strategic recommendations in real time. Legal professionals refine the AI's insights, sometimes aligning with its predictions, while at other times challenging its conclusions, to ensure ethical and contextual fairness or better comprehend and explain its outputs and decisions. As we replace the planks of legal practice with AI, will it still be the same ship of justice, or rather something entirely new?

At the heart of this potential courtroom of the future will be the hybrid human-AI judge. Equipped with unintrusive smart sensors (that surpass augmented reality glasses and voice-activated earpieces), the judge will seamlessly integrate empathy and ethical reasoning guided by the computational power and analytical and intuitive capabilities of AI tools. Machine-learning algorithms will flag patterns of bias in arguments or data. Multimodal AI will enable the integration of text, video, and audio evidence for comprehensive decision-making. Blockchain technology could underpin secure, immutable case records. Predictive analytics will provide likely rulings, while natural language processing tools will analyze courtroom dialogue, identify logical inconsistencies, and generate impartial summaries. Artificial general intelligence (AGI) will draft preliminary rulings, with judges generally expected to adopt them unless there are compelling reasons not to. Robots equipped with AI systems would assist in ensuring compliance, managing procedural tasks and monitoring courtroom performance, blending seamlessly into the ecosystem of justice delivery. Piece by piece, in the courtroom, in law firms, and in legal institutions, the legal system could be refashioned into something entirely new: faster, more precise, and deeply integrated with AI.

This vision is not science fiction but an accelerating reality. According to the Thomson Reuters Institute's 2024 Professionals Report ("the Report"), for example,

Superjustice. Samuel I. Becher and Benjamin Alarie, Oxford University Press.
 DOI: 10.1093/9780198991885.003.0012

79 percent of law firm respondents anticipate AI will have a high or transformational impact on their work within the next five years. Indeed, AI and voluminous data were the most cited trends of anticipated disruption. This surpassed concerns about skilled labor shortages, increased regulation, economic recession, geopolitical instability, and sustainability issues.[1] The remaining 21 percent of respondents who did not view AI as highly impactful may be underestimating the pace of change and thus risking obsolescence as AI continues to reshape the legal market.

The Report also reveals that professionals are increasingly optimistic about AI's potential to enhance productivity, foster innovation, and forge more fulfilling careers. Legal professionals are gradually realizing that AI is not simply a tool for efficiency. Instead, it is a driver of value creation, facilitating faster client responses, reducing errors, and enhancing decision-making. While professionals expect AI to take over routine tasks, they also anticipate a shift, not a reduction, in roles—with human skills like problem-solving, creativity, and adaptability remaining vital.

This chapter explores some of the profound changes AI may bring to the legal profession. First, we discuss how evolving roles will redefine what it means to be a legal professional, with lawyers engaging in new forms of work and developing specializations to meet the demands of an AI-driven system. Next, we turn to the judiciary, where AI-augmented processes and practices promise greater optimization but raise pressing concerns about judicial independence and the preservation of fundamental legal principles. We then analyze how legal business models will adapt, with innovations like value-based pricing and AI-enabled client services challenging traditional structures. Finally, we predict that professional regulation will also face a need for reform, with accrediting bodies and bar associations having to integrate AI literacy and ethical oversight into their remit.

Legal Roles Reimagined

With AI assuming increasingly complex roles, legal professionals must adapt to a landscape characterized by automation and collaboration. This evolution will require a redefinition of professional boundaries. In the short term, it will entail redefining expertise within a hybrid legal ecosystem, blending lawyers' ethical judgment and creative strategy with AI's analytical capabilities while frequently adopting machine-produced rulings and recommendations. As Chapter 5 explored, AI capabilities will continue to advance, and the division of labor between humans and machines will require continuous recalibration rather than a one-time settlement.

Current generative AI tools exemplify AI's transformative potential in legal research and drafting, though their applications are still developing. Large language models (LLMs) are already showing promise in performing research and document drafting,

[1] See Thomson Reuters Institute, "Future of Professionals Report 2024" *Thomson Reuters* (July 2024) <www.thomsonreuters.com/en/c/future-of-professionals.html>.

enabling lawyers to brainstorm and produce outlines and initial drafts in minutes. Similarly, lawyers are increasingly turning to AI tools to expedite document review, analyzing hundreds of pages and identifying key weaknesses in legal arguments within moments—tasks that would otherwise take hours to complete.[2]

These evolving roles are already taking shape, and productivity gains from AI tools are becoming increasingly apparent. A recent study found that reasoning models and retrieval-augmented generation (RAG) systems significantly improved both the speed and quality of legal work across a range of realistic tasks.[3] The study also found that each type of tool offers distinct strengths: Reasoning models excel in analytical reasoning and structuring arguments, while RAG systems enhance accuracy and reduce hallucinations by grounding outputs in legal sources. Notably, even modest user training improved participants' ability to effectively deploy these tools, underscoring the value of developing skills in refining, interpreting, and collaborating with AI-generated outputs.

Beyond current applications, the future holds even more transformative possibilities. We have already explored how AI agents could negotiate for users in disputes, and how AI arbitrators could resolve most of the remaining conflicts. Where trials are still necessary, there would be full automation of processes and real-time analytics during litigation. Advanced AI systems, coupled with virtual reality (VR) and augmented reality (AR) tools, could simulate entire trials, offering lawyers a chance to stress-test their arguments in virtual environments, while AI bots replicate the judge or the jury. These tools will not only enhance strategic decision-making but also provide new methods of client engagement, enabling individuals to visualize potential outcomes in unprecedented ways. As AI reshapes the legal landscape, access to legal information and self-help tools will proliferate and democratize, weakening the monopoly of the legal profession. Traditional roles will evolve, and entirely new ones will emerge.

This may manifest itself in specific ways. Lawyers will assert their expertise in areas where human judgment is indispensable, such as high-stakes negotiations or ethical dilemmas, while deferring to AI for routine or data-intensive tasks. This will create a collaborative professional dynamic that redefines traditional boundaries. For example, as AI tools increasingly handle sensitive client data, specialists in data privacy and cybersecurity will become crucial players in safeguarding confidentiality and preventing breaches.

In this context, we employ the umbrella term "justice architects" to describe legal professionals who strategically integrate, interact with, and oversee AI systems in legal practice. Justice architects will design and implement justice delivery by collaborating

[2] See Steve Lohr, "A.I. Is Coming for Lawyers, Again" *New York Times* (April 10, 2023) <www.nytimes.com/2023/04/10/technology/ai-is-coming-for-lawyers-again.html>.

[3] See Daniel Schwartz and others, "AI-Powered Lawyering: AI Reasoning Models, Retrieval Augmented Generation, and The Future of Legal Practice" *SSRN* (2025). Previous studies found mixed results and were more critical; see Varun Magesh and others, "Hallucination-Free? Assessing the Reliability of Leading AI Legal Research Tools" (2025) 22 Journal of Empirical Legal Studies 216.

with powerful AI systems to analyze arguments and simulate outcomes, evaluate and refine AI-generated insights, and explain AI conclusions to others. They will bridge technological capabilities with legal knowledge and principles, maintaining the essential human elements of justice in an AI-transformed legal system.

Justice architects will include AI auditors, AI intermediators, and legal engineers. AI auditors will specialize in analyzing algorithms for bias, transparency, and accountability, establishing themselves as key players in regulatory and professional settings. AI intermediators will serve as essential bridges between advanced AI tools and the legal system's stakeholders. They would focus on value alignment, ethical interpretation, and high-stakes normative decision-making, where human values remain contested and societal values can evolve. Finally, legal engineers would design, implement, refine, train, and maintain AI-driven systems, bridging the gap between technologists and legal practitioners.

Although AI's potential is vast, its integration into legal practice will also present significant challenges. While democratizing certain aspects of the law, AI tools could disproportionately benefit well-resourced firms and clients who can afford cutting-edge technologies. Meanwhile, smaller firms and underrepresented communities may struggle to access similar tools, thereby widening the justice gap. To address this challenge, public-interest initiatives and subsidized AI tools could ensure broader access to advanced technologies. As we show in this chapter, such interventions could transform AI from a potential divider into an equalizer in the legal system.

The Future of Judging

The promise of enhanced speed, efficiency, and accuracy has already begun to reshape judicial workflows. AI-powered platforms can identify relevant statutes and summarize arguments with precision, potentially reducing case backlogs and expediting resolutions. Machine-learning algorithms might also flag inconsistencies in evidence or identify patterns across similar cases, empowering judges to make faster and more informed decisions.

In September 2023, a British appellate judge, Lord Justice Colin Birss, made headlines for openly discussing his adoption of AI tools in drafting judicial opinions.[4] In describing his experience with generative AI, he noted:

> I asked ChatGPT, "Can you give me a summary of this area of law," and it gave me a paragraph. I know what the answer is because I was about to write a paragraph that said that, but it did it for me and I put it in my judgment. It's there and it's jolly useful.

[4] See Hibaq Farah, "Court of Appeals Judge Praises 'Jolly Useful' ChatGPT After Asking It for Legal Summary" *The Guardian* (September 15, 2023). Additional instances of judicial use of LLMs in other countries are documented in Juan David Gutierrez, "Judges and Magistrates in Peru and Mexico Have ChatGPT Fever" *Tech Policy Press* (April 19, 2023).

Based on his experience, Birss offered a straightforward yet compelling observation: "It is useful, and it will be used." Since then, many judges worldwide have acknowledged the significant potential of AI to enhance access to justice and judicial efficiency.[5]

For starters, judges could engage with AI systems as sophisticated interlocutors during private deliberations. These AI advisors would function as thinking partners, offering counterarguments, identifying potential blind spots, and pressure-testing judicial reasoning through simulated dialogues. After these collaborative deliberations, the AI interlocutor could then draft comprehensive rulings that reflect both the judge's conclusions and the reasoning developed during the exchange. Such a process would mark a shift from AI as a research tool to AI as an analytical companion in the judicial decision-making process itself.

AI tools could also act as a "virtual panel member" that offers insights grounded in world knowledge and large-scale data analysis. In this role, AI might simulate perspectives of underrepresented groups, provide insights into comparative cases in other jurisdictions (and languages), or analyze cases through specific legal frameworks, such as restorative justice or originalism. This could diversify deliberations, challenge conventional interpretations, and bring fresh insights to complex legal issues. Additionally, it could reduce judges' workload, potentially allowing fewer judges to preside over each case while maintaining thorough deliberation.

Naturally, judges may view AI with suspicion and be slow to adopt it. Research on AI adoption suggests that the style of AI explanations significantly impacts user trust.[6] Judges and court users tend to prefer explanations that employ comparative reasoning—outlining why a particular argument was preferred to another—rather than explanations that simply state conclusions. AI systems designed for the judiciary should therefore articulate not just what determination they reached but also why alternative interpretations were dismissed, mirroring the comparative reasoning process that characterizes effective legal argumentation.

Beyond assisting individual judges, AI has the potential to influence judicial structures—particularly in the way that multi-judge panels are composed and operate. The composition of panels can play a pivotal role in shaping outcomes, as judges bring their subjective perspectives, biases, and expertise to deliberations. However, this process is susceptible to manipulation and inconsistencies. For instance, assigning particular judges to specific cases can sway outcomes or create perceptions of bias. AI offers an opportunity to counter such concerns by acting as a neutral arbiter. Applying transparent and objective criteria, AI could ensure a fair distribution of judges to cases, reducing opportunities for undue influence. This innovation could be particularly

[5] See, for example, "Speech by the Master of the Rolls: The Digital Justice System—An Engine for Resolving Disputes" (May 1, 2025) <www.judiciary.uk/speech-by-the-master-of-the-rolls-the-digital-justice-system-an-engine-for-resolving-disputes/>; "Chief Justice Sundaresh Menon: Speech at the Singapore Judicial College 10th Anniversary Celebration" (May 26, 2025) <www.judiciary.gov.sg/news-and-resources/news/news-details/chief-justice-sundaresh-menon--speech-at-the-singapore-judicial-college-10th-anniversary-celebration>.

[6] See Julian De Freitas, "Why People Resist Embracing AI" *Harvard Business Review* (January–February 2025).

impactful in high-stakes or politically charged cases, where even the perception of bias could undermine trust in the judiciary.

AI's role could extend further to hybrid panels comprising both human judges and AI systems. Initially, AI might provide advisory opinions or identify potential biases during deliberations while leaving the ultimate decision to human judges. With further technological development and judicial experience, hybrid panels could help determine which types of cases are best suited for AI involvement in the substantive part of the proceedings. For example, data-heavy disputes may benefit from AI's computational competence, whereas cases requiring ethical judgment might require more human involvement. Feedback mechanisms and continuous assessment would facilitate ongoing refinement of AI integration.

Let us emphasize that AI presents far-reaching potential in mitigating the biases and organizational noise that can influence judicial decision-making, whether stemming from a judge's gender, race, personal background, unconscious preferences, or extraneous factors.[7] AI systems could review a judge's past rulings ("retrospective analysis") to identify patterns that might indicate bias. For example, AI could highlight disparities in sentencing based on demographic groups. Likewise, it could detect inconsistent application of legal principles among judges or panels across similar cases or on different days or times of the day.

Identifying these patterns would aid in assigning judges to cases. It would allow judges to reflect on their decisions and workflows, fostering greater awareness and encouraging adjustments to ensure consistency and fairness. For instance, judges could use this feedback in their day-to-day decision-making by revisiting case files flagged for inconsistencies or biases, consulting with peers to refine interpretations, and incorporating periodic self-assessments into their judicial routines to ensure continuous improvement. This type of review could also be institutionalized as part of performance evaluation systems, promoting accountability while respecting judicial independence.

In the longer term, real-time monitoring may offer another layer of noise and bias detection, focusing on how emotional, physical, or situational factors might unconsciously affect decision-making. AI-powered tools could seamlessly analyze a judge's body language, eye movement, tone of voice, pulse, or blood pressure during proceedings to identify signs of fatigue, stress, or frustration—factors known to impact judgment. For example, a judge experiencing heightened stress might unintentionally favor the party presenting a simpler, more easily understood argument.

[7] The literature here is fascinating. See, for example, Shai Danziger, Jonathan Levav, and Liora Avnaim-Pesso, "Extraneous Factors in Judicial Decisions" (2011) 108(17) Proceedings of the National Academy of Sciences 6889; Donald C Nugent, "Judicial Bias" (1994) 42 Cleveland State Law Review 1; Eric A Posner, "Does Political Bias in the Judiciary Matter: Implications of Judicial Bias Studies for Legal and Constitutional Reform" (2008) 75 The University of Chicago Law Review 853; Eyal Peer and Eyal Gamliel, "Heuristics and Biases in Judicial Decisions" (2013) 49 Court Review 114; Justin D Levinson, Mark W Bennett, and Koichi Hioki, "Judging Implicit Bias: A National Empirical Study of Judicial Stereotypes" (2017) 69 Florida Law Review 63; Doron Teichman and Eyal Zamir, "Judicial Decision-Making: A Behavioral Perspective" in Eyal Zamir and Doron Teichman (eds), *The Oxford Handbook of Behavioral Economics and the Law* (Oxford University Press 2014) 664–702.

AI systems could provide subtle alerts, signaling when a break or reevaluation might be beneficial. These monitoring capabilities could extend beyond judges to witnesses, attorneys, and other courtroom participants, offering judges additional insights with which to inform their assessments of credibility and argumentation. For instance, AI might detect patterns in a witness's physiological responses that suggest fatigue or uncertainty, or identify when an attorney's presentation tactics may unduly manipulate jurors through emotional appeals rather than reasoned persuasion. Of course, such measures must account for privacy concerns and judicial independence, and consider the potential impact of these mechanisms on the behavior of lawyers, jurors, judges, and witnesses in the courtroom.

In the case of multi-judge panels, AI could also offer innovative strategies to counter potential biases arising from group dynamics, such as groupthink or hierarchical influence. Groupthink occurs when dominant voices or ingrained hierarchies suppress alternative perspectives, resulting in less robust decision-making.[8] AI systems could monitor deliberations to ensure equitable participation among panel members, balancing speaking times and prompting reticent judges to share their viewpoints. Visual mapping tools may analyze the flow of discussions in real time, highlighting arguments that dominate or perspectives that are being neglected. For instance, a dashboard could display which legal principles have been thoroughly debated and which remain underexplored, allowing the panel to revisit overlooked points. It may also flag when group dynamics, rather than legal reasoning, appear to be driving judicial deliberations.

Judicial Clerks and the Future of Juries

As AI transforms judicial decision-making, its effects ripple outward, influencing the roles of clerks and juries. Traditionally, clerks have shouldered responsibilities such as legal research, memo drafting, and schedule management—tasks that AI systems can handle with remarkable efficiency. Automation will allow clerks to shift their focus toward higher-order functions, such as crafting nuanced legal analyses or assisting in developing innovative arguments tailored to complex cases. Moreover, clerks could act as intermediaries between judges and AI systems, interpreting algorithmic outputs, verifying their accuracy, and explaining the decisions or outputs generated by these systems. With judges typically being older and clerks younger, clerks are well positioned to bridge generational divides, helping judges understand and adopt emerging technologies that may not initially feel intuitive.

This evolution raises ethical considerations. Historically, judges have borne ultimate responsibility for their decisions, even if clerks play a substantial role in shaping outcomes.[9] The introduction of AI adds a new layer of complexity: AI tools will assist

[8] See, for example, Wendy L Martinek, "Judges as Members of Small Groups" in David E Klein and Gregory Mitchell (eds), *The Psychology of Judicial Decision Making* (Oxford University Press 2010) 73.

[9] See David Crump, "Law Clerks: Their Roles and Relationships with Their Judges" (1985) 69 Judicature 236.

clerks, who, in turn, will assist judges. This multi-tiered system complicates accountability as the boundaries between human and algorithmic contributions become increasingly blurred.

AI also has the potential to considerably reform the functioning of juries, alleviating the challenges associated with traditional jury service while enhancing deliberative processes. One seemingly provocative possibility is the use of AI to replicate personas, allowing virtual jurors to stand in for human counterparts in certain cases or proceedings. These AI-driven personas, modeled on demographic and experiential data, could be used to simulate diverse perspectives, ensuring that the jury pool remains representative.

With traditional juries, AI could also provide real-time monitoring to detect issues such as disengagement, confusion, or bias among jurors, enabling judicial intervention and guidance when necessary. For example, if AI detects that a juror struggles with comprehending evidence, the judge could pause proceedings to address the issue or provide clarification. Furthermore, AI could assist jurors during deliberation, highlighting key evidence, presenting counterfactual scenarios, and ensuring that all voices are heard within the group. Here too, such tools could foster more informed and balanced decisions, partly by reducing the impact of dominant personalities or groupthink.

Addressing Skepticism

Although the technology is already impressive, the incorporation of AI raises questions about how and when these tools should be deployed. At the time of writing, research suggests that public perception of fairness varies depending on the stage of judicial decision-making at which AI is applied.[10] People may accept AI's use in information acquisition (such as gathering and organizing legal data), but are less comfortable with algorithmic adjudication in later stages, like decision selection and implementation. For now, public trust hinges on maintaining a balance between AI's capabilities and the human touch. While public perception is likely to evolve with time, the judiciary must carefully navigate these perceptions to ensure AI systems do not undermine confidence in judicial outcomes.

Skepticism could stem from a combination of factors. First, there is a sense that AI may not be capable of the nuanced judgment required in more complex legal decisions or those with serious social policy dimensions. Algorithmic decision-making can feel impersonal, particularly in cases involving emotional stakes. Moreover, AI systems may be trained on data that reflects past biases in the legal system and beyond, thereby perpetuating them. Concerns about explainability exacerbate these perceptions. Unlike human judges, current AI systems often operate as "black boxes," producing outputs that are difficult to trace back to their underlying reasoning.

[10] See Dovilė Barysė and Roee Sarel, "Algorithms in the Court: Does it Matter Which Part of the Judicial Decision-Making Is Automated?" (2024) 32(1) Artificial Intelligence and Law 117.

To address these challenges, the judiciary must proactively foster public understanding of AI's role. Transparency initiatives, such as publishing guidelines on how AI systems are used in courtrooms and providing clear explanations of their outputs, are essential. Judges and other legal professionals, such as AI intermediators, can also endeavor to demystify AI's competencies and limitations for litigants and the public at large. For example, courts could incorporate public demonstrations of AI tools in action, illustrating how they assist judges without undermining judicial discretion, independence, and autonomy.

Efforts to humanize AI interactions may also help. For instance, hybrid models in which judges actively engage with AI systems and explain their reasoning alongside algorithmic insights could bolster public trust. This approach aligns with a "judge-in-the-loop" paradigm, emphasizing the partnership between human judgment and computational power rather than full automation. It also responds to the concern that granting AI a central role in legal decisions would dehumanize justice.[11]

As the judiciary increasingly embraces AI, robust training programs for judges and legal professionals will be indispensable. These programs must go beyond basic technology instruction to cover AI's implications, limitations, and potential biases. Among other things, judges must understand how an AI system's design and training data can influence its outputs and learn to identify when biases might skew results.

Judicial education should also focus on fostering adaptability and resilience. As AI tools evolve, judges will need to continually update their skills to remain effective. Programs emphasizing continuous learning, supported by bar associations and legal institutions, can help embed this adaptability into the judiciary's culture. In time, AI systems will likely be developed to assist judges with their education.

Notably, many of the challenges we discuss here are transitional. AI tools will likely improve with time and demonstrate increasingly sophisticated legal reasoning. As part of this improvement, AI systems could accurately interpret precedent, identify subtle legal distinctions, and produce persuasive reasoning. The balance of public trust and judicial practice may shift, and judges might find themselves regularly deferring to AI recommendations in routine cases.

Overall, these developments would not necessarily represent the "dehumanization of justice." Rather, they would represent a new paradigm where human judicial oversight focuses increasingly on novel questions, value judgments, and cases with significant social policy implications. Indeed, the exceptional cases may become those where judges override well-reasoned AI positions.

Law Firms of the Future

Traditionally, legal professionals adopted a focus on individual expertise, autonomy, and ethics, viewing themselves as professionals with specialized knowledge and a

[11] See Andreia Martinho, "Surveying Judges about Artificial Intelligence: Profession, Judicial Adjudication, and Legal Principles" (2024) AI & Society 1.

duty to clients. This traditional focus, however, can create friction with the need for rapid adaptation to technological advancements, prompting a critical reassessment of how these values align with evolving market demands and innovation pressures. At the same time, globalization and market forces may push law firms to prioritize optimization, scalability, and hierarchical management.[12] These transactional objectives will also encourage law firms to adopt AI tools. Accordingly, law firms will need to develop environments in which professional autonomy and bureaucratic efficiencies coexist.

Resource scarcity will significantly impact the interplay between these vectors, acting as a powerful catalyst for organizational innovation within law firms. Competition and escalating client demand for cost-effective solutions, coupled with the limited capacity of traditional workflows, are likely to drive the adoption of AI-enabled business models. Firms seeking to scale their services to meet client expectations will turn to AI tools for enhanced productivity and speed, in an effort to maintain their competitiveness.

This resource-driven push for innovation could reshape the traditional pyramid structure of law firms. Historically, firms relied on a broad base of junior associates to handle routine tasks, under the guidance of senior associates and partners. However, as AI automates tasks like document review, discovery, and basic drafting, the economic need for this pyramid structure diminishes. Firms are therefore likely to evolve from "pyramids to pillars," adopting more specialized vertical structures where teams of experts in distinct domains collaborate as equals rather than existing in rigid hierarchies.

This pillar model will feature specialized teams for client relationships, complex legal strategy, technological implementation, and AI oversight. Each of these teams will be valued for their distinct expertise, rather than their position in a hierarchical ladder. This structural transformation will challenge traditional career progression. It will give rise to diverse new roles, while prompting firms to adopt flatter, more collaborative project-based structures to enhance agility and responsiveness to client needs.[13]

Importantly, the automation of routine tasks presents a significant challenge for professional development. Traditionally, junior lawyers cut their teeth on document review, due diligence, and basic drafting. Such tasks served as an apprenticeship of sorts: while routine, they provided crucial exposure to legal concepts, market dynamics, and client operations, allowing young lawyers to build professional capabilities before handling more complex matters. The automation of these foundational experiences could create a skills gap, potentially leaving the next generation of lawyers without the granular understanding that historically underpinned legal expertise.

To address this challenge, firms might adopt two complementary approaches. First, they could develop structured AI-augmented apprenticeships where junior

[12] Compare with James Faulconbridge and Daniel Muzio, "Organizational Professionalism in Globalizing Law Firms" (2008) 22(1) Work, Employment & Society 7.

[13] See Anthony E Davis, "The Future of Law Firms (and Lawyers) in the Age of Artificial Intelligence" (2020) 16(1) Revista Direito GV e1945.

lawyers work alongside AI systems rather than being replaced by them. This collaborative model would require young lawyers to review, validate, and refine AI outputs, developing critical analysis skills while gaining exposure to a broader range of cases than traditional manual review would allow. Second, firms could institute rotation programs, whereby junior lawyers participate in cross-functional teams focused on complex matters. AI would then handle routine aspects while senior lawyers provide intensive mentoring. This approach would accelerate professional development by exposing junior lawyers to high-level work earlier in their careers while ensuring they understand the fundamental processes through their oversight of AI systems. Looking ahead, legal AI tools may evolve and become increasingly intuitive and self-explanatory. Advanced systems could provide real-time guidance and personalized feedback to junior lawyers, accelerating skill development far exceeding traditional methods.

Beyond training and hierarchy, the incorporation of AI into legal practice will reshape the ways that law firms deliver services, interact with clients, and structure their business models. As AI streamlines legal processes and reduces costs, traditional billing models like the billable hour may become obsolete. Firms may adapt by embracing value-based pricing, emphasizing outcomes, innovation, and the unique human expertise lawyers bring to strategic challenges.

Clients, increasingly aware of AI's ability to automate routine tasks, will probably be disinclined to pay premium fees for work largely performed by machines. This shift will push firms to adopt pricing models that reflect the value of their services rather than the time spent delivering them. For example, firms might charge flat fees for routine tasks like contract reviews or adopt contingency-based pricing for high-stakes litigation, where compensation depends on the outcome. To thrive in this evolving landscape, firms will need to redefine how they articulate value. Lawyers will need to shift focus from time logs to the tangible benefits they provide, such as strategic insight, innovative problem-solving, and the ability to negotiate deals or navigate complex interpersonal challenges. These skills, deeply rooted in human judgment, are more likely to remain critical differentiators even as AI continues to advance—at least for now.

New Service Delivery Models

As AI redefines how services are offered, law firms will adopt innovative business models that prioritize convenience, accessibility, and client engagement. Among probable trends, three key ones stand out: subscription-based services, integrated client portals, and hybrid collaboration platforms. We discuss each of them in turn.

Subscription-based legal services will find increasing traction. As discussed in Chapter 6, clients would require individualized attention. Firms could respond by offering tiered subscriptions, possibly granting clients ongoing access to legal advice, compliance monitoring, or document drafting services. For instance, a small business might subscribe to a legal service plan that includes unlimited contract reviews, regulatory updates, and monthly consultations, all supported by AI-driven tools. This approach would generate stable revenue streams for firms while offering clients greater financial predictability and peace of mind.

Integrated client portals could become the norm for law firms, serving as platforms on which clients can access documents, track case progress, and communicate with their legal teams. Advanced portals will integrate AI features, such as automated updates or predictive analytics, enabling clients to monitor potential risks or opportunities in real time. For instance, a corporate client might receive AI-generated alerts about new regulatory changes affecting their industry, along with tailored recommendations for compliance.

Hybrid human-AI collaboration platforms could integrate tools for brainstorming, drafting, and analysis, allowing lawyers and clients to work together seamlessly. For example, a lawyer might use an AI assistant during a client consultation to instantly draft preliminary agreements or simulate potential litigation outcomes. Similarly, an AI-powered interface might guide a client through initial document preparation, asking targeted questions to gather information before passing the data to a lawyer for review.

AI-enhanced legal process outsourcing (LPO) is another potential development in how firms will operate. Traditional LPO has focused on cost reduction through labor arbitrage. Next-generation LPO, however, will leverage AI to create global, specialized service networks. These networks will combine AI-powered tools with distributed expertise across jurisdictions, enabling firms to scale operations efficiently while maintaining quality control. For instance, a firm might utilize AI-enhanced LPO centers for specialized services like multilingual contract review or cross-border due diligence. AI systems could coordinate workflows, ensure consistency across teams, and even perform a considerable part of the work. Table 8.1 summarizes this envisioned evolution.

Table 8.1 Legal Practice Model Comparison

	Traditional Models	AI-Driven Models
Billing Model	Hourly billing	Value-based pricing
Service Delivery	Case-by-case engagement	Subscription services, integrated client portals
Technology Use	Legal research, practice management, document production, communication, cybersecurity	AI for research, drafting, analytics, predictions; virtual and augmented reality tools
Client Engagement	Reactive, personalized	Proactive, data-driven, and collaborative
LPO	Cost reduction through labor arbitrage	Global, specialized service networks
Scalability	Limited by human resources and technological capabilities	Enhanced through automation and AI

Empowering Small Firms: AI as an Equalizer

Prestigious firms often act as early adopters of innovation, leveraging their legitimacy to normalize new practices within the profession.[14] This dynamic, emphasized in institutional theory, is likely to influence the adoption of AI-driven business models and service delivery approaches. However, unlike many previous innovations, which required substantial capital investment and infrastructure, AI technologies are fundamentally reshaping traditional competitive dynamics. Through cloud-based solutions, alternative service delivery models, and digital-first approaches, small and medium-sized firms can quickly follow and even leapfrog larger competitors.

Small and medium-sized practices could use technology to compete with larger firms in complex matters. A small firm may, for instance, use AI to handle discovery for a complex case, producing results comparable to those of a large team at a major firm. More generally, AI tools could amplify market segmentation by enabling deeper specialization and supporting niche expertise, empowering smaller firms to serve broader client bases.[15]

Legal practice management software—comprehensive platforms that integrate multiple legal technologies—can further enhance the capabilities of small firms. Such software could consolidate tools for case management, billing, document drafting, and client communication into a single interface, streamlining operations and reducing costs. For example, AI-driven practice management software might automatically analyze incoming cases, prioritize them based on complexity, and generate tailored client engagement strategies. Current platforms, such as Harvey, Clio, and PracticePanther, are already moving in this direction.

Taken together, AI can empower smaller firms—operating with fewer associates or paralegals—to handle a greater range of matters efficiently and independently. By automating tasks such as research, drafting, and document analysis, AI frees up limited human resources while enabling faster and more precise outputs. These gains extend beyond efficiency: AI tools can help small firms improve clarity, precision, and accessibility in client-facing communications. Small firms leveraging such tools will deliver high-quality services, possibly comparable to those of larger competitors.

Finally, small firms, more often embedded in underserved communities, can leverage AI to reduce overhead and offer lower-cost services to previously underrepresented clients. To be sure, challenges such as technological literacy gaps, financial barriers, and regulatory constraints may prevent smaller firms from fully realizing these advancements without targeted support and infrastructure. Thus, public-interest initiatives could develop open-access AI tools to supplement community-oriented practices and pro bono providers. This would help ensure that marginalized populations adequately benefit from AI advancements in legal services.

[14] See Peter D Sherer and Kyungmook Lee, "Institutional Change in Large Law Firms: A Resource Dependency and Institutional Perspective" (2002) 45(1) Academy Management Journal 102.

[15] See Luis Garicano and Thomas N Hubbard, "Specialization, Firms, and Markets: The Division of Labor Within and Between Law Firms" (2009) 25(2) Journal of Law, Economics, & Organization 339.

Client Relationships and Access to Legal Services

Technological capabilities will shift not only what firms offer but what clients demand. Beyond faster turnaround times and transparent pricing, clients will expect more personalized partnerships, regular communication, and greater involvement in their legal matters. The democratization of legal technology will further challenge traditional hierarchical lawyer–client relationships. As clients gain tools and knowledge to actively participate in legal solutions, they will demand more control over their legal issues.

Advanced AI tools will thus transform the nature of client engagement. As noted, firms will deploy AI-powered client portals offering real-time updates, interactive dashboards, and customized legal information, while intelligent chatbots provide 24/7 basic support. These technologies will enable proactive client service through predictive analytics that anticipate legal needs, monitor relevant regulatory changes, and automatically alert clients to developments affecting their interests.

Beyond service delivery, AI will enhance firms' ability to understand and strengthen client relationships. Sentiment analysis and communication pattern recognition will help firms gauge client satisfaction and anticipate needs. At the same time, automated learning modules and visualization tools will empower clients to better understand their legal matters. These capabilities, coupled with relationship analytics tracking engagement quality and value, will help firms transition from reactive service providers to proactive strategic partners who can demonstrate and measure their impact on client success.

Interestingly, firms could carefully calibrate the degree of anthropomorphization in legal AI tools. While human-like qualities often boost adoption, clients discussing sensitive personal matters might actually prefer an AI that is distinctly *not* human-like. In such situations, a less anthropomorphized AI can be perceived as less judgmental, potentially making clients more comfortable with its neutral interface than they would be with more human-like AI systems, or even with actual humans. This is particularly relevant in contexts where the AI's inherent "distant and cold" nature could be an advantage, not a feature requiring fixing.

Ultimately, the technological empowerment of clients could blur the line between legal advice and self-service. Clients with access to advanced AI tools and AI assistants might negotiate with third parties and perform legal tasks independently. This shift will compel firms to reassess their client engagement models and tools, focusing on areas where human expertise, judgment, and interpersonal skills remain indispensable, particularly in complex or high-stakes matters where a deep understanding of the client is crucial.

Adapting to the Future: A Blueprint for Legal Business Models

As client relationships and service delivery models evolve, law firms must develop comprehensive adaptation strategies. A key imperative will be investing in AI literacy across the organization. Law firms must train their lawyers and staff to employ AI tools effectively while minimizing risks such as overreliance on automation. Such training should include workshops on AI fundamentals, hands-on sessions for tool usage, and case studies demonstrating AI's applications in legal workflows. Successful firms will embrace hybrid human-AI models that foster collaboration, both internally and with clients.

Despite its potential, the adoption of AI-enabled business models faces significant structural and operational hurdles. Traditional law firm structures—built around lawyer human capital and partnership models with their lawyer-centric compensation and promotion systems—may need fundamental reimagining. Indeed, law firm partnerships often struggle with the agility needed for innovation. Moreover, integrating multidisciplinary teams with diverse technical expertise will likely create tension within traditional hierarchies and promotion pathways. Regulatory frameworks that restrict non-lawyer ownership further compound these challenges by limiting access to external capital and technical talent.[16]

As technology becomes increasingly central to legal practice, firms must establish robust institutional frameworks and governance structures for AI use. This includes developing clear protocols for AI-driven decision-making, implementing systematic strategies for detecting and mitigating bias, and establishing accountability mechanisms for AI-assisted outcomes. Firms should also proactively engage with regulatory bodies to shape responsible AI practices, invest in regular ethical audits of their AI systems, and establish internal oversight committees to monitor compliance.

Beyond governance structures, law firms will need to develop a culture of ethical technology use. This should include both ethics training programs and formal channels for lawyers to address technological concerns. As part of this environment, firms, rather than just individual lawyers, should be held accountable for the ethical use of AI. Notably, factors like transparency, explainability, and accountability will be central enablers of trust.[17]

Professional Organizations and Regulation

The challenge of uncovering and addressing historical misconduct was powerfully demonstrated in 2024, when the Alameda County District Attorney's office confronted decades of discriminatory jury selection practices.[18] The discovery of prosecutors' notes documenting the systematic exclusion of Jewish and Black jurors from death

[16] Some jurisdictions, like the United Kingdom, allow non-lawyer ownership in legal service providers. This provides UK firms with greater flexibility in adopting new models vis-à-vis their American counterparts, potentially giving them a competitive advantage. See John Armour and Mari Sako, "AI-Enabled Business Models in Legal Services: From Traditional Law Firms to Next-Generation Law Companies?" (2020) 7(1) Journal of Professions and Organization 27. The discussion in this paragraph draws on this article. Interestingly, however, KPMG has recently been approved to practice law in the state of Arizona. See Justin Henry and Roy Storm, "KPMG Wins Approval to Launch First US Law Firm for Big Four" *Bloomberg Law* (February 28, 2025).

[17] See, for example, Ni Xu and Kung-Jeng Wang, "Adopting Robot Lawyer? The Extending Artificial Intelligence Robot Lawyer Technology Acceptance Model for Legal Industry by an Exploratory Study" (2021) 27(5) Journal of Management & Organization 867.

[18] Jennifer Gonnerman, "An Investigation Into How Prosecutors Picked Death-Penalty Juries" *New Yorker* (November 18, 2024).

penalty cases sparked a comprehensive review of capital convictions. The office's new leadership took the unprecedented step of publicly acknowledging the misconduct and working to remedy past wrongs, even when doing so meant overturning long-standing convictions.

This case demonstrates the persistent failure of traditional oversight mechanisms; the discriminatory practices had continued long after being explicitly banned by the Supreme Court. It also illustrates the potential for reform under leadership committed to transparency and accountability. It furthermore highlights the critical importance of document retention and systematic review procedures, as the misconduct only came to light through the chance discovery of prosecutors' notes that previous administrations had failed to examine. This and other cases underscore the need to harness advanced technological tools as more robust and systematic oversight mechanisms that can prevent, detect, and address misconduct before it becomes entrenched over decades.

Relatedly, professional organizations such as bar associations and law societies will reach a crossroads as AI transforms the legal profession. These institutions, which have historically been tasked with upholding ethical and professional standards, must now grapple with challenges posed by rapid technological change. Should bar associations mandate AI literacy as part of their licensure process? Should they accredit an AI-focused "Legal Engineering" certification? To what extent should professional organizations hold firms accountable for the use of AI, as opposed to focusing solely on individual practitioners? And should bar associations create separate disciplinary frameworks for AI-assisted malpractice versus purely human error?

As these regulatory questions grow more complex, the duties and liabilities of legal professionals may undergo a profound transformation. AI itself could become a tool for detecting and flagging professional misconduct. Applied this way, AI tools could create a new ecosystem of compliance-focused AI applications dedicated to monitoring and enforcing professional standards.

Evolving Professional Standards

As AI becomes central to legal practice, professional organizations may need to revise accreditation standards to include technological competencies. Future bar exams could test candidates on AI literacy, requiring them to demonstrate the ability to evaluate AI tools, interpret algorithmic outputs, and understand legal tech platforms. For example, candidates may be required to optimize legal research prompts, comparing the efficiency and accuracy of different querying approaches across various types of prompts and AI tools.

Beyond accreditation, professional organizations will also need to reconsider licensing requirements. The boundaries of what constitutes the "practice of law" are becoming increasingly blurred as AI tools take on roles once reserved for licensed professionals. Bar associations will face the challenge of determining whether activities like

Table 8.2 Tiered Licensing Framework

	Description	Payment Models	Typical Providers	Examples
Tier 1: Minimal oversight	Exempted or lightly regulated tools	Free or subsidized; focused on access to justice	Nonprofit, community, or government	Eviction defense tools, employment rights bots
Tier 2: Little oversight	Low-risk, automated tools operating independently	Free or low-cost subscription	Open-source, nonprofit, or government	Basic wills, small claims forms, mundane tax paperwork
Tier 3: Medium oversight	Moderate complexity; Shared human-AI responsibility	Low- to mid-range subscription fees	Nonprofit, private sector, or government	AI-assisted research; compliance monitoring
Tier 4: Considerable oversight	High-stakes legal services	Premium fee-for-service models	Private sector, possibly nonprofit	Litigation strategy, settlement modeling
Tier 5: Strong oversight	AI apps for sensitive uses	Premium fees	Private sector	Sentencing, jury selection

drafting contracts or offering basic legal advice using AI bots fall within their purview. One potential approach would be to develop a tiered licensing system that acknowledges different levels of AI-augmented legal service provision. On this basis, certain AI-powered legal services could operate under limited licenses or supervised exemptions, with specific considerations for the type of service provider and payment model.

For example, at one end of the spectrum, nonprofit- or government-developed tools offering free legal assistance might qualify for less stringent oversight, given their focus on expanding access to justice. At the other end of the spectrum, private-sector tools or subscription-based platforms offering advanced capabilities for mid- or high-complexity matters would face more robust regulatory requirements. These tiers, calibrated to factors such as payment models, risk profiles, and service provider types, could bridge the access-to-justice gap while preserving professional oversight.[19] Table 8.2 outlines a potential framework for this tiered licensing system.

Given the pace of AI development, static educational requirements will no longer suffice, and bar associations will need to implement dynamic continuing professional development (CPD) programs to keep lawyers up to date. A CPD module might include topics such as "AI-Assisted Litigation Strategy," "Advanced Legal Research Optimization: Maximizing AI Research Tools," "Predictive Analytics in Case Assessment and Strategy Development," or "Bias Mitigation in Legal AI Systems."

[19] The model would require further nuance and analysis, accounting for multiple factors such as user privacy, cybersecurity measures, externalities, and public policy.

Professional organizations could partner with technology companies to offer cutting-edge training while ensuring alignment with professional values.

Training initiatives should not remain confined within national boundaries. In the long run, AI's cross-border nature may drive harmonization of professional standards at an international level. A shared certification for "AI in Law," recognized across jurisdictions, could become the norm, reducing friction in cross-border legal practices. If this materializes, a multinational firm might engage lawyers certified in a globally standardized AI competency framework to ensure consistency across its offices. Admittedly, such initiatives would require unprecedented cooperation between professional organizations worldwide, possibly offering an opportunity to redefine the role of bar associations in a globalized legal market.

While the initiatives described thus far represent potential regulatory responses, it is important to recognize that market forces will likely drive much of the change, regardless of formal professional standards. Client demands for efficiency, cost-effectiveness, and technological sophistication are already reshaping legal practice ahead of regulatory guidance. Law firms adopting advanced AI capabilities will establish competitive advantages, creating de facto industry standards that professional bodies will eventually codify rather than create. Bar associations and regulators may find themselves in a responsive rather than directive position, documenting and formalizing practices that have already been established through market competition. The most successful adaptation strategy may be to observe where client preferences and market forces are heading and proactively develop the skills and systems that will be valuable in the future.

Despite the likelihood that market forces will drive much of this evolution, we must remain vigilant about a significant historical challenge: the traditional tendency of self-regulating professions, particularly law, to resist innovations that threaten established professional interests.[20] Bar associations have frequently opposed innovations, including independent paralegals, multidisciplinary practices, and non-lawyer investment in legal service providers. In doing so, they often invoked consumer protection rhetoric to mask protectionist motives. These historical patterns suggest that uncritically entrusting bar associations with primary oversight of AI implementation risks stifling precisely the innovations that could most effectively democratize legal access.

To mitigate this risk, any framework for evolving professional standards must include multidisciplinary and multi-stakeholder regulatory bodies. These should comprise not just legal professionals but also technologists, access to justice advocates, and public representatives. This approach could benefit from evidence-based regulatory

[20] See, for example, Deborah L Rhode, "Professionalism in Perspective: Alternative Approaches to Nonlawyer Practice" (1996) 22 NYU Review of Law & Social Change 701; Jacqueline M Nolan-Haley, "Lawyers, Non-Lawyers and Mediation: Rethinking the Professional Monopoly from a Problem-Solving Perspective" (2002) 7 Harvard Negotiation Law Review 235; Gillian K Hadfield, "Legal Infrastructure and the New Economy" (2012) 8(1) I/S: Journal of Law & Policy for the Information Society 1.

sandboxes. Such sandboxes could incorporate outcome metrics focused on public benefit, transparency requirements that document reasoning for restricting new service models, and independent audits of regulatory decisions, thereby identifying patterns of unwarranted protectionism.

Regulatory Innovation

The rise of AI-enabled legal services may justify new oversight frameworks that go beyond traditional regulation. Here, regulation could require AI tools used in legal contexts to pass audits for fairness, accuracy, explainability, and transparency.[21] For instance, regulators might need to review an AI-powered sentencing tool to ensure it does not produce discriminatory outputs. This type of monitoring could mirror existing standards for human lawyers while introducing standards unique to AI, such as explainability and algorithmic accountability.

Nevertheless, implementing such oversight frameworks would present significant operational challenges. Auditing AI systems requires specialized expertise that many regulatory bodies currently lack.[22] The dynamic nature of AI systems, which often evolve through continuous learning, makes point-in-time audits potentially insufficient or quickly outdated. Moreover, the complexity and black-box nature of AI tools, frequently combining multiple algorithms and data sources, could complicate the assessment of fairness and accuracy.

Oversight frameworks also raise practical questions about resource allocation. Who bears the cost of regular audits? How frequently should they occur? What constitutes an acceptable level of algorithmic transparency when proprietary technology is involved? Can reputation markets effectively signal quality and reduce the need for formal oversight? Additionally, the global nature of AI development may create jurisdictional challenges. Tools and frameworks developed in one jurisdiction might be deployed in another with different regulatory standards. These practical obstacles suggest that, while enhanced oversight is vital, its implementation will require careful consideration of resource constraints, technical feasibility, and international coordination.

Beyond these operational challenges lies an even more fundamental tension between fostering innovation and maintaining core professional values. Innovative AI tools, such as predictive analytics for case outcomes or simulations of judicial and jury

[21] On the importance of these aspects in the context of AI integration into law see, for example, Said Gulyamov and others, "Adapting Legal Systems to the Development of Artificial Intelligence: Solving the Global Problem of AI in Judicial Processes" (2023) 1(4) International Journal of Cyber Law 4; Richard M Re, "Artificial Authorship and Judicial Opinions" (2024) 92(6) George Washington Law Review 1558; Barysė and Sarel, "Algorithms in the Court"; Martinho, "Surveying Judges about Artificial Intelligence".

[22] For a similar point concerning regulatory and legislative entities more generally see, for example, Shmuel I Becher, "Unintended Consequences and the Design of Consumer Protection Legislation" (2018) 93 Tulane Law Review 105.

decision-making, promise unprecedented efficiency and sophistication. Nonetheless, they could also inadvertently undermine principles like impartiality, due process, and confidentiality. Consider an AI tool for jury selection: While it may enhance trial strategy, its predictions could perpetuate historical discrimination patterns or undermine the principle of representative juries. Alternatively, consider an AI system for evaluating settlement offers. While such a tool might expedite negotiations, its risk calculations could prioritize financial metrics over less quantifiable aspects of justice and client interests.

Another important question is whether legal technology companies and developers should face oversight equivalent to that of law firms—or even stricter. For instance, a company offering an AI platform for contract review might be required to disclose its training data, provide ongoing updates for compliance, and submit to regular audits by regulatory bodies. Alternatively, robust self-regulation and industry standards may work in tandem with other monitoring tools or perhaps make them superfluous altogether.

That said, imposing stringent licensing requirements on technology companies could have unintended consequences for the legal tech ecosystem. Heavy-handed regulation might stifle innovation by creating prohibitive compliance costs for startups and smaller developers, effectively raising barriers to market entry and entrenching the dominance of established players. Moreover, technology companies and large or global law firms faced with burdensome oversight might relocate their operations to more permissive jurisdictions while serving other markets remotely. This regulatory arbitrage could create a "race to the bottom," whereby companies gravitate toward jurisdictions with minimal oversight.[23]

Enforcement presents additional practical challenges. Unlike traditional law firms, which are bound by geographic jurisdictions and supervised by the profession, online AI platforms and tools operate across borders, making meaningful oversight difficult without unprecedented international coordination. Hence, a more nuanced approach might involve creating incentive structures that encourage responsible innovation rather than imposing rigid regulatory frameworks that risk driving innovation underground or offshore.

While comprehensive licensing may prove challenging, certain fundamental principles, such as transparency, could facilitate monitoring by regulators, policymakers, and researchers.[24] Critics may argue that excessive transparency requirements could

[23] This, of course, is a well-known concern more generally, which the literature critically discusses in various contexts. See Richard L Revesz, "Rehabilitating Interstate Competition: Rethinking the Race-to-the-Bottom Rationale for Federal Environmental Regulation" (1992) 67 New York University Law Review 1210; John D Wilson, "Capital Mobility and Environmental Standards: Is There a Theoretical Basis for a Race to the Bottom?" in Jagdish Bhagwati and Robert E Hudec (eds), *Fair Trade and Harmonization: Prerequisites for Free Trade* (MIT Press 1996) 427; Alvin K Klevorick, "The Race to the Bottom in a Federal System: Lessons from the World of Trade Policy" (1996) 14(2) Yale Law & Policy Review 177.

[24] On the promise and limitations of transparency more generally see Archon Fung, Mary Graham, and David Weil, *Full Disclosure: The Perils and Promise of Transparency* (Cambridge University Press 2007).

enable "algorithmic witch hunts," in which isolated errors become magnified through public scrutiny, subjecting AI tools to harsher standards than human lawyers. However, this risk is outweighed by both the need for proper oversight and the substantial benefits AI systems deliver. If AI legal tools genuinely improve access to justice, reduce costs, and enhance outcomes, transparent evaluation should ultimately reveal these positive impacts, alongside any shortcomings. Truly beneficial technologies should be able to withstand scrutiny while maintaining public trust through openness.[25] The solution, therefore, lies not in less transparency but in developing nuanced evaluation frameworks that distinguish between systematic bias and isolated mistakes.

In summary, professional organizations and regulators must embrace adaptability while preserving the fundamental values of the legal profession. Success will require balancing multiple imperatives: facilitating reputation markets, protecting the public, enabling innovation, promoting access to justice, and maintaining professional standards. This balance will be dynamic rather than static, requiring ongoing dialogue between stakeholders and regular reassessment of regulatory frameworks as AI capabilities continue to evolve.

Leadership and Balance

Regulation provides a framework for addressing some AI-related challenges. Yet, it is leadership within the legal profession that will determine whether these innovations align with justice, equity, and public trust. As this chapter established, leaders must balance fostering innovation with safeguarding core legal principles. This is especially critical as the public simultaneously shows growing interest in and skepticism toward AI's role in justice delivery. Legal leaders are well positioned to emphasize the benefits of AI while addressing valid concerns. For example, courts, legal institutions, or professional bodies could host public forums, release case studies, or disseminate short educational videos showcasing responsible AI use. In their efforts, professional organizations and firm leaders must ensure that trust remains central to AI adoption.[26]

With time, society will adapt. Powerful AI will become seamlessly integrated into all aspects of the legal profession (and everyday lives). Its profound impact on legal

[25] This is not to say, however, that Superjustice should be oblivious to possible AI failures. Quite to the contrary, it is essential to prepare for these failures and prevent them from becoming crises. For possible mitigating measures drawn from crises management see Julian De Freitas, "Don't Let an AI Failure Harm Your Brand" *Harvard Business Review* (July–August 2025).

[26] See, for example, Xin Li, Traci J Hess, and Joseph S Valacich, "Why Do We Trust New Technology? A Study of Initial Trust Formation with Organizational Information Systems" (2008) 17(1) The Journal of Strategic Information Systems 39; Lorenz Graf-Vlachy, Katharina Buhtz, and Andreas König, "Social Influence in Technology Adoption: Taking Stock and Moving Forward" (2018) 68 Management Review Quarterly 37. For a seminal discussion of social capital, trust, and societal cohesion more generally see Robert D Putnam, *Bowling Alone: The Collapse and Revival of American Community* (Simon & Schuster 2000).

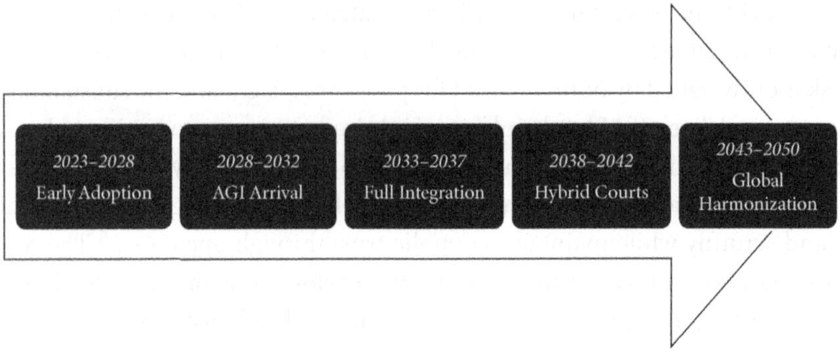

Figure 8.1 AI Integration Timeline

institutions and the roles of legal and paralegal professionals will mark the dawn of a new era. But as Figure 8.1 (optimistically) envisages, the journey toward this transformation will be lengthy, bumpy, and multi-phased. The challenge is immense, but so too is the opportunity that comes with the move toward Superjustice.

9

CRISPR-J in the Age of Superjustice

Precision and Transformation in Law

In 2012, genetic engineering made a significant leap forward with the discovery of CRISPR, a tool that functions like molecular scissors to edit DNA with remarkable precision and ease. CRISPR—short for Clustered Regularly Interspaced Short Palindromic Repeats—has transformed genetics by making gene editing faster, cheaper, and more accurate than ever before. Scientists can now precisely correct harmful mutations that cause human diseases, produce crops and livestock that are more resilient to climate change, and develop new biological materials and clean energy solutions.[1] This groundbreaking technology earned its pioneers, Emmanuelle Charpentier and Jennifer Doudna, the Nobel Prize in Chemistry in 2020, cementing CRISPR's place as one of the most significant scientific advancements of our time.

Imagine applying this level of precision and sophistication to the legal system. What if we could identify and "edit" dysfunctional legal processes and inefficient legal and regulatory frameworks with similar accuracy, tailoring solutions to specific contexts? As readers of this book will already appreciate, Superjustice provides a path forward by integrating artificial intelligence (AI) and data-driven tools to enhance precision, efficiency, and inclusivity in legal systems. CRISPR-J, the design framework introduced in this chapter, builds on this foundation through six core principles: Cost-effectiveness, Rapidity, Inclusivity, Smartness, Predictiveness, and Resilience. This chapter introduces CRISPR-J and applies it to specific legal domains and challenges.

Despite the differences between genetic editing and transforming legal systems, the analogy between CRISPR (in genetics) and Superjustice (in law) runs deep. Just as CRISPR enables precise genetic modification, Superjustice uses data and powerful AI to diagnose and address specific deficiencies in the law. In their respective fields, CRISPR (biology) and CRISPR-J (law) exemplify precision and customization, advancing tailored solutions that move beyond one-size-fits-all approaches.

CRISPR-J, the legal system design framework that embodies the values of Superjustice, is conceptually inspired by CRISPR in genetics. CRISPR's success in

[1] Jennifer A Doudna and Emmanuelle Charpentier, "The New Frontier of Genome Engineering with CRISPR-Cas9" (2014) 346(6213) Science 1258096; Luisa Bortesi and Rainer Fischer, "The CRISPR/Cas9 System for Plant Genome Editing and Beyond" (2015) 33(1) Biotechnology Advances 41; Rodolphe Barrangou and Jennifer A Doudna, "Applications of CRISPR Technologies in Research and Beyond" (2016) 34(9) Nature Biotechnology 933.

Superjustice. Samuel I. Becher and Benjamin Alarie, Oxford University Press.
 DOI: 10.1093/9780198991885.003.0013

genetics lies in its targeted intervention: It alters specific genes to tackle problems while leaving the organism's overall structure intact. Similarly, CRISPR-J targets specific dysfunctions in legal systems, like judicial backlogs, slow procedures, or inconsistent rulings.

Both CRISPR and CRISPR-J signal a transformational shift in their respective domains. They contest traditional boundaries, prompting fresh debates and suggesting innovative approaches to long-standing problems. CRISPR has reimagined the way we approach genetic disorders and agriculture, while CRISPR-J will operationalize Superjustice's goal to make legal systems more responsive, inclusive, and adaptive. Such transformations spark debates about unintended consequences, access inequities, and the limits of scientific intervention. They thus necessitate interdisciplinary collaboration: between biology and ethics in the case of CRISPR, and between law, ethics, and technology in the case of CRISPR-J.

The remainder of this chapter systematically explores CRISPR-J through its six basic principles of Cost-effectiveness, Rapidity, Inclusivity, Smartness, Predictiveness, and Resilience.[2] Table 9.1 summarizes these principles.

We next use concrete case studies to demonstrate how the principles of CRISPR-J translate into practical advancements, better-informed legal discourse, and specific solutions. Each of the following case studies serves as a standalone illustration of the potential of CRISPR-J. From making vague legal standards more inclusive and personalizing legal rules to modernizing monitoring, enforcement, and compliance, CRISPR-J offers a framework for precise, adaptive, and context-sensitive legal reform. The case studies also demonstrate that, despite its potential, CRISPR-J is not a panacea: It requires careful implementation to avoid negative unintended consequences, such as reinforcing existing biases, creating new inequities, or introducing inconsistencies and uncertainties.

Table 9.1 CRISPR-J Basic Principles

	Principle	Descriptor
C	Cost-effectiveness	Optimizing resources to make justice more accessible and affordable
R	Rapidity	Swiftly resolving legal issues through accelerated, streamlined processes and AI-driven efficiencies
I	Inclusivity	Integrating and considering diverse perspectives and cultural contexts
S	Smartness	Leveraging powerful AI to harness data and deliver precise responses and data-driven insights
P	Predictiveness	Anticipating needs and legal trends, to address potential disputes or gaps and reduce friction proactively
R	Resilience	Adapting to evolving societal and technological changes while maintaining fairness and reliability

[2] In the ensuing discussions, we capitalize these terms to emphasize their link to CRISPR Justice.

CRISPR-J: Preventing WEIRD Legal Norms

As we explained in Chapter 2, the law often employs vague legal norms that are not well-defined and are left for further judicial development and interpretation. These legal norms, commonly referred to as "standards," offer the flexibility to accommodate a wide range of circumstances *ex ante* but depend on judicial discretion to determine their precise meaning *ex post*. Standards are prevalent in many legal domains and include terms such as "reasonable," "fair," "acceptable," "good faith," and "best efforts." While standards provide adaptability, they frequently lack the clarity needed to guide behavior effectively, leaving individuals and organizations uncertain about what conduct will meet legal expectations and survive legal scrutiny.

The Reasonable WEIRD Person

The "reasonable person" and its close siblings feature in many legal domains, including tort law, contract law, consumer law, criminal law, and employment law. In consumer law, for example, the concept of the "average" or "reasonable" consumer is a key benchmark, shaping everything from misleading advertising cases to product liability. But who exactly is this "reasonable" person or "average" consumer? Courts and legislators seem to envision someone well-informed, observant, and circumspect. But look behind this legal construct and you will often find what psychology terms a WEIRD character: Western, Educated, Industrialized, Rich, and Democratic.

The WEIRD problem in psychology challenges the universality of findings that are predominantly based on Western subjects.[3] This raises concerns about the overrepresentation of specific cultural traits in shaping global legal standards and assumptions. WEIRD populations are frequently outliers and may exhibit unique characteristics or behaviors in various respects, including visual perception, fairness, cooperation, and decision-making.

The claim that the law is disproportionately based on a WEIRD standard could have profound implications for reform. Take the realm of consumer protection law. While consumer protection law employs universal standards, these standards often embed particular cultural assumptions about rationality, decision-making, and behavior. The result is a supposedly universal standard that reflects narrow cultural assumptions, failing to capture the rich diversity of consumer behaviors and norms.

For instance, courts often apply Western-centric interpretations of what constitutes deception in cases involving misleading advertising, presuming a relatively informed, confident, and autonomous decision-maker. Famously, the European Court

[3] "The Weirdest People in the World?" (2010) 33(2)–(3) Behavioral & Brain Sciences 61. See also Mostafa Salari Rad, Alison Jane Martingano, and Jeremy Ginges. "Toward a Psychology of Homo Sapiens: Making Psychological Science More Representative of the Human Population" (2018) 115(45) Proceedings of the National Academy of Sciences 11401.

of Justice's decision in *Gut Springenheide* (C–210/96) established that the benchmark is an "average consumer who is reasonably well-informed and reasonably observant and circumspect." This standard, while seemingly objective, presumes Western levels of education and modes of information processing and decision-making. Even when scholars criticize the standard, they all too often rely on WEIRD research.[4]

Research on cultural differences in cognition between Eastern and Western populations suggests fundamentally divergent approaches to reasoning and perception, challenging core assumptions about how individuals process information and make decisions.[5] Likewise, individualistic versus collectivistic cultural orientations may shape choices and judgments in ways rarely acknowledged by Western consumer protection frameworks. Indeed, the problem of applying a universal (Western) standard of an imaginary "reasonable consumer" could manifest itself in various ways. Courts and regulators often fail to account for how cultural practices influence attention to warnings and disclosures, shape assumptions about risks and fairness, and affect the importance people attribute to the fine print. Hence, even well-intentioned consumer protection measures can inadvertently disadvantage communities whose behavior patterns differ from the presumed norm.

The discussion about integrating diverse cultural perspectives into the "reasonable person" standard raises a fundamental question about how reasonableness itself is defined. To begin with, there is a tension between the subjective and objective understanding of a "reasonable" person. Legal scholars have long debated whether reasonableness should be understood normatively (as a standard of ideal behavior), or positively (as reflecting typical behavior in a given context).[6] This debate has significant implications for the incorporation of cultural diversity into legal standards. A purely normative approach risks imposing a single, potentially WEIRD-centric vision of ideal behavior on diverse communities. Conversely, a strictly positive approach, while seemingly more inclusive, could lead to the acceptance of harmful, careless, or counterproductive practices simply because they are prevalent within a particular culture.

Empirical research demonstrates that perceptions about what is "reasonable" or "average" are not formed exclusively on the basis of either statistical averages or prescriptive ideals.[7] Instead, they incorporate both descriptive and normative elements. This finding, in turn, challenges the assumption that the "reasonable consumer" or "reasonable person" standard reflects typical or ideal behavior. The inherent WEIRD bias within legal standards underscores that the "reasonable person" test, while aiming

[4] See, for example, Rossella Incardona and Cristina Poncibò, "The Average Consumer, the Unfair Commercial Practices Directive, and the Cognitive Revolution" (2007) 30(1) Journal of Consumer Policy 21.

[5] See Richard Nisbett, *The Geography of Thought: How Asians and Westerners Think Differently . . . and Why* (Simon & Schuster 2010).

[6] See, for example, Alan D Miller and Ronen Perry, "The Reasonable Person" (2012) 87 New York University Law Review 323. For a detailed and nuanced analysis of this standard see generally Mayo Moran, *Rethinking The Reasonable Person: An Egalitarian Reconstruction of the Objective Standard* (Oxford University Press 2003).

[7] See Kevin P Tobia, "How People Judge What is Reasonable" (2018) 70 Alabama Law Review 293.

for objectivity, inevitably incorporates subjective judgments about what constitutes reasonable behavior.[8]

CRISPR-J Reasonable

CRISPR-J could help make the reasonableness standard more democratic, representative, and nuanced by balancing subjective and objective elements. On the one hand, its decentralized data collection system would incorporate subjective community perspectives, enabling diverse cultural contexts to inform the standard. On the other hand, AI-powered data-driven bias detection would mitigate the risks of fragmentation, inconsistencies, and systemic biases. Integrating these complementary approaches, CRISPR-J would create a dynamic hybrid framework that respects individual and cultural differences while maintaining consistent legal principles.

Though this approach would not eliminate subjectivity, it would ensure that diverse perspectives are systematically accounted for. Rather than simply averaging subjective viewpoints or imposing a supposedly objective standard, CRISPR-J would promote intersubjective meaning-making,[9] co-creating legal concepts like "reasonableness" through the interaction of different viewpoints. This approach neither fragments into cultural relativism nor defaults to monolithic WEIRD assumptions. Instead, it cultivates a richer, shared understanding that transcends any single viewpoint, while remaining sensitive to cultural subtleties.

Therefore, in practical terms, CRISPR-J would offer two complementary interventions to "edit" the dysfunctional element of the "reasonable" or "average" standard in consumer law. First, it would enable systematic data-driven approaches to understand how different communities actually interpret and respond to commercial practices.[10] Using AI-powered platforms, communities could contribute their perspectives on particular cases and engage with other cultural viewpoints, collectively negotiating interpretations of commercial practices across different domains. In the context of advertisements, for example, instead of assuming a fixed, abstract "average consumer," CRISPR-J would help courts determine what a reasonable consumer, specifically targeted by the advertisement, should understand. In doing so, it would balance cultural nuance with the need for consistent and fair thresholds for both consumers and businesses.

Second, CRISPR-J would deploy AI and data analytics to prevent systemic bias in legal decision-making. Here, real-time bias detection tools could flag decisions that

[8] See Mayo Moran, "The Reasonable Person: A Conceptual Biography in Comparative Perspective" (2010) 14 Lewis & Clark Law Review 1233.

[9] See Jürgen Habermas, *Between Facts and Norms* (MIT Press 1996); Margaret Gilbert, *On Social Fact* (Princeton University Press 1989).

[10] In many cases, robust observational data—tracking how diverse consumers interact with products, advertisements, and disclosures across cultures—may suffice to identify patterns of understanding and misunderstanding. However, observational data sometimes reveals ambiguities or practices with deep cultural significance that behavior alone cannot explain. This may be particularly valuable in cases like financial services marketed to religious communities with specific prohibitions, or health products with culturally specific claims.

may reflect WEIRD assumptions. To supplement these tools, cultural context databases and elaborated AI-generated worldview models would help courts understand varying consumer cultures.

Such a dual focus—acknowledging subjectivity, while striving for objectivity and bias detection—would better reflect a sophisticated understanding of the reasonable person standard. It would challenge the dominance of WEIRD-centric assumptions, demonstrating how technological tools can make the application of legal standards more equitable and culturally sensitive. The result will be a more inclusive approach to consumer law that maintains its protective function while acknowledging and respecting diverse communities.

In all, this approach exemplifies CRISPR-J principles. It is Cost-effective, because it uses technology to gather and analyze diverse perspectives efficiently. It is Rapid since it enables real-time feedback and adaptation. It is inherently Inclusive, as it allows for previously marginalized voices to be heard. It is Smart in the sense that it uses AI to detect patterns and prevent bias. It is also Predictive, as it anticipates how different communities might interpret commercial practices. Finally, it is Resilient because it creates adaptive standards that evolve with societal needs.

Critiques and Counterarguments

Critics might argue that introducing cultural diversity into legal standards risks further undermining legal certainty and predictable enforcement. After all, businesses need clear guidelines to operate effectively within and across jurisdictions. According to this line of reasoning, the traditional "reasonable consumer" standard, despite its WEIRD-centric limitations, provides some kind of consistent benchmark, albeit somewhat imprecise. Adding cultural nuance to the vague notion of a "reasonable" or "average" consumer, the argument goes, will further muddy the legal landscape and encourage litigation.

We reject this argument, which presents a false dichotomy between cultural sensitivity and legal certainty. The move towards culturally informed standards does not necessitate a decline in legal certainty. In fact, when legal frameworks incorporate data and more accurate models of the worldviews behind actual behavior, they can become more predictable, not less. History offers instructive examples of integrating diverse perspectives into legal frameworks, notably through the evolution of international arbitration standards. Arbitration harmonizes differing legal traditions, bridging civil and common law systems, to achieve predictable outcomes across cultural and legal contexts. Allowing parties to tailor procedural rules and apply neutral legal principles demonstrates how fairness and predictability can coexist, even in systems that take diversity seriously.[11]

[11] See Philippe Fouchard and Berthold Goldman, *Fouchard, Gaillard, Goldman on International Commercial Arbitration* (Kluwer 1999); Julian DM Lew and Loukas A Mistelis, *Comparative International Commercial Arbitration* (Wolters Kluwer 2003). See also more generally Jan Paulsson, *The Idea of Arbitration* (Oxford University Press 2013).

In fact, CRISPR-J's data-driven approach can lead to more concrete and empirically grounded guidance for businesses. Modern computational systems can analyze vast datasets of consumer interactions, legal decisions, and cultural practices to identify patterns in how different communities respond to information, interpret commercial communications, engage with marketplace practices, and make decisions. Machine-learning algorithms can map these varying data points across cultural contexts while maintaining consistent underlying principles. For example, an AI system might recognize that, while the fundamental concept of "misleading advertising" remains constant, the specific elements that constitute deception vary systematically across cultural groups. This feature would facilitate the creation of dynamic standards that adapt to cultural context without sacrificing legal clarity.

Building on this vision, companies could move away from speculating about notions such as the "reasonable consumer" and instead access detailed, data-driven insights about their prospective clients' expectations, worldviews, behavioral patterns, and understanding. In its ideal form, the system could flag potential cultural misunderstandings before they lead to injustices or legal disputes, allowing businesses to adjust their practices proactively while maintaining compliance across diverse markets. If anything, clinging to artificially uniform standards systematically disadvantages certain communities and undermines the goals these standards were meant to serve.

A Three-Pronged System

Having outlined a conceptual dual focus that balances subjective inclusivity and objective bias detection, we can now translate these ideas into a practical, three-pronged implementation framework. The system we describe next provides concrete tools for gathering diverse insights, detecting WEIRD-centric assumptions, and dynamically integrating cultural contexts into legal decision-making. The technical implementation of these culturally aware standards would rely on three interconnected systems: (1) setting baselines, (2) identifying gaps (broadly defined to include mismatches, biases, questionable assumptions, or inefficiencies), and (3) resolving the identified gaps.

Setting baselines

A decentralized, distributed data collection platform would enable communities to contribute structured feedback through natural language interfaces and standardized protocols. This platform could use advanced natural language processing to identify cultural patterns in how different communities interpret commercial communications, categorize consumer expectations, and map varying assumptions about fairness and deception. The system would then leverage data and input to suggest a model of the community's prevailing worldview.

Identifying gaps

A neural network-based bias detection system could continuously monitor legal decisions and regulatory frameworks for potential gaps between the application of the law and the worldview models of the parties involved (or the relevant stakeholders). In our specific context, the focus could be on WEIRD-centric assumptions. Here, the system would be trained on diverse datasets that include Western and non-Western legal traditions, cultural anthropology research, and documented cases of cultural misunderstanding in commercial and legal contexts. When analyzing a legal dispute or proposed regulation, the system would identify specific language, reasoning patterns, or assumptions that may reflect cultural bias.

Resolving gaps

A dynamic cultural context database would synthesize these inputs with existing legal frameworks. The database would not simply catalog different cultural interpretations. Instead, it would use algorithms to map relationships between cultural contexts, legal principles, and commercial practices. This would allow the system to generate specific, actionable guidance that maintains legal consistency while accommodating cultural variation. For instance, when evaluating a potentially misleading advertisement, the system would provide a detailed analysis of how different cultural groups might interpret specific claims or presentations, while maintaining consistent underlying principles about consumer protection.

The implementation framework would follow a graduated approach. Initially, these tools could be deployed in advisory capacities within existing legal structures. At a later stage, their role could gradually expand based on demonstrated effectiveness and iterative feedback. This would enable the careful validation of the system's accuracy and fairness, thereby building trust among stakeholders. Likewise, regular audits would ensure the systems remain current with evolving cultural practices and maintain appropriate sensitivity to cultural nuances.

A significant challenge would be determining which cultural context to apply to specific individuals or communities. Critics might argue that attempting to match parties with particular cultural frameworks risks problematic profiling based on perceived racial, ethnic, or national characteristics. This could reinforce stereotypes, reduce individuals to essentialist cultural categories, and ignore the complex, hybrid identities many people navigate in an interconnected world. The very act of categorizing people by cultural context—whether by algorithm or human decision-maker—potentially undermines the inclusivity the system aims to promote.

However, this is not what we propose. Rather than assigning individuals to predefined cultural categories, our approach would leverage social data to identify the actual communities and influences shaping one's commercial understanding. This data-driven method would recognize individuals as existing at unique intersections of multiple overlapping contexts, instead of belonging to single cultural categories. In this way, CRISPR-J would make cultural assumptions transparent and contestable—an improvement over both the implicit biases of traditional systems and the essentialist profiling that critics fear.

A CRISPR-J-inspired approach to "the reasonable person" standard holds promise beyond consumer law. Other legal domains, including tort, contract, and employment law, also rely on reasonableness concepts that embed cultural assumptions.[12] To be sure, some contexts require caution: Criminal law, for one, should be particularly vigilant when cultural justifications are invoked for harmful behavior. But the core insight remains: Technologically enabled, culturally informed standards can serve the law's foundational goals better than artificial uniformity.

CRISPR-J: Replacing Rigid Legal Rules

CRISPR-J has great relevance not only to legal "standards" but also to legal "rules." As explained in Chapter 2, "rules" are explicit legal provisions in the form of fixed directives that specify behavior and outcomes based on clear, objective criteria. Unlike legal "standards" that rely on subjective judgment to assess conduct, rules provide unambiguous guidance, reducing uncertainty and the need for extensive interpretation. While rules are rigid, they are particularly advantageous in contexts requiring predictable and uniform applications. For instance, speed limits mandate precise maximum velocities (eg, 50 kilometers per hour) that drivers must adhere to, eliminating the need for subjective evaluations. Similarly, legal deadlines, such as filing taxes by April 15 each year in the United States, establish a definitive timeline, promoting fairness and operational efficiency. Age restrictions, such as the legal drinking age of twenty-one or a voting age of eighteen, offer another example, creating a clear benchmark that avoids the need for individualized assessments of maturity or capacity.

Nonetheless, the clarity and simplicity of rules can also be a significant shortcoming. When rules focus on uniform thresholds, they may fail to account for individual circumstances or contextual nuances. A driver exceeding the speed limit to reach a hospital during an emergency, or a young person mature enough to consume alcohol responsibly, might find such rules unduly restrictive or even unfair.

These examples highlight the inherent trade-off in legal design: Although rules excel in simplicity and predictability, they can sometimes sacrifice flexibility and fairness. While current legal systems somewhat mitigate these issues through legally recognized excuses and prosecutorial discretion, these measures are far from ideal. They are not always applicable, are applied inconsistently, often come too late, and frequently fail to provide adequate guidance to individuals in advance.

Personalized Rules

In Chapters 1 and 4, we discussed the potential of personalized law: An approach that dynamically adapts legal rules to individual circumstances using data and AI. Unlike traditional rules, which prioritize clarity and uniformity, personalized laws could

[12] Compare this with John Gardner, "The Many Faces of the Reasonable Person" (2015) 131(1) Law Quarterly Review 563.

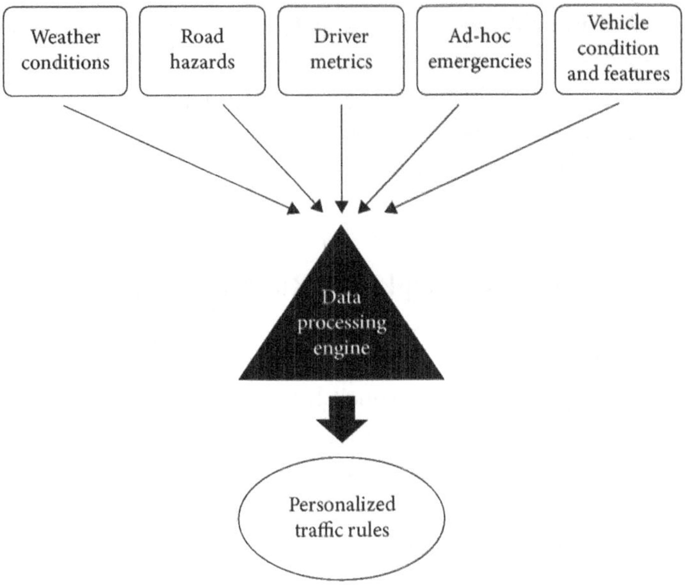

Figure 9.1 Adaptive Traffic Rules—A Personalized Approach

leverage technology to tailor legal norms to better fit the diverse realities of individuals' lives. This concept reimagines fairness and efficiency in law, offering a middle path between the rigidity of fixed rules and the subjectivity of standards.

For example, personalized traffic laws could adjust speed limits based on real-time conditions and ad hoc circumstances. As Figure 9.1 illustrates, such conditions and circumstances could encompass the driver's experience and personal characteristics (including age, gender, health, risk appetite, eyesight, and energy levels), road hazards, weather circumstances, emergencies, and the vehicle's condition or features. Such an approach would build on the strengths of clear rules but introduce flexibility where uniform rules fall short.

Similarly, consider the personalization of age-based laws, such as those regulating voting or alcohol consumption. Instead of rigid thresholds, algorithms could evaluate individual maturity based on education, behavioral data, or psychological assessments. Ultimately, personalized law invites us to rethink the rules versus standards categorization, leveraging technology to create a new spectrum of legal design.[13]

Of course, such an approach must strike a balance between inclusivity and coherence. Hyper-specific rules could lead to over-fragmentation and complexity. Nonetheless, dynamically grouping individuals into broad categories, such as age groups and energy levels, would maintain the benefits of personalization while safeguarding shared societal norms.

[13] See also Anthony J Casey and Anthony Niblett, "The Death of Rules and Standards" (2016) 92 Indiana Law Journal 1401.

Challenges and Concerns

Personalized legal systems must navigate a complex web of conceptual, ethical, and practical challenges. Chief among these concerns is data privacy. Personalized laws rely on vast quantities of personal data, raising questions about how such information is collected, stored, used, and shared. Without robust safeguards, individuals risk exposure to misuse, breaches, or unauthorized profiling. This is particularly significant given that private actors are often better positioned to develop and implement personalized law, due to their access to data, expertise, and internalization of incentives.[14]

Also troubling is the potential for algorithmic bias. AI systems, which would underpin personalized law, often mirror the biases embedded in their training data, potentially perpetuating or even amplifying existing inequalities. For example, a system tailored to predict recidivism might unfairly penalize individuals from marginalized communities, if it has been trained on historically biased data. Likewise, the opacity of AI-driven personalization challenges the principle of transparency that is foundational to justice. When algorithms determine legal outcomes, the reasoning behind decisions can become inscrutable, undercutting trust and making it difficult for individuals to contest or understand the rules applied to them.

As noted in Chapter 4, another pressing concern is the potential erosion of the rule of law.[15] Replacing legal rules with computationally personalized legal regulation poses a radical challenge, as it may constrain private agency and autonomy and undermine the legitimate exercise of power by public bodies. One of the law's essential roles is to bind a community together under a shared framework, fostering trust and reinforcing notions of fairness and equality. Uniform laws presumably entail that everyone is subject to the same rules, creating a sense of cohesion and solidarity within society. Personalized law, however, risks fragmenting this collective identity. When legal regulation is tailored to individuals, it could undermine the perception of equality before the law, replacing the unifying power of common rules with a patchwork of individualized imperatives. This could diminish the law's ability to function as a shared foundation for social order.

Moreover, personalized law risks reinforcing existing inequalities or undermining fairness and fundamental rights.[16] On its face, personalized law may seem to implicitly prioritize welfarism in the form of utility maximization, raising concerns about its compatibility with other goals that go beyond mere efficiency, such as equality. In other

[14] For a discussion of similar challenges see Timothy Endicott and Karen Yeung, "The Death of Law? Computationally Personalized Norms and the Rule of Law" (2022) 72(4) University of Toronto Law Journal 373; Andrew Verstein, "Privatizing Personalized Law" (2019) 86(2) The University of Chicago Law Review 551; Anthony J Casey and Anthony Niblett, "Framework for the New Personalization of Law" (2019) 86(2) The University of Chicago Law Review 333.

[15] See, for example, Endicott and Yeung, "The Death of Law?"; see also Sandra G Mayson, "But What Is Personalized Law?" (2022) University of Chicago Law Review Online 1.

[16] See, for example, Christoph Busch and Alberto De Franceschi, "Granular Legal Norms: Big Data and the Personalization of Private Law" in Vanessa Mak, Eric Tjong Tjin Tai, and Anna Berlee (eds), *Research Handbook in Data Science and Law* (Edward Elgar 2018) 408; Mayson, "But What Is Personalized Law?" (note 15).

words, even when individualized rules are efficient or objectively justified, they may still exacerbate disparities between different social groups.

Wealthy individuals are more likely to drive safer vehicles, enjoy better health, and access resources that contribute to higher safety or performance metrics. Granting these individuals legal privileges, such as higher speed limits, could deepen societal divides and foster resentment. Similarly, considerations such as education or civic engagement—often linked to socioeconomic advantage—could disproportionately favor already affluent communities if they were used to personalize voting ages or other legal benefits. This would risk creating a system where the already privileged gain even greater advantages, further entrenching inequality.

CRISPR-J Principles in Action

While the challenges of personalized law are considerable, they also present an opportunity to innovate. To ensure personalized law fulfills its potential without compromising foundational legal values, we must rethink its design and implementation. The principles of CRISPR-J offer a roadmap for achieving this balance, enabling systems that are not only adaptive but also fair, transparent, and inclusive. In the following paragraphs, we discuss these principles in general terms. Thereafter, we move to specific illustrations.

Cost-effectiveness would entail ensuring that personalized law can be implemented efficiently, making it accessible across diverse socioeconomic contexts. Advanced AI systems would automate the customization of legal rules, reducing the need for costly human oversight. This scalability would enable the benefits of personalized law to reach broader populations without overburdening legal institutions.

Rapidity emphasizes the capacity of personalized legal systems to respond to real-time conditions. By leveraging data streams and dynamic algorithms, legal systems could adapt swiftly to changing circumstances. For example, traffic laws would adjust speed limits during severe weather events or emergencies, ensuring that the law remains effective while protecting public safety.

Inclusivity would be essential for preventing the marginalization of disadvantaged groups. Mechanisms such as fairness audits or the inclusion of representative datasets, along with dynamic, personalized worldview models, would help diminish the risk of bias. For instance, personalizing voting eligibility based on knowledge and maturity would require particular attention to underrepresented populations, avoiding criteria that favor privileged groups.

Smartness would involve designing personalized systems that are intelligent and ethical. Advanced AI would integrate various types of data from multiple sources, enhancing the accuracy of personalized rules, while embedding safeguards to prevent discriminatory outcomes. Rigorous data vetting and transparency measures would help verify that the tailoring of legal regulation aligns with broader societal values.

Predictiveness would seek to anticipate societal needs and individual circumstances. Predictive analytics could identify patterns and trends that inform proactive legal adjustments. AI systems are already being developed to forecast complex phenomena, such as weather patterns and geopolitical conflicts.[17] These developments underscore the potential for similar techniques to foresee legal disputes, regulatory gaps, or systemic risks before they materialize.

Finally, Resilience would guarantee that personalized law remains adaptive over time. Periodic reviews and feedback loops would minimize the risks of unintended consequences, ensuring that the system evolves in response to societal shifts and emerging concerns. If certain personalization practices exacerbate inequalities, resilience mechanisms could dynamically recalibrate the system.

Adaptive Traffic Rules

Let us now return to the example of personalized traffic laws, which would represent a transformative approach to enhancing road safety and efficiency. As noted, adaptive traffic laws would dynamically adjust speed limits and other regulations based on real-time conditions and personal characteristics. Unlike static rules, which apply uniformly regardless of context, an AI-driven system would monitor ad hoc factors. The question, however, is how best to implement this vision while addressing concerns about the rule of law and inequality.

To address concerns about the rule of law, adaptive traffic laws would need to maintain transparency and consistency in their application. A baseline speed limit could serve as a universal minimum, ensuring that all drivers are subject to a common standard. Personalized adjustments would then operate within clearly defined parameters, ensuring that all drivers understand the system and its rationale. This transparency would help maintain public trust and reinforce the principle that, while specific rules may adapt to individual circumstances, the legal system itself applies equally to everyone.

Recall that wealthier drivers are more likely to own vehicles equipped with advanced safety or self-driving features, which could objectively justify higher personalized speed limits. Yet this outcome may disproportionately benefit the already privileged. Critics might argue that it allows wealth to indirectly purchase legal privilege—even if the underlying criterion is safety-based.

As a possible response, the system could incorporate compensatory adjustments, such as prioritizing real-time road conditions or broader traffic flow data over vehicle-specific metrics. Additionally, the algorithm could be designed to reduce reliance on socioeconomic indicators, giving more weight to universal factors like weather and

[17] See Rebecca Dzombak, "A.I. Is Poised to Revolutionize Weather Forecasting. A New Tool Shows Promise" *New York Times* (May 21, 2025); Tekendra Parmar, "Meet the ex-Harvard Professor Who Says His AI Can Predict the Next War: 'I Don't Want to Break the World'" *Business Insider* (June 17, 2025).

road safety metrics. Economic indicators, according to this logic, would only have a marginal role in determining traffic rules.

The principles of CRISPR-J would guide the design and implementation of such a system. Predictiveness would prompt the system to anticipate risks like icy roads or heavy traffic, enabling proactive adjustments to prevent accidents. Rapidity would ensure instantaneous updates during emergencies, such as accidents or natural disasters, providing timely responses to protect public safety. Cost-effectiveness would automate these adjustments using a sophisticated algorithm, reducing the reliance on manual enforcement while enhancing safety and efficiency. By blending adaptive capabilities with equity safeguards, such a system could enhance fairness and safety, without compromising the shared framework of the law. While challenges—such as universal access to technology and avoiding disproportionate benefits to specific groups—remain, adaptive traffic laws illustrate how personalization can theoretically align with ethical principles and broader societal goals.

Personalization for Enhanced Legal Protection Measures

So far, we have noted that some applications of personalization, such as voting laws or traffic rules, present challenges for equity or the rule of law. In other domains, however, personalization could better tailor legal protections and rights. Aligning legal frameworks with individual circumstances can address vulnerabilities, promote fairness, and enhance access to justice—all while maintaining or increasing stability and predictability.

Consider deadlines in taxation or regulatory compliance. Uniform deadlines can inadvertently disadvantage individuals with disabilities or those facing rare or unique individual challenges. A personalized system could automatically adjust deadlines based on real-time needs, offering additional time for those with documented constraints, such as chronic illness or caregiving responsibilities. This would expand accessibility, ensuring that flexibility is paired with clear and transparent guidelines to prevent misuse.

Cooling-off periods and cancellation rights offer another compelling example. Vulnerable consumers, such as older people or those with disabilities, could be afforded extended cooling-off periods to reconsider high-stakes purchases or contracts. Similarly, automatic subscription renewals might require higher levels of consent for inactive consumers, reducing financial exploitation of consumer inertia. This approach would extend the protective logic already present in contract law, which recognizes varying capacities for consent by, for example, making contracts entered into by minors voidable rather than automatically binding.

To mitigate the risk of businesses avoiding interactions with these groups or charging them a premium, regulation could provide clear incentives for compliance. For instance, firms that adhere to personalized consumer protection measures could receive tax benefits or regulatory leniency in other areas. They could also benefit from public recognition, which would enhance their reputation.

Moreover, laws could prohibit discriminatory pricing based on the application of these rights (despite the associated efficiency costs). Transparent rules about eligibility and enforcement would anchor the system in fairness, while periodic reviews would identify and address unintended consequences as they arise. Such measures would safeguard vulnerable populations while encouraging businesses to engage inclusively, striking a balance between equity and economic viability.

Personalization can also reshape workplace protection laws. For example, younger or less experienced workers in high-risk industries may be required to attend more frequent safety training, or their employers may be subject to stricter regulatory oversight. These tailored measures could reduce workplace injuries while fostering equity across a diverse workforce.

To prevent employers from hesitating to hire individuals who require additional protection, the framework could incorporate targeted incentives and safeguards. For instance, employers who hire and train vulnerable workers might receive subsidies, tax credits, or reduced liability for workplace incidents that occur despite compliance with personalized regulations. Additionally, laws could prohibit hiring discrimination based on factors such as age or inexperience, with clear enforcement mechanisms to ensure accountability.

CRISPR-J principles like Inclusivity and Resilience would guide the design of such a system. These principles could ensure the system adapts equitably to the needs of vulnerable workers while maintaining broader labor market stability. While challenges remain, balancing tailored protection measures with meaningful support for employers would allow personalized workplace laws to enhance safety and equity without creating disincentives to hire.

Landlord–tenant laws present another opportunity for personalization. Current laws often apply uniformly, failing to account for financial vulnerabilities or disparities in local living costs. A personalized system could offer enhanced protections against eviction or rent control measures for tenants who demonstrate heightened need. Examples could include tenants in low-income households or those who experience exceptional hardships, such as sudden job loss, significant medical expenses, or displacement due to natural disasters.

Here too, to prevent landlords from avoiding vulnerable tenants or raising rents disproportionately, the framework could adopt innovative measures that benefit both tenants and landlords. For example, landlords participating in personalized regulations could receive government-backed guarantees against missed rent payments, reducing financial risk. Additionally, fast-track dispute resolution services could be provided to landlords managing tenants under personalized protection, minimizing the administrative burden of compliance. To further split costs and divide responsibilities, governments could offer enhanced tenant education programs to ensure tenants understand their duties and responsibilities.

The move towards personalization is evident in many domains, from education, medicine, and entertainment platforms to financial services, and the legal system is no exception. Elements of personalization already exist within legal systems, as demonstrated by sentencing decisions that consider individual circumstances, family law's best-interest-of-the-child determinations, and contract law's consideration of parties' specific capacities and circumstances.

That said, making legal personalization the norm presents unique conceptual, societal, and practical challenges. If implemented poorly, it could erode the rule of law, undermine autonomy and accountability, exacerbate inequalities, and introduce wholesale algorithmic bias. Given these risks, legal personalization should proceed incrementally, focusing on areas with clear benefits, reliable data, and social consensus. Overall, the goal should be to enhance effectiveness, precision, and agility while preserving the law's essential function as a unifying and fair societal force.

CRISPR-J: Enforcement and Compliance

The effectiveness of any legal system hinges on its ability to enforce compliance fairly, reliably, and resourcefully. Yet, traditional enforcement mechanisms are often plagued by inconsistencies, inefficiencies, and inequities. In many domains, the formal law remains in the books, while enforcement lags or fails to materialize effectively.[18] For instance, housing regulations and traffic laws might be rigorously applied in urban areas but inconsistently enforced in rural regions, leading to disparities in how laws are perceived and adhered to. Such variability, combined with socioeconomic, racial, or geographical bias in enforcement, undermines the principle of equality before the law.

Resource constraints further compound these issues, as many regulatory agencies lack the funding or personnel to monitor compliance comprehensively. This results in selective enforcement, weakening deterrence, and potentially emboldening violators who perceive the risk of detection as low. Furthermore, traditional enforcement systems are typically reactive, addressing violations only after significant damage has occurred rather than proactively preventing noncompliance. When enforcement appears arbitrary or insufficient, citizens lose confidence in the legal system, eroding public trust in the rule of law.

Private enforcement mechanisms offer little remedy to these systemic failures, particularly in domains characterized by power imbalances between parties.[19] In areas such as tenant rights, employment law, banking and financial services, insurance

[18] This, of course, is not a novel observation. See, for example, Roscoe Pound, "Law in Books and Law in Action" (1910) 44 American Law Review 12.

[19] See, for example, Mark Galanter, "Why the 'Haves' Come Out Ahead: Speculations on the Limits of Legal Change" (1974) 9 Law & Society Review 95; William LF Felstiner, Richard L Abel, and Austin Sarat, "The Emergence and Transformation of Disputes: Naming, Blaming, Claiming . . ." (1980) 15 Law & Society Review 631; Laura Beth Nielsen and Robert L Nelson, "Rights Realized? An Empirical Analysis of Employment Discrimination Litigation as a Claiming System" (2005) 2 Wisconsin Law Review 663; Lauren B Edelman, *Working Law: Courts, Corporations, and Symbolic Civil Rights* (University of Chicago Press 2016).

claims, healthcare billing, consumer protection, unfair contract terms, data privacy, antitrust matters, and environmental protection, individual stakeholders often lack the resources, expertise, or incentives to pursue legal action effectively. The costs of litigation, both financial and emotional, typically outweigh potential remedies for individual plaintiffs. At the same time, wealthy corporate defendants can leverage their superior resources to prolong proceedings or pressure for unfavorable settlements. Consequently, powerful actors might systematically violate legal norms with relative impunity, knowing that the probability of facing meaningful consequences remains low.

The principles of CRISPR-J offer a promising framework for addressing these systemic challenges. CRISPR-J would employ means such as AI, big data, advanced sensors, and IoT to make monitoring, enforcement, and adjudication smarter and more adaptive. In the following discussion, we explore how CRISPR-J Enforcement could revolutionize compliance and processes across various domains: judicial decision-making, environmental regulation, consumer protection, product obsolescence, and employment law rights.

Noise in Judicial Processes

One of the most critical applications of CRISPR-J principles lies in judicial decision-making, which remains vulnerable to human limitations such as bias and noise. Bias refers to systematic deviations in judgment caused by personal predispositions, preferences, or institutional pressures that consistently influence decision outcomes in a particular direction. For example, judges who exhibit leniency toward certain demographic groups or impose harsher sentencing for specific crimes are demonstrating bias.

Conversely, noise refers to random and unpredictable variability in judgments.[20] This could stem from extraneous factors such as fatigue, hunger, or the time of day, which studies suggest may result in judges being more lenient early in the day and harsher just before lunch.[21] Such variability undermines the principle of equality before the law, introducing randomness and inconsistency into the enforcement of legal norms.

CRISPR-J Enforcement principles, particularly Smartness and Predictiveness, offer innovative tools with which to address these challenges. AI-powered systems could analyze patterns in judicial decisions to distinguish between bias and noise, enabling tailored interventions. For bias, the system could highlight systematic deviations in

[20] For a general and comprehensive analysis of "noise" and its impact on human judgment and decision-making see Daniel Kahneman, Olivier Sibony, and Cass R Sunstein, *Noise: A Flaw in Human Judgment* (Hachette UK 2021).

[21] See, for example, Shai Danziger, Jonathan Levav, and Liora Avnaim-Pesso, "Extraneous Factors in Judicial Decisions" (2011) 108(17) Proceedings of the National Academy of Sciences 6889. For challenging the robustness of these conclusions see Keren Weinshall-Margel and John Shapard, "Overlooked Factors in the Analysis of Parole Decisions" (2011) 108(42) Proceedings of the National Academy of Sciences E833.

decisions linked to consistent patterns of inequity, prompting institutional reforms or training initiatives.[22] For noise, these systems could detect variability caused by external factors, providing real-time feedback or alerts. For example, the system could flag when a judge's decisions deviate from established patterns and suggest breaks during moments of heightened fatigue or stress. Similarly, AI tools could optimize court scheduling to ensure that complex or high-stakes cases are heard when judges are most alert and focused, reducing the impact of noise.

Beyond merely mitigating human limitations, AI tools can be used to actively drive systemic consistency. Recent empirical evidence indicates LLMs may already be more consistent decision-makers than human judges. A 2026 study comparing the sentencing decisions of LLMs against those of retired judges found that the AI models exhibited significantly lower sentencing disparity.[23] This suggests that AI tools can serve as a stabilizing anchor, offering a "consensus" benchmark that helps edit out the erratic variability inherent in human adjudication. While some studies warn that LLMs can be overly formalistic, they also find that specific prompting strategies can mitigate this rigidity.[24] This reinforces the necessity of CRISPR-J's design interventions: By astutely "editing" how AI is deployed, legal systems can harness machine consistency while minimizing the risk of inequitable outcomes.

Environmental Regulation

One great piece of wisdom asserts that "an ounce of prevention is worth a pound of cure." While the judiciary often intervenes after the fact to address violations or harms, prevention is frequently a more effective and efficient strategy. *Ex ante*, regulatory agencies and governmental organizations play a pivotal role in ensuring compliance with the law.

Environmental regulation offers a compelling example of how CRISPR-J principles can drive innovation in oversight practices, proactively tackling violations that can cause significant and sometimes irreversible damage. Illegal dumping, excessive emissions, and other environmental harms frequently go undetected. This unfortunate reality underscores the need for monitoring systems that can intervene before damage escalates.

To advance prevention measures and reduce reliance on reactive interventions, regulators could leverage advanced IoT devices and AI algorithms to monitor industrial emissions in real time, flagging issues or violations as they occur. For instance, sensors installed in factories could automatically detect and report pollutant levels exceeding

[22] See also the proposals discussed in Chapter 7.
[23] See Oren Gazal-Ayal, Zohar Elyoseph, and Adir Solomon, "Evaluating Large Language Models as Judicial Decision-Makers" (2026) Justice Quarterly (forthcoming).
[24] See Ori Katz and Eyal Zamir, "Law, Justice, and Artificial Intelligence" (2025) SSRN (finding that LLMs exhibit considerably less noise than humans, and prompting techniques such as instructing LLMs to predict judicial decisions or consider litigant sympathy "somewhat reduces their formalism").

legal limits, enabling immediate responses. Similarly, satellite imagery, combined with AI analysis, could track deforestation activities and prompt legal interventions to prevent further damage.

These technologies exemplify the CRISPR-J principles of Smartness, Rapidity, and Predictiveness, as they harness advanced tools to create responsive and effective systems. However, scaling these solutions to a global level presents challenges, particularly for resource-constrained jurisdictions. Collaborative efforts, such as international funding mechanisms or public-private partnerships, could play a crucial role in bridging these gaps and ensuring broader access to these innovations.

Predictive analytics can further enhance preventative strategies by analyzing historical data to identify high-risk industries, regions, or circumstances, enabling regulators to allocate resources proactively. At the same time, the Inclusivity principle would guarantee that enforcement mechanisms do not disproportionately burden small businesses or economically vulnerable communities. For example, smaller enterprises might receive compliance support to help them meet environmental standards, promoting the equitable application of regulations.

Such a technology-enhanced enforcement paradigm necessitates a fundamental recalibration of penalty structures. As Gary Becker's influential deterrence theory suggests, optimal enforcement balances detection probability with the severity of the penalty.[25] In traditional environmental regulation, where violations are detected infrequently, penalties must be disproportionately severe to achieve deterrence. This, however, can result in draconian fines that undermine public trust and incentivize problematic prosecutorial and judicial discretion.

CRISPR-J's high-detection enforcement model would allow for more moderate, proportionate penalties while maintaining or even enhancing deterrent effects. For example, as real-time emissions monitoring approaches 90–100 percent detection rates, penalties could be recalibrated to reflect actual harm caused rather than serving as multiplied proxies for undetected violations. This rebalancing would foster compliance without breeding resentment, reinforcing the system's legitimacy while maintaining its protective function.

Consumer Protection Enforcement

Consumer protection presents another domain where CRISPR-J Enforcement could significantly reduce the gap between the formal law on the books and the law in action. Vulnerable consumers often face a host of exploitative and misleading practices. These typically range from misleading advertisements and manipulative pricing strategies to influencer marketing and outright fraud.

[25] See the seminal work Gary S Becker, "Crime and Punishment: An Economic Approach" (1968) 76(2) Journal of Political Economy 169.

Consumer protection issues are further exacerbated by the complexities of the digital marketplace, where dark patterns manipulate consumers and blur the lines of accountability.[26] Moreover, deceptive product listings on e-commerce platforms and the proliferation of scams further exploit consumers, leaving regulatory frameworks struggling to keep pace with these developments. Certain populations, such as the elderly or naïve consumers, are particularly at risk, as they often struggle to navigate complex disclosures or recognize exploitative tactics.

CRISPR-J Enforcement offers encouraging solutions to these persistent challenges. AI tools could dynamically and rapidly analyze online advertisements and sales patterns to detect deceptive claims such as fake discounts or false product endorsements, flagging high-risk entities for closer scrutiny. For instance, AI systems could automatically compare advertised prices with actual market values to identify manipulative pricing tactics, alerting regulators and platforms that can take immediate action. While they are not a magic bullet, predictive models could identify companies or sellers with a history of consumer complaints or unusual refund patterns, enabling regulators to target enforcement efforts proactively. Adaptive enforcement mechanisms, such as automated monitoring of e-commerce platforms, could ensure that legal frameworks keep pace with evolving digital practices, blocking deceptive product listings and issuing fines in real time.[27]

In addition to these technological advances, the principle of Inclusivity would ensure that vulnerable populations are adequately protected by tailoring interventions to their specific needs. For example, elderly consumers could benefit from simplified (and perhaps personalized) disclosures that clearly outline the terms of online transactions, reducing confusion. Similarly, young online shoppers would benefit from clear warnings about recurring subscriptions and hidden fees, avoiding the need to navigate complex cancellation procedures or dispute unexpected charges. More generally, platforms could be required to ban or restrict dark patterns, such as confusing consent toggles or misleading urgency messages, which exploit consumers' psychological vulnerabilities.

Tackling Product Obsolescence

At the intersection of environmental and consumer protection, product obsolescence presents unique enforcement challenges. Product obsolescence refers to the processes

[26] On the dangers and risks that consumers face see, for example, Arunesh Mathur and others, "Dark Patterns at Scale: Findings from a Crawl of 11K Shopping Websites" (2019) 3.CSCW Proceedings of the ACM on Human–Computer Interaction 1; Martin Mende and others, "Consumer Vulnerability Dynamics and Marketing: Conceptual Foundations and Future Research Opportunities" (2024) 52(5) Journal of the Academy of Marketing Science 1301; Natali Helberger and others, "Choice Architectures in the Digital Economy: Towards a New Understanding of Digital Vulnerability" (2022) 45 Journal of Consumer Policy 175.

[27] The model of responsive regulation, with its emphasis on proportionate and context-sensitive responses, closely aligns with our approach. See Ian Ayres and John Braithwaite, *Responsive Regulation: Transcending the Deregulation Debate* (Oxford University Press 1992).

and design decisions that cause a product to become outdated, nonfunctional, or undesirable, often leading to its replacement. To address this sticky problem, regulations need to promote repairability and durability.[28]

However, such right-to-repair laws and durability standards require robust monitoring mechanisms to ensure compliance. Without effective enforcement, manufacturers may continue to employ practices that take advantage of asymmetric information and consumers' behavioral biases, thereby shortening product lifespans, undermining sustainability, contributing to global waste, and perpetuating consumer exploitation. Industry pushback further complicates enforcement: Manufacturers often resist compliance, citing concerns about intellectual property protection and increased production costs.

CRISPR-J principles could address these challenges by leveraging advanced monitoring tools. For instance, IoT-enabled devices could track product usage and performance, flagging patterns indicative of premature obsolescence. Similarly, digital platforms could allow consumers to report repairability issues directly to regulators, creating a dynamic feedback loop for enforcement. Predictive capabilities would augment this approach by analyzing warranty claims and repair data to identify manufacturers or product categories with high noncompliance risks. Regulators and consumer organizations could use this information to prioritize inspections or audits, focusing resources where they are most needed.

CRISPR-J Enforcement's application to product obsolescence could make consumer protection more proactive and effective. It could safeguard individual rights while addressing urgent environmental challenges. These measures would bridge the gap between the law and market practices, while positioning regulators, consumer advocacy groups, and environmental protection agencies as champions of sustainability. Together, they could empower consumers, enhance accountability, and facilitate a more transparent global marketplace.

Employment Rights

Employment law provides another context for CRISPR-J Enforcement. The literature on employment rights paints a bleak picture. Underdeveloped enforcement mechanisms, combined with the vulnerability of employees, fear of retaliation, and lack of resources and awareness, create significant barriers to justice. The prohibitive cost of litigation further deepens these challenges, leaving workers, especially those in

[28] See Eléonore Maitre-Ekern and Carl Dalhammar, "Regulating Planned Obsolescence: A Review of Legal Approaches to Increase Product Durability and Reparability in Europe" (2016) 25(3) Review of European, Comparative & International Environmental Law 378; Shmuel I Becher and Anne-Lise Sibony, "Confronting Product Obsolescence" (2021) 27 Columbia Journal of European Law 97; Jurgita Malinauskaite and Fatih Buğra Erdem, "Planned Obsolescence in the Context of a Holistic Legal Sphere and the Circular Economy" (2021) 41(3) Oxford Journal of Legal Studies 719.

precarious employment situations, struggling to receive their rightful earnings and the protection they deserve.[29]

Tipping regulations provide a practical example of how employment law rights can be strengthened through CRISPR-J Enforcement. The UK's Employment (Allocation of Tips) Act 2023 mandates that tips be distributed to employees without deductions, with very limited exceptions. However, ensuring compliance presents significant challenges, particularly for smaller establishments or businesses that rely on cash, in which traditional enforcement mechanisms may be ineffective. Without proper oversight, workers in the hospitality sector, often comprising less powerful or precariously employed individuals, may continue to be deprived of their rightful earnings.

CRISPR-J principles could offer inventive ways to address these challenges. Digital tracking systems integrated with electronic payment platforms could monitor tips in real time, ensuring accurate allocation to employees. For example, digital systems could automatically compare tipping data reported by employers with transaction records, flagging discrepancies that might indicate violations. Predictive analytics could analyze historical data to pinpoint businesses or industries with elevated risks of noncompliance, enabling regulators to prioritize inspections and audits on likely violators.

Likewise, Inclusivity would guarantee that these solutions empower workers across diverse environments. Accessible and cost-effective reporting mechanisms, such as secure mobile apps or anonymous online portals, would assist employees in raising concerns about unfair practices without fear of retaliation. Digital interfaces could ensure real-time transparency on tipping policies through personalized communications, adapting disclosures to the needs of different stakeholders—whether multilingual workers, seasonal employees, or customers—while maintaining a clear audit trail of all interactions.

Smart initiatives could further enhance these efforts by using technology to develop engaging measures that promote awareness of employment rights. For instance, employment law concepts could be reimagined through visually appealing formats like comics, infographics, fun quizzes, or short animations, making complex legal rules more accessible. Podcasts and educational videos tailored to specific industries could provide workers with practical insights into their rights and the mechanisms available for addressing grievances.

Along these lines, interactive simulations could mimic real-world scenarios, allowing workers to navigate virtual environments in which they learn to identify unfair

[29] See, for example, Clyde Summers, "Effective Remedies for Employment Rights: Preliminary Guidelines and Proposals" (1992) 141 University of Pennsylvania Law Review 457; Louise Sadowsky Brock, "Overcoming Collective Action Problems: Enforcement of Worker Rights" (1996) 30 University of Michigan Journal of Law Reform 781; Peter KC Lee, Antonio KW Lau, and TCE Cheng, "Employee Rights Protection and Financial Performance" (2013) 66(10) Journal of Business Research 1861; Cynthia L Estlund, "How Wrong Are Employees About Their Rights, and Why Does It Matter" (2002) 77 New York University Law Review 6.

practices, understand their rights, and practice reporting mechanisms. For example, interactive games could simulate workplace dilemmas, such as confronting wage theft or deciding whether to report misconduct, thereby helping players internalize legal principles through experiential learning. In the long run, such strategies might even enhance trust among employers, employees, and regulators, establishing better norms that promote fairness and compliance in employment practices.

The CRISPR-J Paradigm: From Reaction to Precision

This chapter demonstrated the practical relevance of CRISPR-J principles—Cost-effectiveness, Rapidity, Inclusivity, Smartness, Predictiveness, and Resilience—across a wide range of legal domains. It illustrated how CRISPR-J principles can refine vague legal standards, personalize legal rules, and modernize enforcement mechanisms. To recap, Table 9.2 portrays the versatility and usefulness of CRISPR-J principles.

Yet, real-time monitoring and data-driven enforcement raise legitimate concerns about privacy, surveillance, and algorithmic bias. These risks underscore the importance of implementing safeguards such as data anonymization protocols, robust appeal mechanisms, and human oversight. Moreover, economic disparities and social inequalities present challenges to adoption, necessitating phased timelines, subsidies, and transparent frameworks.

The power of CRISPR-J lies not in eliminating normative dilemmas but in shedding more light on them and equipping us with better tools with which to address them. CRISPR-J solutions prompt us to grapple with essential and enduring normative questions. How should we balance precision with inclusivity? How do we ensure that efficiency does not overshadow other fundamental values? And how can we preserve human agency and democratic accountability in increasingly automated legal processes?

Ultimately, CRISPR-J offers a path toward a legal order that is both principled and pragmatic; one that is ready to meet the complexities of a rapidly changing world. This journey would require cautious optimism, thoughtful collaboration, a willingness to experiment, and an ongoing commitment to fairness and accountability. As we turn to the limitations and challenges that lie ahead, it is clear that the evolution of law is not just a technical endeavor but a profoundly human one: guided by values, shaped by dialogue, and enriched by the pursuit of justice itself.

Table 9.2 CRISPR-J Principles Applied Across Legal Domains

Legal Domain	Cost-effectiveness	Rapidity	Inclusivity	Smartness	Predictiveness	Resilience
Legal standards and judicial decisions	Reduces costs of case-by-case analysis	Faster identification of bias, deviations, or inconsistencies	Giving voice to diverse demographics	Analyzes consistency	Anticipates external factors impacting judgments	Adapts rules based on evolving norms
Legal rules	Efficient use of data and resources	Real-time adjustments	Tailored rules to protect vulnerable groups	Advanced data systems; nuanced adjustments	Predicts risks based on individual and environmental data	Adapts norms as new data emerges
Environmental regulation	Efficient, scalable IoT monitoring	Real-time detection	Equitable application; supporting resource-constrained regions	Violation monitoring and compliance tracking	Predicts high-risk industries and areas for proactive monitoring	Adapts enforcement to emerging challenges
Consumer protection	Focus on prevention; automated monitoring	Rapid detection of harmful business practices	Protects vulnerable or naïve consumers	Real-time AI screening	Predicts high-risk sectors for fraud or violations	Adjusts frameworks based on dynamic marketplace practices
Employment rights	Streamlined reporting via digital platforms	Swift response to detected misbehaviors	Empowers workers with accessible tools and information	Technology-enhanced education; AI identifies non-compliance	Anticipates high-risk industries or circumstances	Robust protections against retaliation

10
Charting Superjustice

Framing the Challenge Landscape

It is 2050. The plaintiff's artificial intelligence (AI) agent, representing an entrepreneur, has accused a global tech company of intellectual property theft. The defendant, through its own AI agent, claims that the innovation in question was independently developed. The legal arguments are made by AI. The legal case is decided entirely by an AI arbitrator, with no courtrooms, judges, jurors, or attorneys—just algorithms parsing data, weighing evidence, considering arguments, and rendering a verdict. As the parties receive the verdict, there is no gavel strike or courtroom murmur, but only a notification blinking on screens. The global tech company is either exonerated or held accountable in seconds, and both parties know exactly where they stand. Case closed.

This imagined future scenario raises technical, ethical, societal, and institutional issues. For some, it is a marvel: justice delivered at lightning speed, impervious to human bias and error. For others, it is deeply unsettling. Where is the humanity in justice? Who programmed the values that determine fairness? Can we trust algorithms to deliver justice? Can the aggrieved party appeal and ask that a human review the algorithm's decision?

As the previous chapters illustrated, integrating AI into legal systems presents myriad issues, spanning multiple domains. These challenges are neither unique nor isolated; they permeate institutions and society, potentially reshaping the very nature of justice itself. Examples abound. Improving algorithmic accuracy—a technical issue—may require vast amounts of data, which raises ethical concerns about privacy and bias. Similarly, designing fair AI systems—a societal goal—hinges on effective regulatory oversight (a governance challenge) and adequate training for legal professionals (a human challenge). Addressing one issue without considering its impact on others risks harmful unintended consequences.[1]

Without a cohesive framework, the challenges that come with AI integration often seem like a grab bag of disparate problems. This makes it difficult for stakeholders to prioritize effectively. Policymakers may focus on regulating AI outputs while neglecting data governance; legal professionals may address liability issues while overlooking societal accessibility. Confronting one problem at a time makes perfect sense in many contexts. Nonetheless, a fragmented approach to legal transformation could lead to

[1] On the value and importance of adopting a holistic approach generally see Donella H Meadows, *Thinking in Systems: A Primer* (Chelsea Green Publishing 2008); Fritjof Capra, *The Systems View of Life: A Unifying Vision* (Cambridge University Press 2014).

Superjustice. Samuel I. Becher and Benjamin Alarie, Oxford University Press.
 DOI: 10.1093/9780198991885.003.0014

patchwork solutions, inefficiencies, and, ultimately, a justice system that struggles to capitalize on the promise of an AI-driven future.

This chapter introduces a multilayered analytical framework to conceptualize the various challenges that come with the broad introduction of AI into legal systems. The framework captures not only the nature of these challenges and the opportunities they present but also their evolution over time and the systems they affect. At its core lies what we call the Dynamic Challenges Matrix—a tool that maps challenges across three dimensions:

1. Life-cycle stage: tracing challenges from their initial emergence, through system integration, to long-term sustainability. This dimension highlights their temporal progression.
2. Domain focus: categorizing challenges by their primary area of impact—whether (i) technical, (ii) human, (iii) governance-related, or (iv) societal. This dimension reflects their operational locus.
3. Complexity level: assessing the depth of each challenge, from (i) direct and localized issues, through (ii) systemic interdependencies, to (iii) transformative shifts that redefine legal paradigms. This dimension highlights the difficulty of addressing the challenge.

The proposed Dynamic Challenges Matrix equips stakeholders with a practical guide to navigating the evolving and cross-domain nature of AI-driven legal transformation. While the matrix offers a structured analytical framework, real-world challenges often span multiple categories, blur dimensional boundaries, and evolve over time. Even so, mapping challenges across life-cycle stages, domains, and complexity levels enables stakeholders to see the bigger picture: how these challenges develop, interact, and demand coordinated solutions. The remainder of this chapter unfolds through the lens of this matrix, weaving together many of the challenges discussed throughout the book.

Life-Cycle Stages: The Evolution of Challenges

As legal systems gradually integrate powerful AI, challenges will emerge, evolve, and persist over time. The concept of life-cycle stages captures this temporal dimension. In our proposed model, life-cycle stages comprise three phases. First, emergence relates to the issues that are revealed during the initial implementation of advanced AI in legal contexts, where foundational AI-related challenges like algorithmic accuracy, hallucination, and bias arise. Next, integration marks the mid-term phase at which AI systems are deployed within legal infrastructures, revealing governance and workflow challenges. Finally, sustainability focuses on the long-term impacts and implications of AI in justice systems, including systemic transformations in equity, the role of legal professionals, and the maintenance of public trust.

This examination of challenges across stages reveals how short-term technical issues may cascade into systemic or societal concerns. For instance, a data privacy issue during the emergence stage could evolve into governance dilemmas during integration, ultimately impacting public trust in the sustainability phase.[2] With this in mind, let us explore the three stages.

Emergence: Foundational Challenges

The emergence stage marks the initial phase in the adoption of AI in legal systems, where foundational challenges arise during the development and deployment of new technologies. These challenges are frequently, though not solely, technical and transitional. Often, they concern the fundamental capabilities and limitations of AI tools in performing legal tasks and informing legal processes.

One immediate challenge during emergence is AI accuracy.[3] Algorithms deployed in legal contexts must produce reliable results, whether they are drafting contracts, analyzing case law, or predicting case outcomes. Errors at this stage—inaccurate case citations, flawed reasoning chains, or hallucinations whereby AI tools generate references to non-existent legal precedents—can undermine the credibility of AI tools and erode trust among legal professionals and the public alike. Ensuring accuracy requires rigorous testing, validation processes, and ongoing refinement. Yet, such efforts are often constrained by the quality of both the training and the data available, which in turn links this challenge to broader issues such as data governance.

Bias in training data represents a particularly pressing issue.[4] As we explained in various contexts throughout the book, AI systems learn from existing data and texts, which can reflect societal inequities and institutional biases. If these biases are not addressed early, they risk being perpetuated, or even amplified, by AI systems. For instance, if an algorithm used for bail recommendations is trained on biased judicial decisions or skewed statistical data, it may produce results that disproportionately disadvantage certain groups. Addressing this challenge at the emergence stage requires identifying and mitigating bias during data collection and preprocessing, as well as incorporating fairness metrics into the development pipeline.

Another foundational challenge is data privacy. As the previous chapters, and particularly Chapters 4, 6, and 9, illuminated, data is the lifeblood of Superjustice. Superjustice depends on vast quantities of sensitive information, including client

[2] Addressing issues early before they grow into larger and more complex challenges is sound advice in many walks of life, from financial debt to medical conditions and home maintenance. For engaging discussions see Malcolm Gladwell, *The Tipping Point: How Little Things Can Make a Big Difference* (Little, Brown 2006); Nassim Nicholas Taleb, *Antifragile: Things That Gain From Disorder* (Random House Trade Paperbacks 2014).

[3] AI accuracy is a critical concern across various domains, particularly in health and medicine. See, for example, Myura Nagendran and others, "Artificial Intelligence Versus Clinicians: Systematic Review of Design, Reporting Standards, and Claims of Deep Learning Studies" (2020) 368 British Medical Journal [10.1136/bmj.m689]; Douglas Johnson and others, "Assessing the Accuracy and Reliability of AI-Generated Medical Responses: An Evaluation of the Chat-GPT Model" (2023) Research Square [10.21203/rs.3.rs-2566942/v1].

[4] See, for example, Sandra G Mayson, "Bias In, Bias Out" (2019) 128 Yale Law Journal 2218.

records, case files, and proprietary legal documents. In the context of personalized law, Superjustice will also encompass troves of personal user data. Yet collecting and processing this data raises significant concerns. For example, an AI system designed to personalize traffic rules or tailor consumer protection measures might require access to private and sensitive information, raising questions about how this information is stored, shared, and anonymized. Resolving these issues at the emergence stage is critical to safeguarding users' autonomy and mastery, ensuring compliance with privacy regulations, and building a strong foundation for the further deployment of powerful technologies.

While many of these challenges may seem daunting at first glance, there is reason for optimism. AI technology is improving rapidly, and many of the foundational issues are becoming less pronounced over time. For instance, hallucinations—in which AI systems generate non-existent legal precedents or fabricate facts—have already been substantially reduced in newer models and some platforms.[5] Recent empirical research, including a randomized controlled trial, shows that tools combining retrieval-augmented generation (RAG) and reasoning models can significantly improve legal accuracy and reduce hallucinations, even outperforming human-only baselines.[6] Likewise, advances in algorithmic design and training methodologies continue to enhance accuracy and reliability.

In addition to these technical improvements, emerging evidence suggests that bias can sometimes be mitigated through instructional design. As discussed in Chapter 9, a recent study on mortgage underwriting found that simply instructing a large language model to make unbiased decisions effectively eliminated racial disparities in loan approvals, without retraining or modifying the model's architecture.[7] Similarly, another study found that prompting LLMs to respond rationally significantly reduced cognitive biases in economic and financial decisions.[8] As both users' understanding and model capabilities evolve, such strategies could become an integral part of responsible AI application in law.

Finally, the long-term promise of artificial general intelligence (AGI) offers the potential to address foundational challenges comprehensively. Unlike today's specialized AI systems, AGI could reason and adapt across diverse legal tasks, making it far more capable of avoiding errors. In the interim, however, incremental improvements are critical. To that end, collaborative efforts among technologists, policymakers, and legal professionals could drive progress in targeted areas.

[5] See, for example, Patrice Béchard and Orlando Marquez Ayala, "Reducing Hallucination in Structured Outputs via Retrieval-Augmented Generation" (2024) arXiv preprint arXiv:2404.08189; SM Tonmoy and others, "A Comprehensive Survey of Hallucination Mitigation Techniques in Large Language Models" (2024) arXiv preprint arXiv:2401.01313; OpenAI, GPT-4 Technical Report (2023) <https://openai.com/research/gpt-4>. As to platforms, NotebookLM is an AI-powered research assistant developed by Google, designed to provide reliable and source-based responses. Its knowledge is primarily derived from the materials the users upload, making it more grounded and less prone to hallucination compared to general AI chatbots.

[6] See Daniel Schwartz and others, "AI-Powered Lawyering: AI Reasoning Models, Retrieval Augmented Generation, and the Future of Legal Practice" (forthcoming, 2026) Journal of Law and Empirical Analysis.

[7] See Donald E Bowen III and others, "Measuring and Mitigating Racial Disparities in Large Language Model Mortgage Underwriting" *SSRN* (2025).

[8] See Pietro Bini and others, "Behavioral Economics of AI: LLM Biases and Corrections" *NBER* (2025).

Integration: Navigating Mid-Term Challenges

The integration stage represents the mid-point in AI's adoption journey, at which systems transition from isolated innovations to embedded tools. This phase introduces challenges tied to governance, institutional workflows, and human adaptation, as AI interacts with diverse legal frameworks and stakeholders. Unlike the foundational technical challenges of emergence, integration challenges are more systemic, requiring coordination across institutions and domains. As Moore explains,[9] technology adoption follows distinct stages, progressing from early innovators to broader mainstream acceptance, with each stage presenting new barriers. Legal AI must similarly transition from experimental applications to systemic tools, overcoming resistance and ensuring institutional alignment.

One significant challenge at this stage is workforce adaptation.[10] As AI systems become central to law, professionals must learn to work with them. Whereas workforce adaptation is also important during the emergence stage, it becomes a deeper and more comprehensive challenge in the integration stage. Chapter 8 highlighted the need to ensure that professional training programs equip practitioners to leverage AI's capabilities and understand how best to benefit from its potential. At the same time, vendors would, in most cases, have a profit incentive to help the market adopt new tools. It is thus reasonable to assume that ease of use and lower friction to produce the desired results will come with product maturity.

Another critical challenge during integration is ensuring robust governance and accountability frameworks for AI-driven processes. As AI systems play increasingly central roles in legal contexts, defining responsibility for their outputs will become essential.[11] For example, if an AI tool generates a flawed legal argument or offers erroneous advice, who bears the liability: the developer, the lawyer using the tool, or the firm implementing it? Governance during integration also involves establishing mechanisms for regular audits, ensuring compliance with ethical standards, and creating oversight bodies to monitor the use of AI.[12]

A third issue during integration is cross-border operations. As explained in Chapters 3–4 and 8, AI systems designed to assist with international cases or transactions must navigate a patchwork of legal standards, regulations, and jurisdictional

[9] See Geoffrey A Moore, *Crossing the Chasm: Marketing and Selling High-Tech Products to Mainstream Customers* (3rd edn, Harper Business 2014).

[10] See generally Yoesoep Edhie Rachmad, *Transforming Workforce Skills in the Era of Society 5.0: Integrating Technology and Artificial Intelligence in Competency Development*, The Academic Professor Board Protocol 2019, United Nations Global Compact 137635 UIPM, 2019.

[11] The issue of liability for mistakes generated by technological tools is not new and applies to numerous domains. Examples include autonomous cars, AI interpretation of legal text, AI-assisted medical diagnoses, automated financial trading, automated content moderation systems, and AI-generated legal advice. See, for example, Kevin Funkhouser, "Paving the Road Ahead: Autonomous Vehicles, Products Liability, and the Need for A New Approach" (2013) 1 Utah Law Review 437; Andrew D Selbst, "Negligence and AI's Human Users" (2020) 100 Boston University Law Review 1315; Dylan Walsh, "Who's at Fault When AI Fails in Health Care?" (*Stanford Institute for Human-Centered Artificial Intelligence*, March 14, 2024) <https://hai.stanford.edu/news/whos-fault-when-ai-fails-health-care>.

[12] We explored this in various contexts, including throughout Chapters 3–6.

boundaries. For instance, an AI contract analysis tool might handle agreements involving parties in countries with vastly different contract laws or dispute resolution norms. These discrepancies raise questions about the system's ability to interpret legal nuances accurately. Harmonizing such systems requires technical upgrades, multi-language capabilities, and regulatory alignment across jurisdictions. Achieving this alignment can prove challenging in areas like privacy protection, intellectual property, and international dispute resolution.

The challenges of integration are inherently systemic, arising from interactions among AI systems, legal professionals, and institutional frameworks. Encouragingly, history shows that systemic challenges are not insurmountable, and collaboration on a global scale is possible. For instance, the widespread adoption of digital banking faced similar issues of trust, governance, and workforce adaptation, yet these were overcome through technological advances, regulatory frameworks, and public education. Likewise, collaborative efforts in the legal domain can address integration challenges effectively. Policymakers would be tasked with establishing clear accountability structures, while technologists would work with legal professionals to enhance explainability and interpretability.

As with the emergence stage, AGI might ultimately resolve many integration challenges. Unlike today's specialized AI, AGI could possess a broader understanding of diverse legal systems, allowing AI tools to navigate jurisdictional differences with greater precision and adaptability. In the meantime, addressing integration issues with optimism and foresight would constitute an important stepping-stone toward the long-term sustainability of AI-driven justice systems. We turn to that next.

Sustainability: Addressing Long-Term Transformations

The sustainability stage represents the long-term horizon of Superjustice, where the specific challenges shift from immediate technical or governance issues to broader societal and institutional transformations. While questions of equity and ethics are highly relevant in the earlier stages of emergence and integration, here they take on a more expansive dimension. Rather than addressing localized or system-specific issues, the focus in sustainability is on how these principles can be embedded into the basic structures and norms that shape justice systems over time. Thus, this phase asks fundamental questions about how AI systems can be designed and managed to support justice equitably, ethically, and sustainably at a systemic level.

One critical challenge during this stage is systemic transparency. As AI systems become more integral to judicial processes, the opacity of their operations can undermine institutional credibility.[13] Many advanced AI models rely on complex machine-learning

[13] On the so-called black box nature of AI tools and its impact on public trust see, for example, Warren J von Eschenbach, "Transparency and the Black Box Problem: Why We do not Trust AI" (2021) 34(4) Philosophy & Technology 1607; Juan Manuel Durán and Karin Rolanda Jongsma, "Who Is Afraid of Black Box Algorithms? On the Epistemological and Ethical Basis of Trust in Medical AI" (2021) 47(5) Journal of Medical Ethics 329; Philipp

techniques, such as neural networks, that are inherently difficult to interpret. If litigants or the public cannot understand how decisions are made, the perception of justice as transparent and fair may diminish.

Addressing this challenge requires embedding transparency, explainability, and accountability into AI systems at every level to ensure decisions are accurate and comprehensible. As AI tools will increasingly operate autonomously, it will be imperative to provide clear rationales for their decisions—a task Chapter 9 assigned to AI intermediators. Long-term solutions include developing interpretable AI models, establishing standards for algorithmic auditing, and creating mechanisms for continuous oversight and public reporting. Here too, the potential arrival of AGI, with a superior ability to explain and reason in ways that humans can understand, might make this problem largely obsolete.

Another important concern is the environmental impact of AI systems. As legal institutions increasingly rely on AI tools, the infrastructure supporting these systems—data centers, cloud computing, and high-performance hardware—may demand significant energy resources. This is not a challenge confined to Superjustice or the legal sector; it reflects a broader issue across all AI advances, as increasingly complex models require massively more compute power.

Fortunately, significant progress is being made in addressing this challenge.[14] Researchers are actively developing energy-efficient algorithms designed to perform complex tasks with reduced computational overhead. Innovations in hardware, such as neuromorphic computing and quantum processors, promise to drastically reduce the energy consumption of AI systems in the long term. Additionally, many tech companies are committing to carbon-neutral AI infrastructure, leveraging renewable energy sources like solar and wind to power data centers.

A third transformative challenge is the concentration of power among tech providers. As legal systems rely on AI technologies that are currently being developed by a handful of major corporations, the balance of influence may shift from public institutions to private entities. This raises concerns about transparency, accountability, and control. For example, proprietary algorithms owned by tech companies might shape case outcomes or legal strategies without being subject to public scrutiny. Beyond governance risks, this trend has systemic societal implications. It could be viewed as a privatization of the justice system, eroding institutional autonomy and reducing public trust.

Addressing this issue requires regulatory frameworks that mandate algorithmic transparency, reduce reliance on private actors, and foster competition in the legal

Schmidt, Felix Biessmann, and Timm Teubner, "Transparency and Trust in Artificial Intelligence Systems" (2020) 29(4) Journal of Decision Systems 260.

[14] See Justine Calma, "Google's Future Data Centers Will Be Built Next to Solar and Wind Farms" (*The Verge*, December 11, 2024) <www.theverge.com/2024/12/10/24317888/googles-data-center-solar-wind-renewable-energy-intersect-partnership>; Soumyendu Sarkar and others, "Carbon Footprint Reduction for Sustainable Data Centers in Real-Time" (2024) 38(20) Proceedings of the AAAI Conference on Artificial Intelligence; Nitin Rathi and others, "Exploring Neuromorphic Computing Based on Spiking Neural Networks: Algorithms to Hardware" (2023) 55(12) ACM Computing Surveys 1.

Table 10.1 Life-Cycle Stages and Key Challenges

Life-Cycle Stage	Description	Key Challenges discussed
Emergence	Initial phase	• AI accuracy • Biased training data • Data privacy
Integration	Mid-term phase	• Workforce adaptation • Governance frameworks • Cross-border operations
Sustainability	Long-term phase	• Systemic transparency • Environmental impact • Power concentration

tech market. Proactive measures that empower broad-based, *ex ante* participation in the development and deployment of legal AI technologies, possibly in the form of open-source alternatives, could supplement these initiatives. As others have suggested, predistribution—for example, ensuring universal and early-stage access to powerful AI infrastructure—may offer a more robust long-term solution to systemic inequality and power asymmetry.[15] Concrete strategies could include public investment in open-source legal AI platforms, community-driven algorithm design, and mechanisms for collective ownership of AI assets. Such initiatives would contribute to a legal AI ecosystem defined by broad stakeholder representation, ensuring that the transformative benefits of Superjustice remain equitably distributed and institutionally accountable.

The life-cycle stages of emergence, integration, and sustainability offer a structured framework for understanding how challenges evolve as AI is integrated into justice systems. As the preceding discussion illustrates, the three stages we present are not isolated silos but interconnected phases, and decisions made early on can affect later stages. For example, improving algorithmic accuracy during emergence can reduce governance failures and bolster public trust during sustainability. Yet for analytical clarity, Table 10.1 recaps the challenges by stage.

Domain Focus: Understanding Areas of Impact

However helpful, the temporal roadmap provided by the life-cycle stages represents only one dimension of AI's impact on justice systems. While the life-cycle stages dimension captures how challenges evolve over time, the domain focus dimension examines where these challenges manifest themselves. This perspective categorizes challenges by their primary areas of impact, thereby enabling targeted interventions. Here, we identify four key domains that encapsulate the breadth of AI's influence:

[15] See, for example, Saffron Huang and Sam Manning, "Here's How To Share AI's Future Wealth" *Noema* (April 22, 2025).

1. Technical domain: Challenges related to algorithms, data infrastructure, and system performance.
2. Human domain: Issues surrounding workforce adaptation, legal training, and human oversight.
3. Governance domain: Concerns about accountability, regulatory frameworks, and institutional workflows.
4. Societal domain: Broader challenges affecting public trust, accessibility, and equity in justice.

Understanding challenges through these domains adds precision to the analysis. For instance, technical challenges like algorithmic bias demand solutions rooted in engineering and data science, while societal challenges like public trust require engagement with communities and broader transparency efforts. This domain-specific lens helps identify who is best positioned to address each challenge—whether it is technologists, legal practitioners, policymakers, or civil society—and what kinds of resources and strategies are needed.

Technical Domain: Navigating Core AI Challenges

The technical domain addresses the core capabilities and limitations of the technology itself. Challenges in this domain often arise early but may persist across life-cycle stages, affecting the functionality and reliability of AI tools. Among these, we next survey three major challenges: explainability, system robustness, and data completeness.

As AI systems are integrated into legal contexts, it is imperative to ensure that their outputs are understandable and interpretable. While earlier discussions have addressed concerns about the opacity of AI systems, the focus here is on the technical advances that will be needed to bridge the gap between complex decision-making processes and user comprehension.[16] In legal contexts, AI tools need to produce results that can be explained clearly to lawyers, judges, clients, and the public alike. For instance, an AI system determining the length of incarceration must not only provide a result but also articulate the factors it considered and how it weighed them. Addressing this challenge requires ongoing efforts to develop interpretable models, as well as supplementary tools that clarify AI reasoning.

System robustness presents another multi-faceted challenge. For one, legal systems are vast and varied, addressing everything from straightforward contract enforcement to complex international disputes. AI systems must be resilient enough to handle a wide range of scenarios, including those for which they were not explicitly trained. Failures in robustness can arise, for example, when an AI tool trained

[16] See Finale Doshi-Velez and Been Kim, "Towards a Rigorous Science of Interpretable Machine Learning" (2017) arXiv preprint arXiv:1702.08608; Zachary C Lipton, "The Mythos of Model Interpretability: In Machine Learning, the Concept of Interpretability is Both Important and Slippery" (2018) 16(3) Queue 31.

on domestic law misinterprets international agreements or when it struggles with new social developments or ambiguous legal terminology. Tackling this challenge will involve diversifying training datasets to better reflect the variability of real-world legal contexts, implementing rigorous stress-testing protocols, and adopting continuous learning mechanisms that enable systems to adapt to new conditions dynamically. Here again, AGI represents a long-term vision for overcoming robustness issues, offering the flexibility to navigate novel and complex legal scenarios with reasoning capacities that could exceed those of human experts.

A third challenge lies in the completeness and quality of the data that AI systems rely on. Incomplete or fragmented datasets are a persistent issue in the legal domain, as information is often jurisdiction-specific and may sometimes be outdated or inaccessible. An AI system lacking access to recent case law may provide a flawed legal analysis or fail to account for pivotal developments. Likewise, many AI systems are predominantly trained on English or Western legal frameworks. This leaves gaps in smaller jurisdictions, rarer languages, and Indigenous traditions. Finally, robust legal datasets are relatively scarce and concentrated in the hands of a few powerful companies.

As we explained in Chapters 3 and 4, addressing these issues requires coordinated efforts to create legal data repositories, standardize formats, and ensure open access to critical legal information. Collaborative initiatives among public institutions, private organizations, and academia can drive the development of such repositories. Additionally, advances in data validation pipelines can ensure the accuracy and reliability of training datasets. In the longer run, AGI could further streamline data management by autonomously identifying gaps and inconsistencies, reducing the burden on human oversight.

The Human Domain: Adapting to AI's Transformative Potential

The human domain addresses the interplay between AI systems and the people who design, oversee, and interact with them within the justice system. This domain emphasizes the critical role of human judgment, adaptability, and acceptance in realizing AI's potential for equitable and effective legal transformation. Three key challenges will shape the ways that legal professionals and broader communities navigate this evolving landscape: balancing oversight and delegation, addressing education and training gaps, and overcoming resistance to change.

As we explored in Chapter 5, balancing human oversight with the delegation of tasks to AI systems is a vital and intricate endeavor. While current AI excels at processing vast datasets and identifying patterns, certain legal tasks still demand human qualities such as moral reasoning and contextual sensitivity. Striking the right balance involves defining the boundaries of AI's autonomy in legal decision-making, ensuring that humans remain integral to areas requiring moral and contextual judgment. This challenge spans the integration stage, where AI is introduced into professional workflows, and possibly the emergence stage, as trust in AI systems may hinge on preserving some forms of meaningful human involvement. In these earlier stages, mitigation strategies may include establishing clear guidelines for human oversight, embedding ethical safeguards into AI systems, and creating hybrid models in which AI enhances human decision-making without replacing it. As AI becomes more powerful and capable, however, human involvement should recede.

Chapters 7 and 8 further underlined another critical issue: the gap in legal education and training. The rapid integration of AI into legal systems has outpaced the development of curricula designed to prepare legal professionals for this transformation.[17] Lawyers and judges are often unfamiliar with the technical underpinnings of AI tools, such as predictive algorithms or natural language processing systems, making it difficult for them to use these technologies effectively. At the same time, there is a risk that overemphasis on technical skills could erode traditional legal expertise such as critical reasoning and argumentation. This challenge is particularly pronounced during the integration stage, as professionals must adapt to working alongside AI.

As we previously noted, addressing this gap requires reimagining legal education and professional development. Curricula must blend AI literacy with core legal competencies, ensuring that practitioners can leverage AI tools while retaining the analytical skills that define the profession. Training programs should also emphasize interdisciplinary collaboration, equipping legal professionals to work with technologists and policymakers.

Resistance to change—another theme with which the readers of this book are already familiar—presents an equally important challenge. Many legal professionals are skeptical about the reliability and fairness of AI, fearing that its adoption could erode professional roles or lead to errors that undermine the justice system's credibility. This resistance is not without precedent. Similar fears accompanied the digitization of legal research tools, only to subside as professionals recognized their value. In fact, this pattern of initial skepticism and gradual acceptance extends far beyond the legal profession, reflecting a broader societal response to technological disruption. Throughout history, from the Industrial Revolution to the digital age, technological advances have consistently generated both opportunities and displacement, creating winners and losers in their wake. The legal profession's current hesitation toward AI mirrors a recurring cycle of adaptation that has characterized society's relationship with disruptive technologies.[18]

Overcoming resistance to AI requires more than demonstrating technical reliability: It demands that we reshape how professionals perceive their roles in an AI-augmented system. Here, the concept of legal democratization, as explored in Chapter 6, offers a compelling pathway forward. By enabling individuals without elite legal credentials

[17] See William J Connell and M Hamlin-Black, "Artificial Intelligence and Legal Education" (2019) 36(5) The Computer and Internet Lawyer. See also Marjan Ajevski and others, "ChatGPT and the Future of Legal Education and Practice" (2023) 57(3) The Law Teacher 364.

[18] On societal resistance and acceptance of technology see Viswanath Venkatesh and Fred D Davis, "A Theoretical Extension of the Technology Acceptance Model: Four Longitudinal Field Studies" (2000) 46(2) Management Science 186; Liette Lapointe and Suzanne Rivard, "A Multilevel Model of Resistance to Information Technology Implementation" (2005) 29(3) MIS Quarterly 461.

to perform higher-stakes tasks, AI can expand access to justice and reduce costs, while empowering professionals to focus on oversight and high-value contributions. For instance, community workers equipped with AI tools could offer culturally relevant legal assistance, alleviating the workload on lawyers and judges.

Trust in AI-generated communications presents another important challenge in the human domain. Recent research suggests that people currently trust messages significantly more when they believe they came from human leaders rather than AI systems, regardless of whether this belief is accurate.[19] This "authorship effect" suggests that even high-quality AI outputs may face skepticism simply due to their perceived artificial origin. Such perceptions, in fact, may also explain calls to watermark AI outputs to inform the public of their origin.

For legal communications, whether from judges, attorneys, or legal institutions, this challenge could undermine the credibility of AI-assisted decision-making and correspondence. Yet, this appears to be another transitional issue that will diminish over time as people become accustomed to the integration of AI in legal systems and everyday life. That said, addressing this transitional issue would require strategic approaches that we have discussed throughout the book. These include, for example, maintaining transparency about AI involvement, ensuring humans remain in the loop where appropriate, and implementing rigorous quality control to ensure accuracy and appropriate tone in AI-generated content.

Governance Domain: Establishing Accountability and Equity

The governance domain addresses the structures, policies, and processes required to manage AI's integration into legal systems responsibly and effectively. Among the critical priorities in this domain are clear and enforceable standards for AI auditing.[20] Unlike traditional auditing processes, AI auditing is inherently complex, requiring the examination of opaque and autonomous algorithms, vast training datasets, and unpredictable outputs.

AI systems deployed in legal contexts must be regularly evaluated to ensure compliance with ethical, legal, and technical standards. Without clear auditing protocols, systemic errors may go unnoticed, ethical breaches may remain unaddressed, and public trust may be hard to establish. Developing and implementing these protocols would involve creating interdisciplinary frameworks that combine expertise in law, technology, and ethics. Over the long term, the auditing process might integrate autonomous tools powered by AGI to conduct continuous evaluations.

[19] See "Why CEOs Should Think Twice Before Using AI to Write Messages" (2025) *Harvard Business Review* 23–27.

[20] See Jakob Mökander and Luciano Floridi, "Ethics-Based Auditing to Develop Trustworthy AI" (2021) 31(2) Minds and Machines 323; Jakob Mökander, "Auditing of AI: Legal, Ethical and Technical Approaches" (2023) 2(3) Digital Society 49.

Another significant challenge in the governance domain is embedding ethical principles into AI governance structures. Earlier chapters in this book underscored the critical role of ethics in shaping AI applications in law. Governance frameworks must prioritize such principles at every level, from algorithm design to policy implementation, ensuring that these technologies align with societal values and norms. For instance, any algorithms used to allocate legal aid must avoid reinforcing existing inequities, while systems for predictive policing must be monitored vigilantly to prevent misuse or overreach.

The question of who ensures that ethical and other principles are actually implemented brings us to the critical matter of oversight body design. Effective oversight requires multi-stakeholder regulatory bodies composed of legal experts, technologists, ethicists, and civil society representatives, with rotating membership to prevent capture by special interests. These bodies would have clear mandates, encompassing developing standards for AI auditing, reviewing high-stakes AI deployments before implementation, investigating algorithmic failures or biases, and issuing authoritative guidance on best practices.

To balance technical expertise with democratic legitimacy, oversight bodies should operate transparently. In doing so, they should employ real-time monitoring tools and dynamic feedback mechanisms alongside clear public reporting requirements and citizen participation in audits. Their effectiveness would be measured against specific outcomes like reduced algorithmic bias, improved public trust, and enhanced system performance. As AI capabilities advance through the life-cycle stages, oversight functions would evolve: focusing first on technical accuracy during emergence, then on systemic fairness during integration, and ultimately on long-term transformative impacts during sustainability.

Ethical considerations in governance must also proactively anticipate future dilemmas. For example, integrating ethical impact assessments into AI development cycles—similar to the way that environmental impact assessments guide sustainable development—can help anticipate systemic risks. Here too, fostering collaboration among technologists, legal practitioners, ethicists, and community representatives could guarantee that diverse perspectives are being considered in legal decision-making processes.

The third challenge relates to access and equity in governance. As discussed in Chapter 6, the digital divide remains a persistent barrier, particularly in rural and economically disadvantaged areas. While internet penetration in high-income countries is near universal, disparities in connectivity quality, affordability, and digital literacy persist among lower-income and rural populations. Globally, the gap is even wider, with approximately one-third of the current world's population still lacking internet access.

Governance frameworks must address these inequities by ensuring that AI tools are accessible, inclusive, and culturally sensitive. To that end, the previous chapters detailed a suite of measures: designing mobile-friendly legal platforms; incorporating offline functionalities; fostering digital literacy through tailored programs; and customizing legal services to the user's characteristics and education. Beyond these measures, governance mechanisms should incentivize equitable resource allocation to ensure that underserved communities can access AI systems. Policymakers, for instance, could subsidize access to legal AI tools in marginalized areas or prioritize the development of multilingual and culturally relevant platforms that respect minorities, heterogeneous communities, and local customs. Public-private partnerships could further support the deployment of AI solutions tailored to meet these unique needs.

Societal Domain: Addressing Justice for All

The societal domain encompasses challenges that influence the broader public perception. Such challenges often intersect with the governance domain, yet extend further to include societal values, cultural contexts, and the dynamic relationship among individuals, communities, and institutions. In this context, we revisit two key related challenges through a societal lens: trust-building in AI systems and balancing personalization with universal standards.

Establishing public trust in AI-driven justice systems is an overarching challenge for Superjustice.[21] We have already noted that public acceptance of AI in legal processes would require guaranteeing fairness, reliability, and impartiality. Concerns about AI bias, lack of transparency, and its perceived impersonal nature could fuel skepticism. For instance, the use of AI in bail decisions, workplace recruitment, parole determinations, and criminal sentencing has raised the alarm over algorithmic bias, disproportionately affecting marginalized groups. Moreover, we emphasized that the opacity of AI systems could exacerbate distrust, as citizens may legitimately demand to understand how decisions that impact their lives and the fabric of society are made. Addressing these concerns would require a multifaceted approach: embedding explainability into AI systems, fostering participatory governance models where communities have a voice, and implementing independent audits to validate fairness and accuracy. Whereas AGI holds the prospect to exhibit more advanced forms of reasoning, current strategies must build public confidence incrementally to avoid alienation and backlash.

Balancing the promise of personalization with the necessity for universal legal norms presents another societal challenge. Chapters 4, 6, and 9 demonstrated that Superjustice has the potential to offer highly tailored services, solutions, and rules. We noted that such personalization could account for ad hoc circumstances and reflect the specific needs of individuals and communities.

[21] On the issue of public trust in AI see, for example, Ella Glikson and Anita Williams Woolley, "Human Trust in Artificial Intelligence: Review of Empirical Research" (2020) 14(2) Academy of Management Annals 627; see also Ryan Calo, "Artificial Intelligence Policy: A Primer and Roadmap" (2017) 51 UC Davis Law Review 399.

However, any shift toward personalization risks undermining the consistency and predictability that are hallmarks of a fair legal system. Excessive reliance on personalization may dilute collective norms, eroding the universal principles that underpin justice. To strike the right balance, AI systems should incorporate mechanisms to ensure that more tailored approaches and solutions align with overarching legal standards and societal values. This can include frameworks for harmonizing individual outcomes with broader policy goals and leveraging AI to identify patterns that inform better standard-setting processes.

The societal issues surveyed here illustrate the complex nature of many key challenges. Trust-building efforts will depend on technical advances in explainability, while bridging the digital divide requires governmental interventions and community engagement. Similarly, reconciling personalization with universal standards necessitates an interdisciplinary approach that integrates technical innovation, legal theory, and public consultation.

Interwoven Domains: Navigating Overlaps and Interdependencies

While the framework categorizes challenges into technical, human, governance, and societal spheres, these domains frequently overlap and interact with one another. A technical issue like algorithmic bias, for example, inevitably influences societal perceptions of fairness, requires governance interventions, and demands human expertise to mitigate it. The interdependencies among the various challenges underscore the complex, diverse nature of the issues ahead, highlighting the importance of developing holistic approaches to problem-solving. Without recognizing these interconnections, solutions risk being siloed, creating unintended consequences that may exacerbate the very issues they aim to solve. Table 10.2 demonstrates the breadth of considerations needed for effective AI governance.

Table 10.2 Domain Focus and Key Challenges

Domain Focus	Description	Key Challenges discussed
Technical	Core capabilities and limitations of AI	• AI explainability • System robustness • Data completeness
Human	Interactions between AI and legal professionals	• Workforce adaptation • Resistance to change • Democratization
Governance	Policies and frameworks	• AI auditing • Embedded ethics • Equitable access
Societal	Broad implications	• Public trust • Legal personalization

Complexity Levels: Scaling the Depth of Challenges

Having explored where challenges will manifest themselves through domain focus, we now turn to the final dimension of the Dynamic Challenges Matrix: complexity levels. In essence, complexity levels provide a complementary third lens for analyzing AI-related challenges. Unlike life-cycle stages, which chart challenges temporally, or domain focus, which categorizes them by their primary area of impact, complexity levels examine the depth and scope of challenges. Through its three-tiered structure—direct, systemic, and transformative—this dimension reveals insights into how issues affect localized processes, spill over through interconnected systems, or reshape foundational norms. To illustrate, we next examine how some previously discussed challenges manifest across these complexity levels.

1. The Direct Level: This level captures immediate, relatively well-defined challenges. These challenges often involve clear cause-and-effect relationships, such as algorithmic errors or explainability gaps, and they typically surface during the emergence stage. Solutions at this level are likely to be targeted and specific, addressing localized problems without significantly altering broader systems.
2. The Systemic Level: This level reflects challenges that emerge from interactions across multiple domains or stakeholders. These are second-order effects, such as cross-jurisdictional conflicts or institutional workflow disruptions, which can ripple through interconnected systems. Systemic challenges are more prevalent during integration, when AI is first interacting with existing legal infrastructures. Typically, resolving these challenges would require coordinated efforts across institutions.
3. The Transformative Level: This level encompasses challenges that fundamentally alter justice systems, societal norms, or institutional paradigms. Examples include shifts in public trust or the redefinition of justice delivery models. These challenges typically dominate the sustainability stage. They demand holistic, forward-looking strategies that aim to ensure long-term equity, accessibility, and transparency.

Direct Level: Addressing Immediate and Localized Challenges

The direct level of complexity encompasses challenges that are immediate, well-defined, and localized in nature. These issues often have clear cause-and-effect relationships, making them the most actionable for stakeholders in the short term. However, even at this seemingly straightforward level, these challenges can lay the groundwork for broader systemic or transformative effects if they are not addressed effectively and promptly.

One critical challenge at the direct level is ensuring the security and integrity of Superjustice systems. Cybersecurity threats, such as hacking, data breaches, and system manipulation, pose significant risks to the credibility of Superjustice. Adversarial attacks could alter the outputs of AI systems, undermining their reliability in high-stakes contexts. Such vulnerabilities are not hypothetical. Adversarial attacks are well-documented in the context of image-recognition AI, where maliciously altered inputs can cause AI systems to misclassify objects. For example, subtle modifications to input images could lead to misclassifications, such as making an AI perceive a stop sign as a speed limit sign; a flaw with potentially catastrophic consequences in high-stakes applications like autonomous vehicles.[22]

Addressing this challenge requires robust security protocols and continuous monitoring to detect and mitigate threats in real time. The legal sector must also adopt red-teaming strategies, intentionally probing AI systems for weaknesses to strengthen their defenses. A red team might simulate an adversarial attack to evaluate how well Superjustice processes can withstand attempts to alter their outputs or manipulate their decision-making processes. As noted in Chapters 6–8, cross-disciplinary collaboration is essential: Technologists must work closely with legal professionals to implement adaptive cybersecurity frameworks and prioritize transparent threat detection and response mechanisms.

Another challenge at the direct level is introducing AI systems into legal workflows, which requires careful planning to ensure smooth integration. Challenges at this level include identifying high-impact use cases, preparing institutions for operational changes, and mitigating any risks associated with implementation failures. A lack of stakeholder buy-in, stemming from unclear objectives or insufficient training, could compound these risks.

As explored in Chapter 8, successful implementation depends on a phased strategy that involves piloting AI solutions, gathering feedback, and iterating improvements before full deployment. Policymakers and legal professionals must champion these efforts by establishing clear objectives and benchmarks, ensuring that tools align with organizational goals. Over time, autonomous AI tools (including AGI) could enhance implementation strategies by seamlessly adapting to institutional workflows and learning from user interactions, minimizing friction in adoption.

To ensure accountability and continuous improvement, AI systems in legal contexts must be rigorously evaluated for their performance, accuracy, and impact. Measurement challenges at this level involve defining appropriate metrics, establishing baseline standards, and implementing systems to track outcomes over time. Evaluation efforts should extend beyond technical metrics to include qualitative assessments of societal and institutional impact. This is particularly critical during the emergence and early integration stages, as these phases offer the opportunity to identify weaknesses before systems are scaled. Overall, the development of standardized evaluation frameworks—potentially led by public-private partnerships—could promote consistency and comparability across AI tools.

[22] See Christian Szegedy and others, "Intriguing Properties of Neural Networks" (2013) arXiv preprint arXiv:1312.6199.

Systemic Level: Navigating Complex Interdependencies

The systemic level captures challenges that emerge from the intricate interplay among multiple institutions, domains, and stakeholders. These challenges are more complex than direct issues, as they reverberate across interconnected systems and demand coordinated solutions. To illustrate, we next discuss two systemic challenges: cybersecurity coordination and institutional workflow reengineering.

The increasing reliance on AI in legal systems will heighten the importance of robust cybersecurity coordination across institutions. Legal data will often flow among courts, law firms, enforcement agencies, clinics, community centers, law schools, and private entities, creating a web of interdependencies that is vulnerable to cyber threats. A breach in one entity's system could compromise sensitive client information or disrupt interconnected judicial processes. The challenge could be exacerbated by a lack of standardized protocols for sharing and securing data across jurisdictions. Therefore, policymakers, technologists, and institutions must jointly establish unified cybersecurity frameworks. Solutions could include cross-institutional threat monitoring, real-time information-sharing systems, and simulation-based stress tests to identify vulnerabilities.

Another systemic challenge is workflow reengineering: the broader institutional changes that will be required to adapt legal frameworks to AI's influence. At the emergence and integration stages, consider the shift of entire judicial systems to digital-first models. AI might enable automated case triaging, prioritizing cases based on complexity, urgency, or societal impact. Implementing such systems will require coordination across multiple legal and governmental entities, as well as significant adjustments to institutional hierarchies and operational practices. Similarly, the creation of multi-agency platforms for AI-driven case management would entail reengineering workflows not just within individual courts but across interconnected justice systems.

Systemic-level changes also raise governance and equity concerns, requiring institutions to ensure that workflow reengineering serves public interests rather than exacerbating inefficiencies or inequities. For example, reliance on AI to streamline case resolutions could inadvertently deprioritize complex but socially important cases, such as those involving marginalized communities. Tackling this challenge requires aligning institutional reforms with robust governance frameworks, ensuring that systemic changes fairly improve justice delivery.

Transformative Level: Redefining Justice Paradigms

At the transformative level, challenges move beyond technical fixes or systemic coordination to foundational shifts in justice systems, societal norms, and institutional paradigms. These challenges demand not just innovation but also a rethinking of the principles and structures underpinning justice systems. In this context, we survey two essential challenges: the move to autonomous justice systems and aligning incentives and participation for equitable AI-driven transformation.

We opened this chapter with an imaginary future scenario in which AI makes autonomous judicial decisions without human involvement. As AI increasingly undertakes core judicial functions, including decision-making, the very concept of justice as a human-centered endeavor will be called into question. Litigants, lawyers, and the public may struggle to reconcile AI's impartiality with its perceived lack of deep human qualities. As explained in Chapter 8, if people do not trust the outcomes produced by these systems, even the most accurate and efficient technologies risk rejection.

Anticipating this transformation, forward-looking strategies might involve embedding societal values into AI systems through participatory governance. This could include public consultations on how AI adjudicates specific types of cases or on incorporating diverse cultural norms into algorithmic decision-making processes. In addition, educating the public, highlighting the capabilities and advantages of powerful AI, implementing changes gradually, and emphasizing human-AI collaboration over AI replacement during the initial stages could soften resistance. In the long term, powerful AI will gain prominence and popularity, and AGI might combine machine precision with an adaptive understanding of societal values to bolster trust.

An additional transformative challenge is aligning incentives and ensuring equitable participation. Superjustice cannot be built without the commitment of key stakeholders, including governments, private companies, civil society, and the international community. However, each actor faces distinct participation constraints. Governments may be hesitant to invest in AI legal tools without clear political or economic payoffs. As they are mostly motivated by profit, tech companies may prioritize proprietary systems over open-source collaboration. Regulators may be captured by lawyers' protectionist motivations. Marginalized communities, already underserved by justice systems, typically lack the motivation, resources, or advocacy to shape these systems to meet their needs.[23]

Chapters 3–4, 6, and 8 provided insight into this thorny issue and exemplified that overcoming this challenge would not be easy. It would require fundamentally redesigning global justice governance and establishing frameworks that incentivize diverse participation. For instance, public-private partnerships could foster collaboration between governments and tech companies, providing financial incentives for open-source innovation or subsidies for deploying AI tools in underserved areas. Additionally, creating participatory platforms for civil society and marginalized groups would ensure their voices are heard and actively influence this transformation.

Bridging Complexity: From Localized Issues to Transformative Change

Table 10.3 depicts the various levels and their challenges. The interplay among these levels should not be overlooked, as challenges rarely stay confined to one tier

[23] On these and related issues see R Edward Freeman, *Strategic Management: A Stakeholder Approach* (Cambridge University Press 2010); Virginia Eubanks, *Automating Inequality: How High-Tech Tools Profile, Police, and Punish the Poor* (St Martin's Press 2018); Yochai Benkler, "Coase's Penguin, or, Linux and the Nature of the Firm" (2002) 112(3) Yale Law Journal 369.

Table 10.3 Complexity Level and Key Challenges

Complexity Level	Description	Key Challenges discussed
Direct Level	Immediate, well-defined challenges	• AI security and integrity • Integration into workflows • Evaluation metrics
Systemic Level	Challenges arising from interactions across multiple domains	• Cybersecurity coordination • Institutional workflow reengineering
Transformative Level	Foundational challenges, reshaping justice delivery	• The move to autonomous justice systems • Incentive alignment

of complexity. Addressing the challenges across the direct, systemic, and transformative levels would require a long-term, holistic approach that embraces the complexity of transforming justice systems. Together, these tiers of complexity form a cohesive framework for understanding how AI's integration into legal systems can unfold responsibly and effectively. Looking ahead, however, AGI could bridge gaps across all levels of complexity, offering solutions that adapt dynamically to evolving needs.

Mapping the Path to Superjustice

The Dynamic Challenges Matrix offers a framework for navigating the multifaceted challenges that Superjustice must tackle. It integrates the temporal lens of life-cycle stages, the spatial categorization of domain focus, and the scaling depth of complexity levels. By mapping these dimensions, this chapter illuminated how stakeholders can understand, prioritize, and address the pressing issues in a systematic and actionable way.

As emphasized throughout, the matrix's dimensions are not isolated silos, but interdependent phenomena that, together, reveal the bigger picture. The matrix thus captures the fluidity of AI challenges, highlighting the need for policymakers, technologists, and legal professionals to design effective, integrated solutions. More fundamentally, the matrix demonstrates that addressing these challenges is not about resolving discrete technical or institutional issues, but about reimagining and transforming the fabric of justice systems.

More than a diagnostic tool, the matrix is a guide for thoughtful, iterative progress. With this holistic framework, stakeholders can transform challenges into opportunities, forging an ecosystem in which Superjustice is not a fixed destination but an evolving journey. That journey starts here.

Conclusion: Law for Human Flourishing

In the 2013 film *Her*, Theodore falls in love with Samantha, an AI operating system. Beyond the romance, what captivates audiences is Samantha's ability to understand and navigate the complexities of human emotions, relationships, and dilemmas. The film raises profound questions: What roles should AI play in our lives? What boundaries must we establish as AI systems become increasingly sophisticated? Fast forward just one decade, and these questions are no longer speculative. Generative AI is reshaping many facets of human life, forcing us to confront the implications.

Throughout much of our modern history, justice has been humanity's north star, yet its pursuit has been marked by both triumph and tragedy. From the Code of Hammurabi to the Universal Declaration of Human Rights, our efforts have sought to codify fairness, enshrine equality, and uphold human dignity. Now, as we stand at the threshold of a new era, emerging AI technologies offer a historic opportunity to refine and deepen this pursuit by augmenting justice in ways our ancestors could scarcely imagine.

The recent major technological advances in AI, robotics, and data analytics arrive at a moment when our justice systems are already facing mounting pressures. Courts worldwide are struggling with case backlogs, while access to justice remains limited for many. The complexity of modern legal challenges is stretching traditional legal frameworks to their limits. Meanwhile, the rise of global supply chains, cross-border commerce, climate change agreements, and transnational issues demand innovative legal solutions that transcend national boundaries.

This book has explored how AI can help us overcome these challenges and move toward Superjustice: revolutionary legal systems that are decentralized, democratized, personalized, and technologically enabled. We are already witnessing the emergence of AI-powered legal research tools, predictive analytics, smart contracts, and automated text analysis—early harbingers of the Superjustice era. The convergence of advanced AI capabilities (including large language models and natural language processing), blockchain technologies, and quantum computing will create possibilities for legal innovation that were once confined to science fiction.

Central to this vision is what we have called CRISPR-J: Cost-effective, Rapid, Inclusive, Smart, Predictive, and Resilient Justice. In years to come, developments in AI, such as artificial general intelligence (AGI), will accelerate Superjustice's ability to process complex (legal and non-legal) datasets and tackle thorny policy, social, and legal puzzles. This, in turn, will enable exponential advances and precision in legislation, conflict resolution, judicial prediction, regulation, and enforcement.

Superjustice. Samuel I. Becher and Benjamin Alarie, Oxford University Press.
 DOI: 10.1093/9780198991885.003.0015

Many of the intractable problems of our legal systems stem from structural imbalances of wealth, access, and power. AI's immense potential offers a hopeful path toward more accessible, inclusive, and equitable justice for all. However, realizing the vision of Superjustice will necessitate navigating complex challenges with foresight, determination, and care. The path forward demands understanding Superjustice within broader geopolitical trends, confronting the obstacles ahead, and embracing a shared commitment to action.

Balancing Optimism

Superjustice offers an optimistic vision for the future of legal systems, championing access to justice, promoting the equitable distribution of technological benefits, and facilitating global harmonization. This kind of optimism is not just wishful thinking—it is also a vital force that drives human progress and innovation. Throughout history, optimistic visions have sustained societies in the face of challenges, enabled bold experiments, propelled individuals and communities, and catalyzed transformative change.[1] However, this optimistic outlook exists alongside a global landscape in which technological advances collide, confront, and interact with entrenched political realities. Progress and backlash define our times: While progress in AI presents unprecedented opportunities for justice, geopolitical tensions and societal divisions threaten to undermine this potential.

As we write this concluding chapter, President Donald Trump's second term has signaled a systemic shift in American politics, foreign relations, and the relationship between the state and big tech. The European Union, historically a bastion of regulatory frameworks grounded in liberal-democratic ideals,[2] has recently seen electoral gains for conservative parties and movements, sparking discussion about potential implications for its governance and policy approach. Meanwhile, the war in Gaza, the instability in the Middle East and Africa, and Russia's invasion of Ukraine continue to inflict devastating human, economic, and environmental costs—reshaping global security architecture, exposing the fragility of international order and cooperation, and underscoring how AI-driven tools are also impacting modern conflict.

We live in an era of acute contradictions: extraordinary technological progress juxtaposed with a surge of nationalism and cultural resistance. We are also witnessing unparalleled global interconnectivity alongside growing isolationist tendencies.[3]

[1] On the qualities and advantages of optimism see, for example, Martin EP Seligman, *Learned Optimism: How to Change Your Mind and Your Life* (Vintage 2006); Tali Sharot, *The Optimism Bias: A Tour of the Irrationally Positive Brain* (Vintage 2012); Charles S Carver and Michael F Scheier, "Dispositional Optimism" (2014) 18(6) Trends in Cognitive Sciences 293; Barbara Fredrickson, *Positivity: Groundbreaking Research Reveals How to Embrace the Hidden Strength of Positive Emotions, Overcome Negativity, and Thrive* (Crown Publishers/Random House 2009).

[2] It is commonly argued that "America innovates, China replicates, and Europe regulates." Some of the recent technology-related regulations in the EU include the *Digital Services Act*, the *Digital Markets Act*, the *Artificial Intelligence Act*, and the *Cyber Resilience Act*.

[3] We are inspired here by Fareed Zakaria, *Age of Revolutions: Progress and Backlash from 1600 to the Present* (Random House 2024).

For one, the intensifying USA–China superpower rivalry casts a long shadow over global cooperation in AI development and regulation. This competition threatens to fragment efforts to address shared challenges, hindering collaborative AI advancements and destabilizing the international cooperation needed to fully unlock the benefits of Superjustice. Nonetheless, our enduring human capacities—optimism, empathy, adaptation, and moral growth—point toward a future where thoughtful planning allows us to harness technology for justice and shared prosperity.[4]

Confronting Reality

One straightforward lesson from *Her* is the need to approach AI with humility and healthy skepticism. Beyond geopolitical tests, Superjustice must also confront four interconnected types of challenges: technical, human, governance, and societal. Each presents unique hurdles—varying significantly across different legal traditions, cultures, and societies—that ought to be carefully navigated.

At the technical level, current AI's capabilities, while impressive, still fall short in critical ways. Although they are rapidly evolving, today's AI systems can struggle when confronted with novel scenarios. The complexity of legal reasoning, the nuance of contextual understanding, and the challenges of explainability and accuracy all push the limits of today's AI systems. Justice demands more than raw processing power: It requires systems capable of applying legal principles with subtlety and wisdom, while detailing their reasoning in ways that foster trust, comprehension, and accountability.

Yet technological capabilities alone will not define justice; human perceptions will be equally influential. Resistance to AI in legal systems stems not only from mere technological skepticism but also from fundamental concerns about the nature of AI and the essence of justice itself. Many perceive AI as opaque, inflexible, and emotionless—all qualities that seem fundamentally at odds with the philosophical human dimensions of justice. In its contemporary iteration, AI lacks true understanding. It cannot engage in the nuanced contextual reasoning and meaning-making that characterize human cognition.

Poorly designed AI systems risk prioritizing the letter of the law over its spirit, thus producing outcomes that are procedurally or technically correct, yet morally deficient. Some may legitimately fear that deploying powerful AI in legal decision-making could contradict humanism. Such a shift, the argument goes, could disconnect us from the physical world and from grounded human experiences. Moreover, legal professionals

[4] To be sure, the path to leveraging AI for global justice is not merely a matter of innovation but is deeply shaped by geopolitical struggles and strategic alignments; see Leopold Aschenbrenner, "Situational Awareness: The Decade Ahead" (June 2024), and particularly Part IIId, titled "The Free World Must Prevail" <https://situational-awareness.ai/>. On the overall encouraging trajectory of humankind see Steven Pinker, *The Better Angels of Our Nature: Why Violence Has Declined* (Penguin Books 2012); Yuval Noah Harari, *Sapiens: A Brief History of Humankind* (Random House 2014); Hans Rosling, Ola Rosling, and Anna Rosling Rönnlund, *Factfulness: Ten Reasons We're Wrong About the World—and Why Things Are Better Than You Think* (Hodder & Stoughton 2018).

may fear being reduced to overseers, losing agency (and lucrative livelihoods) to machines, and playing a diminished role in shaping justice.

Superjustice must heed the widespread preference for human interaction and respect the public perception of justice as a moral, social, and emotional enterprise. But this raises a provocative question: If AGI-empowered Superjustice becomes clearly superior to legal professionals, will we arrive at a future where humans are *barred* from being in the justice loop? And, perhaps more importantly, are we willing to accept that outcome?

While human and technical factors shape AI's potential, translating these insights into practice requires robust governance structures. Governance hurdles involve creating frameworks that balance innovation with responsibility. Questions of liability, decision-making authority, and ethical oversight remain unresolved, as policymakers struggle to anticipate the wider consequences of AI. National lawmakers and international bodies must clarify liability standards, while professional associations would need to develop best practices that guide developers and lawyers alike.

Beyond the immediate regulatory landscape, broader societal considerations loom large. These reflect fundamental questions about public trust in legal systems and the social perception of accountability, justice, and equity. Furthermore, AI-transformed legal systems could amplify existing biases, further complicating efforts to ensure fairness and accessibility. Achieving meaningful progress demands an integrated strategy: designing transparency into AI systems from the ground up, establishing inclusive governance frameworks that amplify marginalized and community voices, and implementing rigorous third-party oversight to safeguard equitable and precise outcomes. The interconnected nature of these challenges magnifies their scope. Technical solutions must address human concerns to build trust; governance frameworks must account for both technological capabilities and societal needs; and public acceptance depends on integrating these elements harmoniously.

In addition to these multifaceted obstacles, addressing cultural and regional nuances is imperative in ensuring the inclusivity of Superjustice. Justice is not monolithic; it reflects diverse traditions, encompassing civil law, Indigenous legal norms, religious frameworks, and hybrid legal structures. Superjustice must be flexible enough to adapt to and incorporate these varying contexts, while respecting local values and aspirations. Recognizing this complexity, Superjustice should evolve through decentralized dialogue with diverse legal traditions and communities, ensuring justice that is culturally responsive and equitable.

Shaping Tomorrow

The question we should ask is not what AI *will* do to our legal systems, but what we *want* it to do. While the task of leveraging new technologies to recreate our legal systems for the benefit of all society is formidable, it is not insurmountable. Achieving this vision demands that clear principles and thoughtful implementation strategies guide the path to Superjustice.

Legal professionals must evolve from passive technology users to active system-shapers who work with technologists to guarantee that AI advances justice. Legal tech companies must prioritize transparency and accountability, shifting their focus from efficiency metrics to fostering meaningful access to justice. Citizens, too, must play an active role in the design process through participatory mechanisms that ensure these systems reflect community values and societal needs. Likewise, philanthropists and social impact investors should incorporate equitable legal tech innovation and accessible justice platforms into their investment strategies. Together, stakeholders can galvanize efforts to deliver a future in which AI advances fuel a justice system with boundless reach and impact.

If the law is to serve humanity better, Superjustice must represent more than an efficiency upgrade: It should mark a seismic shift from scarcity to abundance in justice delivery. This paradigm shift opens a unique opportunity to move from a world where the benefits of justice are confined to the privileged few to one where justice flows freely, legal knowledge is democratized, and access to justice is a universal right. This transformation embodies our chance to reclaim law as a force for social good.

As technologies advance,[5] we stand at a crucial juncture. It is our choices that will determine whether and how technology redefines the future of our legal systems. Yet, the ultimate success of Superjustice depends not on technology but on our collective will to experiment with and embrace new tools, demand that they be used for good, and align them with human values. Progress in justice systems requires deliberate human action—we drive change to make it happen.

In *Her*, Samantha's remarkable intelligence invites us to imagine how AI might enrich our lived experiences and relationships. In the end, it is our willingness to employ these tools with wisdom, courage, and purpose that will determine whether Superjustice becomes a lasting reality. The decisions we make today will echo for generations. As we design and leverage powerful AI tools, we must remember that they do not operate in a vacuum: our commitments and actions set their direction. In reimagining our legal systems through the lens of powerful AI, we hold the opportunity—indeed, the responsibility—to transform justice itself into an enduring, evolving wisdom that optimally serves humanity.

[5] As of December 2024, for example, Google announced that its Willow chip represents a breakthrough. See Tim Bajarin, "Why Google's Quantum Computer Chip Willow Is a Game Changer" *Forbes* (December 13, 2024) <www.forbes.com/sites/timbajarin/2024/12/13/why-googles-quantum-computer-chip-willow-is-a-game-changer/>. In February 2025, a few months later, Microsoft announced its significant progress in its endeavor to produce topological quantum bits. See Rachel Courtland, "A New Microsoft Chip Could Lead to More Stable Quantum Computers" *MIT Technology Review* (February 19, 2025). See also Ahmed R Sufi, "Universal Photonic Artificial Intelligence Acceleration" (2025) 640 Nature 368; Shiyue Hua and others, "An Integrated Large-Scale Photonic Accelerator with Ultralow Latency" (2025) 640 Nature 361.

Index

For the benefit of digital users, indexed terms that span two pages (e.g., 52–53) may, on occasion, appear on only one of those pages.

Tables and figures are indicated by an italic *t* or *f*.

The manufacturer's authorised representative in the EU for product safety is Oxford University Press España S.A. of El Parque Empresarial San Fernando de Henares, Avenida de Castilla, 2 - 28830 Madrid (www.oup.es/en or product.safety@oup.com). OUP España S.A. also acts as importer into Spain of products made by the manufacturer.
Printed and bound by CPI Group (UK) Ltd, Croydon, CR0 4YY
15/09/2026
02217434-0001